PRANA

ONE BREATH, MANY WORLDS

BERNIE CLARK

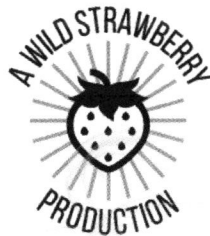

A WILD STRAWBERRY PRODUCTION

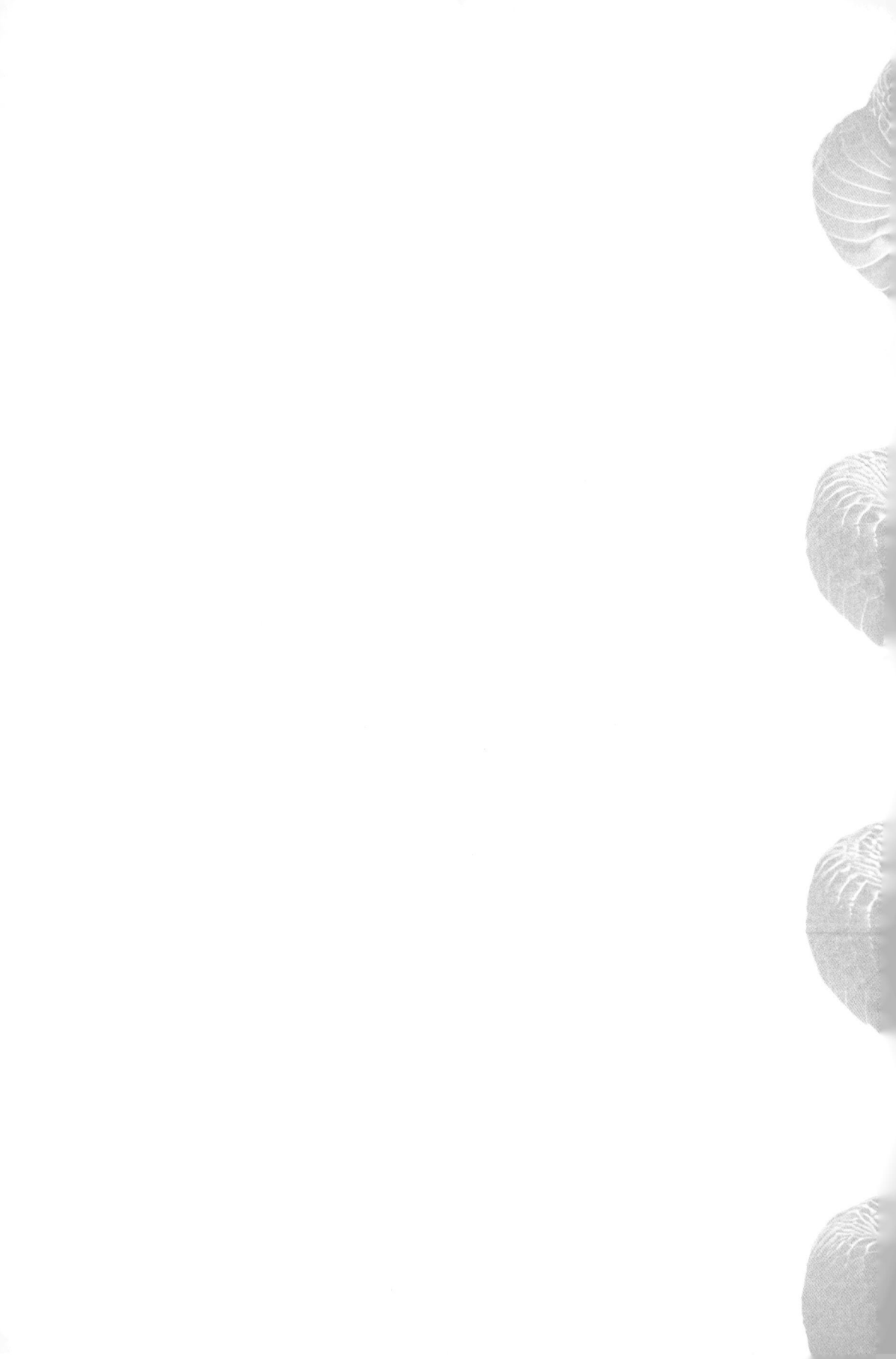

PRAISE FOR PRANA — ONE BREATH, MANY WORLDS

Prana is a luminous and deeply original work—part memoir, part mythic tapestry, part philosophical inquiry—that breathes life into one of the most enduring mysteries of human existence. With rare intellectual range and heartfelt storytelling, it explores the many meanings of breath, life force, and spirit across cultures and centuries. It is a masterful meditation on what it means to be alive—and aware—in the subtle currents that sustain us.

Mark Stephens, author, *Breathing: The Art and Science of Pranayama* and *Yoga Sequencing: Designing Transformative Yoga Classes*

Bernie Clark takes the reader deep inside the mystical, invisible, subtle, yet powerful realms of prana. Through extensive research, combined with personal experience and scientific studies, he sheds light on this intriguing and commonly misunderstood universal force, managing to do so in an engaging and accessible manner.

David Swenson, Author of *Ashtanga Yoga: The Practice Manual*

With *Prana*, Bernie displays what a thorough thinker, heartfelt practitioner, and deeply engaging writer he is of this essential subject at the nucleus of all yoga: prana. Another essential text for all yoga enthusiasts.

Sarah Powers, Co-founder of the Insight Yoga Institute and Author of *Insight Yoga* and *Lit from Within*

Having read all of Bernie's books, this is by far my favorite. It's a wonderful mix of the personal, scientific, and creative that explores not only the earliest origins and history of yoga but its underlying energetic and mystical aspects as well. Many of us as teachers have pondered these deep questions, and Bernie has brought his unique perspective to fleshing them out in ways that illuminate the principles and teachings that make yoga universal.

J. Brown, Host of the *Yoga Talks* podcast

Prana is a key concept in yoga theory and practice. But what is prana? Is prana a god? A physical force? Or the power that connects the immaterial soul to the material body? Is it just an ancient name for bio-electricity, or is it an intelligent life-force that modern science is slowly uncovering? Bernie Clark's new book, *Prana*, explores these questions by tracing the historical uses of the word prana in ancient and modern cultures. He has created masterfully imagined dialogues between ancient yogis, Greek philosophers, Taoist sages, and modern theosophists. His book is interwoven with Bernie's own experiences and culminates with a review of modern scientific investigations and theories. It is well researched, clearly written, and full of references. Read Bernie's book *Prana*. It might make you reconsider what prana is, and how breathing exercises and physical asanas influence it manifestations.

Paul Grilley, Author of *Yin Yoga: Principles and Practice*
and *Chakra Theory and Meditation*

As a science educator, I've long struggled to reconcile the esoteric ideas of "prana" and "chakras" with scientific thinking. In *Prana*, Bernie Clark doesn't resolve that tension—he honors it. Blending myth, history, and modern insight, he invites us not into certainty but into informed wonder. Whether you're a skeptic or a seeker, *Prana* offers a compelling and nuanced map for exploring one of yoga's most elusive concepts, making it a must-read for any yogi.

Matthew Huy, Co-author of *The Physiology of Yoga* and
Co-founder of the Enlightened Yoga Collective

To all my students who have taught me so much
Who sat before me and gave me their trust
To everyone who breathed and felt breath's touch
Who were moved to stillness, as return we must

Inquiries should be addressed to:

Wild Strawberry Productions
2488 West 7th Avenue
Vancouver, BC, Canada
V6K 1Y7

First edition: 2026

Editor: Dania Sheldon. Cover and interior design by Alex Hennig.

Printed in the USA

ISBN 978-1777687328 (paperback)

ISBN 978-1777687335 (e-book)

MEDICAL DISCLAIMER

The contents of this book are intended for general information only and not as specific medical advice. Please check with your healthcare provider before following any suggestions found herein. The guidance given in this book is not meant to replace medical advice and should be used only as a supplement if you are under the care of a healthcare professional. When you are not sure of any aspect of the practice, or feel unwell, seek medical advice.

Contents

Figures

Gratitude

My journey into yoga began when Shakti Mhi opened the door. I walked through that door decades ago, but my mind and heart still recall the kindness and wisdom I received from every teacher I sat before or whose books or videos I devoured. I bow to Shakti, David Swenson, Erich Schiffman, Rod Stryker, David Williams, Saul David Raye, Tim Miller, Doug Keller, Shiva Rea, Fiona Stang, Mike Dennison, Richard Freeman, Sarah Powers, and Paul Grilley. Teachings evolve as our knowledge expands and experience grows. The words I recall in this book may not be what my teachers would speak today. Indeed, I am sure their journey has deepened their own understanding, and their teachings have grown as they integrated their lived practice into their offerings. While I have documented what I recall of those days, if you should happen to be graced by their presence, allow them to share what they know today. Please do not limit them to what they taught me so many years ago.

My gratitude extends to the people who helped me turn the vision of this book into the reality you hold in your hands. Thanks to Dania Sheldon for her editorial expertise. To Mary Wilson for catching the tiny typos that always seem to escape my sight. To Alex Hennig for putting the words into place and formatting the book. To Pillar Wyman for her wonderful index. And a special thanks to the alpha and beta readers who gave so freely of their time and provided feedback on my early drafts. Thank you, Reinhard Pekarek, Nathalie Keiller, Itamar Erez, Sebastien de Castell, J. Brown, Nyk Danu, Matthew Huy, Saul David Raye, David Williams, Erich Schiffmann, David Swenson, Sarah Powers, Mark Stephens, and Paul Grilley.

And, once more, my gratitude to all the students who sat, listened, and asked questions. I never learn more than when I am questioned and find I have no answer to give. That is the sharpest motivation to seek greater knowledge and wisdom.

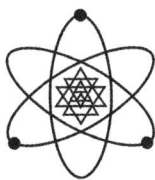

Departure

Hold lightly to your certainties
For maps are always changing.
The beliefs you hold so dearly now
Will soon need rearranging.

The window seat was excellent for viewing but cramped for the long journey ahead. The aisle seat made more sense, but I chose the view. The engines were started and the airplane jerked as we started the push-back from the gate. I was flying from Vancouver, Canada to New Delhi on my first visit to India.

There were two paths I could have chosen: flying via Europe and the Middle East, over the cradle of Western Civilization and the scientific method; or through Asia, over the lands of mystery and history. On later journeys, I tried both routes—blending cultures, timelines, and perspectives.

The journey you are about to embark upon likewise has two paths that ultimately arrive at the same destination. The purpose of the journey is to learn about *prana* and the practice of *pranayama*.[1] While today the word prana is often synonymous with "life force" or "life energy," this is not how it started out. The word "energy" in its modern meaning of the ability to do work was defined by scientists in the nineteenth century. What did prana mean to our ancestors? It was intimately tied to life—but how, exactly? All life had something to do with breath and the air around us. But to consider prana as simply air misses the nuances and depth of this ancient idea. How did people in antiquity understand life? What sustained it—and what happened when it left? Thus, one path we will follow is the historical and philosophical. We will visit ancient times and cultures to see how they thought about life and its source.

The second path takes us along a modern and personal road: a journey of discovery through teachers, traditions, and the hard-won lessons of practice. My own journey began with yoga teacher training and early lessons in modern pranayama. Over time—through practice, missteps, and mentorship—my understanding deepened.

Thus, a second path we will traverse, which will intertwine with the first, is one of personal discovery.

There is, however, a third—not historical or philosophical, and not only personal: the scientific path. It asks not only what prana once meant or how pranayama is practiced today, but what prana might mean in a world still searching for the essence of life. Is prana a metaphor, a biological force, a spiritual reality? Or all of these at once?

Like my own travels to India, sometimes we will journey east and sometimes west. Like woven threads, these stories will sometimes cross, loop, or change direction. Be prepared to switch directions often and sometimes suddenly, but trust the threads.

This book weaves together personal stories, cultural myths, and historical perspectives—part memoir, part history, part philosophical reflection—all circling back to one elusive question: *What is prana?*

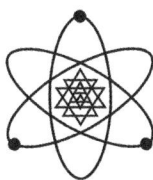

CHAPTER I:

In the beginning

*And the LORD God formed man of the dust of the ground, and breathed
into his nostrils the breath of life; and man became a living being.*
Genesis 2:7

What is Prana?

"Why *prana*?" I asked Shakti soon after taking up yoga.

"What do you mean?" she replied.

"Why did you name your studio the Prana Yoga and Zen Centre? What is prana?"

"Prana is life—it is the energy that gives life."

"Like oxygen?"

"Oxygen is necessary, but prana is more. It's everywhere. It can mean breath, but it's more than that. There is a practice we do called *pranayama*: prana is our life force, and *yama* means control, so pranayama teaches us how to control our life force—enhancing it when weak, containing it when strong. Since *prana* can also mean breath, pranayama works through controlling the breath."

Over the years, especially during my initial teacher training with Shakti in August 1998, I learned more about the various practices of pranayama, and of its dangers and contraindications. Some lessons I learned the hard way—through personal missteps and mishaps in practice.

Distinguishing Spirit from Soul

In Western thought, the words *spirit* and *soul* are often used interchangeably. But in the yogic traditions of South Asia, the distinction is clear: *atman, jiva, purusha*—these refer to the soul, the seer or witness. *Prana, vayu, kundalini*—these are energies of life, but they are not the self. *Atman* is awareness; *prana* is force.

An analogy may help. Imagine a sleek electric car. The body is the vehicle; the soul is the driver. But without electricity—prana—the car won't move. You need both: the soul to direct and the spirit to energize.[2] The electricity in the battery is the spirit, the vital animating force. Prana is not the driver, not the observer or the knower. It moves the system, but it does not see. It is necessary for life but not sufficient. When the driver gets out, the car dies. When the battery is drained, the car stops, and the driver has to exit and walk to another.

"And the Spirit of God moved upon the face of the waters." (Genesis 1:2, KJV)

The Hebrew word translated as "Spirit" is *ruach*, which means wind, breath, or spirit. It is a dynamic, animating force. The word for soul in Hebrew is *nephesh*, denoting life and personal identity. The New Testament book Hebrews contains the description "dividing soul and spirit, joints and marrow," showing a clear delineation.[3] The epigraph for this chapter illustrates that Adam had neither life nor soul until God breathed both into him.[4]

In ancient Greece, philosophers also recognized a difference between soul and spirit. *Pneuma* referred to air or breath—the animating force—while *psyche* denoted the soul, the conscious self or personality. Similarly, in Latin, *spiritus* means breath, while *anima* refers to the soul. This distinction between breath as a requirement for life and soul as the essence of the living is deeply rooted in these philosophical and religious traditions.

From the time of Saint Paul—himself Greek-educated—Christian theology emphasized the role of the Holy Spirit (*pneuma hagion*), the divine breath or presence that animates and sanctifies the soul. Here again, spirit is not the same as soul: the Holy Spirit is the presence of God moving within and upon the soul but is not the soul itself.

The Sanskrit word atman, often translated as soul or self, derives from the ancient Indo-European root *etmen*, meaning "to breathe."[5] It gave rise to terms like Old English *æðm* and Dutch *adem*, all connected to the notion of breath. Likewise, in East Asia, *chi* (or *qi*) in Chinese[6] and *ki* in Japanese reflect the idea of vital energy intimately linked to breath. While the terms soul and spirit do get conflated, and they definitely are related, for the purposes of our investigation, we will define them to be distinct and different: soul is our essence; spirit is the vitality that energizes life.

Most cultures likely noticed that where there was breath, there was life—and when breath left, life did too. Breath, then, became not just air, but a link to something beyond. There was something about the air that entered our bodies that gave and sustained life. And clearly, after breath left the body, the person had also departed.

Where did the person go? What actually left? Those mysteries were answered by stories, myths, and religions. The fact that the departed could be remembered and at times would appear in dreams indicated that something of them still existed, still persisted in a realm that the living could not fully perceive. But in the dead body remaining, whatever essence, force, or energy that had given it life had clearly gone.

That force is what Shakti was calling prana. Across traditions, this vitality—breath, spirit, prana—was seen as the thread between the seen and unseen, between body and soul, between matter and meaning. Sometimes, our prana is full, and we feel energized, vibrant, alive. At other times, it wanes—and the results can be troubling, as I would soon discover firsthand...

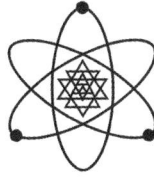

CHAPTER 2:

White Sulfur Springs

I lay in bed, unable to rise. The room didn't spin—at least, not when I stood up. But lying down, the dizziness returned. Confusing? I know. An experience is easy to have but often difficult to describe. Dizziness is how I tried to explain it to Paul and Sarah, but I could see they didn't really understand what I meant. Perhaps light-headed would have been a better term, but it wasn't exactly that either. I couldn't sit up or stand—if I tried, I'd fall.

When I woke up that morning, I immediately knew something was wrong. The 6:30 a.m. morning meditation and following yoga practice would be starting soon. In the main hall, students would be gathering, laying down their mats, setting up their cushions, and sinking into silence. It was Monday morning, January 10, 2005, and I had three days left of a 10-day yin yoga teacher training course at the White Sulfur Springs Resort in the Napa Valley of California with Paul Grilley and Sarah Powers. They took turns teaching the course; Paul would do one morning and Sarah that afternoon, and then the next day, Sarah would begin and Paul would be front and center in the afternoon. What to do in the pre-breakfast "open practice," however, was up to each student. I had been doing my regular ashtanga first series practice, and it felt good. I felt good. Because I felt good, and yesterday had been a day off, I had decided to walk into town to do some laundry.

The resort included 20 buildings spread near the main lodge, just five kilometers from St. Helena. I should have hitched a ride with other students going into the town to do sundry chores and shopping, but I decided to walk. It took longer than I'd expected, and the laundry was busy that day, so I had to power-walk and at times jog to get back in time for Sarah's silent yin yoga practice at 3:30pm. That exertion, combined with my morning yang practices, pushed me over an edge. The price I paid was my immobility the next morning.

I couldn't get up, but my bladder was insisting that I couldn't stay in bed, either. I decided to crawl to the bathroom. After relieving myself, I rolled back into the bed. No morning practice today. I could only hope that I didn't have to spend the whole day in bed. Would anyone notice? Would they come to check? What would I tell them?

This was not the first time I'd experienced this dizzy, lightheaded, faint, weak, cottony-headed feeling—I still don't know the best way to describe it. But it was the worst episode I had ever experienced.

After a couple of hours of lingering in bed, counting breaths, calming my inner fears about what could be wrong, I was able to sit up. I slowly dressed. The weather was cool. Even though this was California, and winters north of San Francisco can get cold, I felt unseasonably cold—and unreasonably so. I put on several layers and shuffled to the main hall. Fortunately, there was a large couch against one wall. That would serve as my yoga mat for the morning. I lay on that couch and watched Sarah lead the morning workshop.

When I appeared, people noticed that I was not as vertical as normal. Paul came over to enquire what was going on. After I explained my situation, he suggested that I go to the hot tub and warm up. I demurred. Ever since catching heat stroke one afternoon in India, I have never done well in heat. I told him that I was too pitta in nature for hot tubs. Paul responded, "Well, you are not pitta now!"

He was right, but so was I. Years later, I figured out why a hot tub would not have been a good idea for me then. Yes, I was very cold, but my blood pressure was also very low. Going into a hot tub could have dropped it into the danger zone.

I listened to my inner guidance and apathy and remained on the couch. Present were around 40 students—a nurse, an acupuncturist, and yoga teachers from around the world—all drawn by Paul and Sarah's pioneering work. The acupuncturist, Kyle Miura, took my pulse and said that it was "very deep," probably indicating chi insufficiency to the endocrine system. But he did not have his needles with him and couldn't suggest much to help. (Today, Kyle is a fully fledged doctor and professor who works in Berkeley, California, and he still offers yoga classes.)

Questions in Flight

A special guest was in attendance: John Ayoub, PhD and past president of the Center for Integrated Human Studies (CIHS) in Encinitas, California. He had been invited to demonstrate a device designed by Paul's teacher and the founder of the CIHS, Dr. Hiroshi Motoyama. The device was called the AMI, or the apparatus for measuring meridian intensities. It could assess meridian flow electrically—just as Kyle had done manually through pulse diagnosis. John measured my state. His diagnosis: my flow of chi through the Urinary Bladder and Kidney meridians was very weak.[7] John suspected adrenal insufficiency and recommended I see a doctor about this when I got back home.

I managed to struggle through the last few days of the training, then the commute back to San Francisco and my return flight to Vancouver, Canada. On the flight home, I had time to obsess: Why was my prana so weak? What exactly *was* prana, anyway? To search for answers, I would have to travel far—into memory, into history, into myth. I began to remember an older teaching, one that came to me like a wind whispering through the trees...

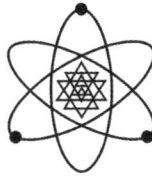

CHAPTER 3:

The Boy Who Could See the Wind

If we would like to uncover the roots of prana, we must excavate deeply into the soil of the past. We have to dig well beneath today's veneer of computers and electricity, down past the layers of steam, metals, and civilizations. We have to reach the strata of our primal ancestors and speculate on how the proto-yogis of prehistory viewed life, breath, and fire. Fire was the key technology then, and trance was the primal shaman's most important inner tool. Every flower has hidden roots buried in the dark earth; so too, prana as we know it today sprouts from an unknowable depth. Perhaps a story will explain this more clearly...

Awnka came too early, and in some ways, far too late. He was the youngest of Ka-ril's seven children. Only two of Awnka's siblings were still alive. Two others had died shortly after being born, and the firstborn, Tarka, well... he also came too early and grew up to be strange. Mansha had taken him away when the rest of the people became frightened. The strange visions that Tarka had suffered were happening to Awnka now. Ka-ril was concerned that Mansha would again be called.

Awnka was a surprise. Ka-ril had been certain she would not bear any more children. Her third mate had proven singularly inept at fathering offspring, and she was getting quite grey and heavy. She thought six births was enough, since her two surviving children were certain to become adults. That's all the people needed. Two adults to replace two adults. She certainly hadn't been planning on more. Late in her life, though, he appeared—but too early, for Awnka emerged at least two moons sooner than expected.

Awnka survived, somehow. Mansha made sure of that. He ministered to the child every day, taking him from Ka-ril after she fed him, to massage his tiny limbs and torso.

Mansha would chew roots, then breathe fumes over Awnka's body. He would bathe the baby in fragrant water. Warm. He always kept Awnka wrapped tightly and near the fire. He made Ka-ril promise to keep Awnka well bound and warm whenever he was not at her breast, for at least six seasons. This retarded Awnka's ability to crawl or walk, and he never seemed to learn to talk properly, either.

Awnka was not like the other children, just as Tarka had not been like them. He would stand stock still for long periods, as if bound, or attending to a world no one else could know. His eyes would glaze over, his head tilted, as if intently listening. He said he was listening. But even though his eyes were half-closed, he said he was also seeing. He was watching the wind. You couldn't watch the wind by looking directly at it. You had to glimpse it from the corner of your eye. The wind had colors; it danced for him, danced around him and through him. Sometimes, he claimed, it took him away, but it always brought him back.

Awnka knew a day before anyone else when the rain would return. He knew before anyone else when the ground would shake. He said they began as tiny seeds. No one understood. When he warned of the stampede, the people believed him and moved their encampment up the hill before the first elephant appeared. But some people claimed Awnka called the elephants, made the rain fall and the earth shudder. They worried he was not a herald but a cause.

Awnka had to go with Mansha to learn how to control his power. Ka-ril could not deny Mansha when he came for her son. Mansha took Awnka away, as he had taken Tarka. But Tarka had perished in the ordeal that Awnka was to undergo. Ka-ril was concerned for her son but equally concerned for everyone else. She could only stand, cry, and watch Mansha lead Awnka away.

Awnka didn't complain. He silently followed Mansha. He knew Mansha, of course. Everyone knew Mansha, even though he seldom visited and rarely stayed overnight. If people were afraid of Awnka, they were terrified of Mansha. But their fear never pre-vented them from seeking his aid when bad luck or bad demons afflicted them. He was the people's protector from the other world, their guide who helped to bring them safely through dark times or recover from a grave illness, usually. He sometimes failed, but only, he said, when there were simply too many demons to fight. He was no one's friend, though. Indeed, no one really knew Mansha.

Mansha led Awnka far from his tribe, to places Awnka only knew from the wind. His feet had never walked these paths before. A small cave was to be his home for three moons. He was not to leave except in the middle of the night to walk in darkness, to strengthen his legs and his senses. Each morning, Mansha would bring some water. For the first fourteen days, Awnka was given no food. Then, with the daily water would be some boiled and mashed roots. After the first month, Awnka appeared drawn, skinny, and constantly tired. It was then, when he could barely stand on his own, that Mansha intro-duced Awnka to fire and smoke.

Mansha built a big fire inside the small cave one night. Awnka was ordered to stay at the back of the cave and absorb the heat. He passed out several times, and only then would Mansha take him out of the cave, revive him, then place him back by the inferno. Close to morning, when the fire had burned down to embers, Mansha showed Awnka how to walk on the coals and eat the glowing embers. It took many weeks for Awnka's burns to heal, but Mansha was always unharmed.

Mansha returned only once a week, reprising the lessons of fire and teaching Awnka to breathe in ways that would stoke his own inner fire. He needed no clothes to stay warm, even on the coldest nights. At this point, they would walk in the forest, discovering the mysteries only available in the dark. Awnka had already known the speech of wind and earth. He discovered that wind and breath are the same, and that people are breath, too. When breath leaves a body, the person leaves the body. Since he could see the wind, he could learn to see breath and follow it, tame it, and bring it back to the body. This was to be his most important power, but there were other languages to learn as well: the languages of fire, smoke, and plants. One day, assuming he survived this ordeal, Mansha would teach him all the languages—of animals, of sky, of the other world and its people, the Ka-mi.

Awnka's mind was strong. He knew how to breathe himself into a trance. Ka-mi were attracted to him. Mansha could see their joy in being around Awnka, and in time, Awnka would see them too, talk to them, sing their songs, and command them.

Awnka learned a powerful secret from Mansha: "The breath can fly, but the body cannot. You must learn to hide and protect your body when your breath goes roaming, for the body is defenseless at those times. It is good to let others think that the body can fly, for the fear others hold is protection for your body. But you must never believe the body can fly. Many apprentices have died trying to fly out of a tall tree. Only the breath is free and has that power."

Mansha was incredibly old and knew he would see only a few more seasons. He was grateful that Awnka had survived his initiation. Successful initiates were rare and thus precious. Tarka had died within the first few weeks. Tarka could not tame fire. It burned and devoured him. Mansha was fire. He taught Awnka to be fire, too.

Mansha means "knower." Mansha is not a name. It is an ancient title. In time, Awnka would be known by this title. After his initiation was complete, after he died and was reborn several times during his training, he would climb the seven great limbs of the central tree of the forest, live for a time in the nest of the eagles at the top, then become an eagle; his breath would fly off and return to the people to watch over them, to fight their unseen battles, and to reap his own rewards. He would grow strong, famed, and feared, and then find the next initiate, as had been done through all time.

The Shaman

The above story is a fantasy based upon years of reading and thinking about life before history.[8] Primal human life is unknown to us, but many have speculated on what it must have been like. Often, human existence is envisioned as comprising myriad tribes hunting and gathering, growing to a limit of maybe 100 or 200 people and then splitting into separate tribes, with each going their own way. Agriculture was probably known, but it was never the overriding way to obtain food. Throughout unrecorded history, the animal world was probably more important than the plant world, even though plants undoubtedly provided much more substance and materials than the animals ever could.

To look at this age, we must do the impossible: we must forget what we know today. No primal shaman had ever heard of concepts like "energy" or "life force": those ideas are far too recent. They would not even have had the concept of prana, but certainly they knew breath, air, and fire. What they thought about life, its cause, and what happens when it ends will forever be pure conjecture on our part, based on stories we create about ancient burials and figurines left behind. But whatever understandings our primal ancestors held became the basis for all that was to follow.

A plant would never chase, kill, and devour a man. Plants stayed put; animals did not. Many could kill you. Small animals could be just as dangerous as the larger ones; a snake could be poisonous, and bees can sting. But animals were also food. In this confusing world, covenants were needed between humans and animals. The covenants took the form of stories, easy to remember and important to learn.

Stories allowed us to understand the world and predict what might happen. The stories gave us the rules to live by. These rules governed the interactions between nature and people, and rules had to be enforced. That was a job for the shaman. Shamans walked the storied bridges between the human world and the realms of plants, animals, and the spirits of earth, water, wind, and fire.

As suggested, shamans have been considered proto-yogis.[9] Through their initiations and training, the shamans mastered the same tools that later yogis would also employ: dance, trance, plants, breath, and ecstasy. But there are differences. It has been bluntly stated that shamans seek to help others, while yogis seek to help themselves. That may seem overly harsh to the yogis, and it should be pointed out that shamans expect to be compensated for their services. They are paid in goods, prestige, social status, power, and even sex. Yogis seek personal gains more directly, hoping to achieve control over their own body and states of mind, magical abilities, and ultimately, spiritual liberation. The tools of the shaman and yogi may be similar, but the aims are quite different.

The First Profession

The role of the shaman was likely the first profession. Here, to differentiate the earliest shamans from the wide variety of modern shamans, the term "primal shaman" will be used when referring to the ancient mystics. Primal shamans were professional healers. Ultimately, death comes to every living thing, but when a person feels unwell, it is natural to seek aid and assistance. For this, our ancestors undoubtedly went to their shaman.

Why and when life's troubles arise is beyond the understanding of any normal person. However, all communities have one or two who are different. The strangeness of a certain individual, one born with an extra finger, a crooked face, a deformed foot, or who acquired strangeness as they grew—strangeness in speech, walk, or other behavior—automatically set them apart. It seems fitting that the one marked as strange within society would be the one to commune with the strangeness beyond it. Perhaps with that communion, the strange within society could be ambassadors to the strange outside the mortal realm, to plead, cajole, demand, or force a capitulation in favor of the human world. The one who knew how to do this would naturally be sought out, honored, feared, and hired.

Life is unpredictable and filled with the undesirable. No one really knows what tomorrow will bring: whether your mother's illness will abate, the tribe will win their next battle, the hunt will be successful, or the rains will return on time. Having recourse to a power that can shed some light on what might happen and how to prepare for it—or, better yet, prevent any bad times ahead—is worth any expense. The person claiming to foretell the future and forestall its dangers was certainly worth listening to. That person was the shaman.

Manvir Singh, a researcher who has investigated shamans around the world, proposed that "shamanism is a suite of practices developed through cultural evolution to convince observers that an individual can influence otherwise uncontrollable outcomes. In particular, the shaman is an individual who violates intuitions of humanness to convince group members that he or she can interact with the invisible forces who control unpredictable, important events."[10]

The successful shaman needs the quality of strangeness to demonstrate that they are not simply human but also part of another world where invisible powers lie that can help or harm us. And the shaman has to be a master of ritual and trance, the tools necessary to go into the other realm and battle on our behalf. Above all, the shaman must be believable and believed in.

Agency, Anxiety, and Pattern Recognition

Through evolution, *Homo sapiens* have attributes, skills, and characteristics allowing us to survive and thrive in an uncertain world. Three particularly important characteristics are agency, anxiety, and pattern recognition.

Imagine one of your ancient ancestors seated in some tall grass beside a copse of trees, talking with friends. He notices movements in the grass near the trees and feels apprehensive. His gaze is now fixed there. Some monkeys are cavorting, seemingly unconcerned, but he still feels tense, afraid. What just happened?

Agency is about cause and effect. Things happen for a reason. The grass near the trees moved, and his sense of agency tells him there was a cause of that action.[11] It is a mystery that needs attention, because the unknown may mask a potential danger. Until he knows for certain that he is safe, anxiety focuses his attention and prepares him for action.[12] We did not evolve for happiness; we evolved to be anxious so we'd be good at surviving.[13] A happy-go-lucky hominid who lacked anxiety did not survive long enough to become anyone's ancestor.

Pattern recognition is a powerful cognitive skill that allows us to make sense of the world and predict how the world will behave. While your ancestor scans the grasses, his mind is correlating the visual inputs into patterns and comparing these with past experiences to see whether they signify danger or are benign. Playful monkeys or foraging birds move the grasses in a particular pattern; stealthy predators have a distinctly different pattern. Here, anxiety and pattern recognition guide him to conclude which agent caused the grass to move. He signals to his friends, and they silently move far away from the trees, then see a pair of hyenas charge the monkeys.

Our minds create stories filled with agents. It matters not whether the stories are true; what matters is that we act "as if" they are true. Who cares whether the grass was moved by the wind or by a silently approaching predator? Grass moves, and we must pay attention.

Feeling and Judgment

We perceive two types of agency: our own sense of control (feeling of agency) and our judgment that others or things have agency (judgment of agency). These perceptions often lead to amusing behaviors. Consider crossing a street at a pedestrian-controlled light: pressing the button gives a sense of control. Even if someone else has already pressed it, you press it again, believing—however irrationally—that your action influences the light. Logically, you know it's on a timer, yet your logical brain will create a plausible cover story for your action: what if the other person didn't press hard enough? Or what if their button doesn't work? It can't hurt to be sure. Thus, it is (you tell yourself) entirely logical for you to have pressed that button. Why did you press it multiple times? Well... I am sure you will come up with a reason for that, too.

Judgment of agency arises when we attribute events to unseen forces. If grass moves, we assume something caused it—an animal, wind, or another invisible force. This cognitive leap led early humans to believe in spirits as explanations for the unknown. Shamans emerged as mediators with these unseen agents, promising healing, protection, or success in uncertain situations. Their influence persisted because they acted where outcomes were ambiguous—before a hunt, during illness, or in battle. Success reinforced their power; failure was blamed on factors beyond their control.[14]

The unseen agents are known as spirits. In primal times, spirits were the cause of all the unexplained things our ancestors experienced. Our ancestors' stories told to explain the world were spiritual stories. Today, belief in unseen forces remains. Whether through ancient spirits, modern rituals, or subconscious habits like pressing a button multiple times, our minds instinctively seek agency in a world that often operates on its own terms.

Shamanic Technologies

Manvir Singh believes that the key technology of the shaman is trance. While in a trance, they can visit the other realms, turn into a spirit or totem animal, converse with or battle demons. Manifestations of trance include displays of "trembling, shuddering, horripilation [a hair-raising experience], swooning, falling to the ground, yawning, lethargy, convulsions, foaming at the mouth, protruding eyes, large extrusions of the tongue, paralysis of a limb."[15] Anyone witnessing these conniptions would likely agree that the shaman is not fully present in the here and now but is somewhere else, doing battle or suffering grave discomfort.

The ability to induce belief in his power is precisely what kept the primal shaman in power. But credibility is determined by cultural norms: if the shaman's story of battling demons fits with society's belief in the reality of demons and spirits, the shaman is likely to be believed. His story makes sense. If society's mythos does not have demons but instead has celestial beings and gods determining our fate, the shaman's story will have to employ these themes. And if the mythos of the times is more rational and scientific, then the shaman will have to couch his power in those terms.

Shamans all over the world use a wide variety of tools and techniques to convince others of their strangeness and then suggest they are capable of overcoming the unseen agents threatening us. Strangeness can come from ascetic practice, refraining from sex, performing otherwise taboo practices, demonstrating immunity to poisons and pain—including walking on or swallowing hot coals—speaking strange languages, and performing a host of magic tricks. Trance can be obtained through plants, chants, fasting, freezing, dancing, drumming, and many more esoteric behaviors.

One surefire way of invoking trance is through changes in the breath. Ritual dancing, drumming, twirling, and running automatically affect the breath, as can drugs, chanting, meditation, and deliberate breathing practices. Breath and fire are two of the most important tools of the primal shaman, and they are two keys to unlocking the mystery and history of prana.

Towards the Present

In primal times, there naturally would have been an awareness of the importance of breath to life. No breath, no life. And fire would also have been seen as an essential part of daily life. Fire keeps us warm, cooks our food, holds back the darkness of night, and protects us from wild animals. But while fire, breath, and spirits would have been common concepts, there probably was not yet an idea of a life force, an élan vital. It is likely that the dualistic idea of a soul, separable from the body, which continued beyond the edge of death, did not exist.[16] With our modern views, it may be hard to conceive that people once believed only in the body and the animating spirit of the breath. If there was a soul, it was a physical part of the body and died when the body died, and that was it! When the breath left the body, the body and its soul were dead.[17] Before the idea that soul and body could be split apart, spirit was the essence of the animals, of water, fire, clouds, trees. All the things that affect people would have spirit.

The boy who saw the wind was a fire-walker and one of the first to follow the breath beyond the veil, but he was not yet a yogi. He was on the path, though. This was not quite the path I would find when I visited the Prana Yoga and Zen Centre.

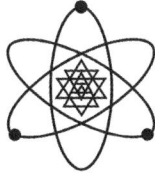

CHAPTER 4:

Prana Yoga

I first saw someone doing yoga in April 1997, at a small studio in downtown Vancouver affectionately known as Prana. Its full name was the Prana Yoga and Zen Centre. If Awnka was my imagined ancestor in the way of breath and fire, it was at Prana that I got my first taste of modern yoga.

I had come to find a group to meditate with. My twenty-year marriage had ended two years earlier, and while friends and Jungian analysis had been helping me get over the distress, it was taking a long time. I had begun meditating in the 1970s, in my early 20s, to handle the stress of a career in sales. But throughout those years, I was always practicing on my own, drawing upon advice gleaned from a variety of books about Zen. Now, in my early 40s, I needed a sangha, a community to practice with. Learning Zen from a book (I had been warned!) is like reading menu after menu while starving for food: the menus may look good, but they don't fill the belly. Self-taught meditations from books were equally unfulfilling. It was time to get serious.

Behind a narrow, glass front door, stairs took me to the second floor, where I found a sparse, open yoga room with white walls, a dark green, plush carpeted floor, about twenty thin, hand-sewn cloth mats in green and yellow arrayed in rows, each with a rectangular burgundy cushion, the kind you might find in a relaxed, laid-back Lebanese restaurant, and a few bamboo paintings of cherry blossoms and birds hanging on the walls. The center had just opened two weeks before, and the owners were limited in financial resources. They could not afford the rubber, plastic, and bamboo yoga mats, bolsters, and cushions that would become standard fare in yoga studios within ten years. On this day, the studio had no students.

I stepped into the room and offered a "hello" to the emptiness. From a back corner I had not noticed, a recessed area leading to an exit, a woman appeared. It is hard to remember what stood out about Ifat when I first met her; there are so many memories. Her attire was not North American modern. She was dressed in a dark blue robe flecked with black and gold, and matching dark blue pants. The lower part of her robe had rows of lighter blue patterns of squares, dots, and swirls. It appeared to be some sort of velvet; it looked heavy and warm, fitting the cool, wet, early spring weather in Vancouver. But her attire was not the most memorable feature. I would grow accustomed to Ifat's unique fashion sense and penchant for custom-tailored, flowing garb. It was not her ageless beauty, either, although I did estimate her to be in her mid-20s, which was a bit disconcerting if she was the Zen teacher; how much experience could she have gained so young? She was likely in her mid-30s—though she certainly didn't look it. No, most memorable were her eyes. Like her hair, they were dark. While her hair was pitch black, her eyes had a glow to them, like coal suffused with a deep heat. The heat in her eyes was accompanied by a warm smile and a rich Israeli accent.

Ifat Erez—or perhaps I should call her Shakti Mhi, as she is more popularly known today, for somewhere in the early 2000s, she changed many things in her life, including her name—was newly arrived in Vancouver. She had alighted a few months earlier, with a newly minted husband, Itamar Erez, and a limited amount of capital, acquired through a strategically timed wedding that had preceded their journey. Weddings, in most cultures, are occasions for gift giving, and Shakti had insisted any gifts to her and Itamar should be strictly cash. She knew this would be her only source of capital until the new center was thriving. I became her first meditation student in Vancouver.

Yoga came a few months later. Initially, I had no interest in yoga; I wanted to tame my mind. My body was fine. Besides, I couldn't relate to the yoga students I would see leaving the studio as I arrived for meditation. They were young, trim, female, and obviously very flexible. That was not me. But Shakti was persistent and persuasive; she wanted me to add yoga to my meditation. After a few months, she hooked me by uttering the magic words, "Yoga will really help your golf game!" *That* I could relate to.

Golf, to me, was Zen. Zen and the art of archery; Zen and motorcycle maintenance; Zen and tennis; Zen could be applied to any activity, including golf. I was an avid golfer; I studied it even more than I played it. There was not much I wouldn't do to improve my golf game. So I took up yoga. And yes, Shakti was right—it improved my golf game. I felt much more relaxed during tournaments, I finally broke par for the first time, I won my club championship, and I even had my first hole-in-one that year. However, yoga fascinated me so much that I quit golf in order to focus more fully on my yoga practice. So, in a way, Shakti lied—yoga killed my golf game. Well, not quite, but it did put my game into hibernation for about 15 years. Today, I am back golfing, and yoga is still helping me keep my scores respectable. But yoga for golfers is a different book, one I am not ready to write just yet.

The curiosity and fascination Shakti awakened drove me to learn as much as I could about the histories and philosophies underpinning yoga, meditation, and their religious and spiritual practices. Through authors like Joseph Campbell, David Gordon White, Thomas McEvilley, and Eliades Mircea, an ancient world opened before me. Yoga, it turned out, had a far deeper and more complex past than I'd ever suspected. What I loved about Joseph Campbell's approach to teaching was his compelling use of stories: myths, which he said were false on the outside, but true on the inside.[18] So as we follow the evolution of shamanism into organized religion, it seems only fitting to do this through a story.

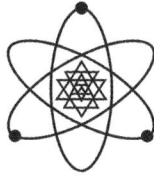

C H A P T E R 5:

The Woman Who Talked to the Stars

To understand how prana evolved in meaning and importance, we must enter a world where breath met brick, where water was more than refreshment—it was life itself. This story begins over 4,000 years ago, in a temple of baked clay and sacred smoke, in a city once known as Lagash. Here, we glimpse not a shaman's trance, but a priestess's ritual. Through her eyes, we witness how the breath of the gods became tied to blood, fire, and the celestial order. This fictional vignette, though imagined, is drawn from actual historical artifacts, inscriptions, and cosmologies of Sumer. It reflects the changing view of life force—from wind and fire to water and blood.

Would he come back?

Nanse had read the signs. Her stellar predictions had always proven true, and the sun had always returned before. But Gudea, king and high priest of Lagash, had muddied the waters. He'd renamed the sun god. No longer was it Utu or even Samas. Now, the sun was called Ningiszida, Gudea's personal god. Nanse, the temple's high priestess, had to adapt. Today was the winter solstice and the dedication of Ningiszida's temple. It was her duty to ensure the sun returned.

She touched the rough outer wall—unfinished brick without plaster or art. Construction had been delayed when workers were diverted to army duties, but the temple was close enough to complete the ceremony. A faint scent of cedar incense drew her inward.

The morning was bright, blue, cool, and cloudless. Inside, despite the numerous oil lamps and tallow candles made from the fat of sheep's kidneys, it was dim. The few windows high above helped, but they were there for the smoke, allowing a way for it to rise to the heavens, and specifically to the moon. Sacred smoke always went to the moon. The single window high in the thick southern wall was angled so that when Ningiszida was at his highest in the sky on the shortest day of the year, his light would shine down upon the altar.

By noon, everyone would know whether Nanse's entreaties were successful. When the ceremony was complete, she would have to stop speaking to Utu or Samas, the former names of the sun. Even the gods change. The gods were known by many names, and it was the duty of the priests to understand them all, cultivate their favor, and avoid any slights that may cause their anger. After all, humans had been created by the gods to be servants, and any servant who serves poorly is doomed.

For many months, Ningiszida sank lower and lower in the southern sky. If he could not be convinced to stop his wayward wanderings, the land would grow colder, darker, and eventually lifeless. As she predicted, over the last three days, the sun had fallen no further towards the southern horizon. She had marked the altar with the lowest point of his light, and today, if Ningiszida was returning, his light would not reach that mark. If her rituals had been done correctly (and of course they were!) and today's sacrifices were acceptable, he would not only return from the southern skies but take up residence here in his new house.

As her eyes adjusted to the indoor light, Nanse looked to the north door, where people were already gathering. None were dressed in fine attire; it was too early for the rich merchants and city functionaries to arrive. Present only were the farmers and soldiers and their families. Gudea had not yet arrived.

From the outside, the temple towered over the other buildings of the complex. Nanse's own residence was the second-largest building, a two-story home. The complex housed a granary, mangers, and sleeping quarters for the workers. Clerics occupied the only other two-story building, but the busiest was the common house, where the sick were tended and the homeless fed.

Ningiszida was the god of fertility, vegetation, life, and now, the rising sun. He ruled the underworld, where he slept at night, but he also lived in the sky. At night, with her finger, Nanse would trace his constellation, Hydra, the winged snake, the longest constellation, reaching from the far south to the north. She felt the earth beneath her feet and realized Ningiszida was there too, in the underworld below.

A temple is not just the house of a god; it is a center of society. Two full fields were set aside by Gudea solely to grow grain to be used by the temple. Ordinary people, after removing their shoes and washing their exposed skin, would stand, kneel, or lie prostate before the altar and the statue of Ningiszida.

On days with no rituals or feasts, the temple was still busy: the complex provided shelter for the homeless, food for the hungry, and healing for the sick. On this special day, however, nothing profane would be allowed near the temple. All the sick, all the women who had recently given birth, and all the men with shrunken penises were ordered outside the city gates. Nothing deemed offensive would be visible to Ningiszida.

Gudea arrived in a simple procession, accompanied by his wife, Ninalla, and their son Ur-Ningirsu. Gudea was dressed as always in simple dark robes and wore a lamb's wool sock hat pulled down over his head, with the bottom rolled up again like a brim as wide as his forehead. His face and head bore no hair; he was shaven and clean. As the high priestess, Nanse too had no hair upon her head. Gudea entered the private sanctuary of the priests, a small, roofless room at the southeast corner of the temple, and replaced his dark robes with the clean, pure, white robes of the priestly caste. Gudea walked with stately grace, hands folded right over left. His upright posture and solemn face bore the confidence of a ruler certain of his power and place.

Seven large urns of barley, seven fish, seven rings of gold, water, wine, beer, oils, and milk—all were ready for the offering. The incense was constantly replenished. Earlier, Nanse had checked on the seven lambs. They were penned, and the red-clad butcher-priests had their copper knives sharpened. The urns used to collect the blood of the lambs as the main offering of life to Ningiszida were ready and the braziers stocked with wood for roasting the meat.

The heart of any sacrifice was fire, the mouth of the gods and the way to the moon, the sky, and the stars. There was a small fire on the altar, into which butter and grain would be fed, but the main fires were located outside the temple. The best cuts of meat would be cooked inside and offered to Ningiszida on the altar.

Noon was approaching. The light of Ningiszida was creeping slowly toward the mark Nanse had made on the altar three days ago. She prayed that at its lowest point the beam of light would be no higher than her mark. Gudea began the ceremony by washing his hands and pouring the first offering of wine into the large, central basin. Around

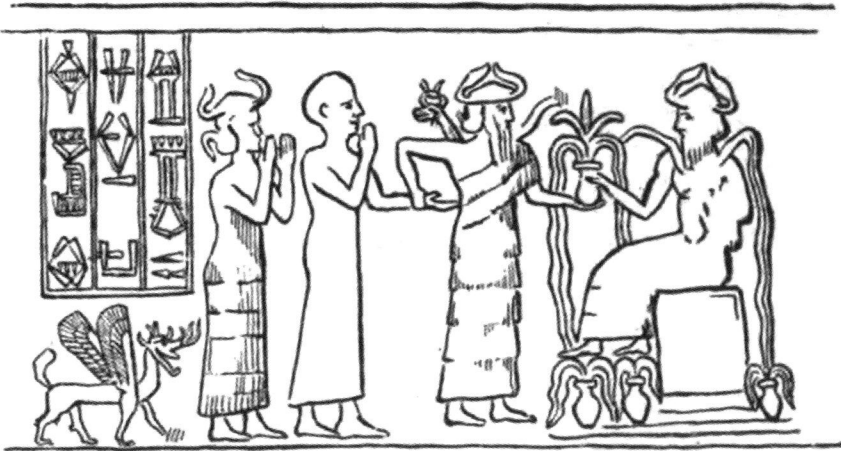

Figure 1: This drawing from a Sumerian seal shows Gudea being taken by his father, Ningiszida, and his mother, Ninsumun, to Ningirsu. It represents Gudea's acceptance as king by the gods. Of note are some of the symbols: the two snake heads coming out of the shoulder of Ningiszida; and the horned crown of the goddess Ninsumun.[19]

the sides of the basin, the artisans had carved a tableau showing Gudea and, to his right, Ningiszida, Gudea's spiritual father. Ningiszida was identifiable by the snake-like heads of dragons that rose from his shoulders. To the left of Gudea was Ninsumun, Gudea's spiritual mother, the nurturing goddess, wearing the horns of a cow. Ningiszida was holding Gudea's arm and presenting him to Ningirsu, showing that Gudea's claim to divine kingship was approved by the gods. On the opposite side of the basin were seven winged goddesses flying above seven maidens with jars overflowing with life-giving water. All were standing, floating upon a river of water, a river of life.

Nanse handed Gudea his libation cup filled with water, which he emptied into the basin. The cup depicting Ningiszida showed a pair of snakes entwined around the staff of life; their tails were joined at the bottom of the staff, and each snake curved and crossed the other six times, until the heads were touching at the top of the staff. Unbeknownst to Nanse, as this symbol diffused into the West, it would be called the caduceus of Hermes, a symbol of commerce. In the East, it would become a symbol of Shakti in her guise as Kundalini, with the snake on the right called *pingala*, the one of the left called *ida*, and the central staff of life named *sushumna*. The points of crossing would be called *chakras*. To the sides of each snake were dragons with the wings and talons of eagles and the bodies of lions. These were the mushussu, the dragons of Hydra.

Nanse chanted her liturgy: she sang of the greatness of Gudea. With each line of praise, she would pass an item to Gudea. He would address Ningiszida and pour the water and wine into the basin. As noon approached, the shaft of light crept downward to the demarcation on the altar. This was the time for the ultimate offering: the blood of the lambs. In the pens, the butcher priests began the sacrifice: one would hold a lamb, keeping the head up and neck extended, while another would insert the sharp

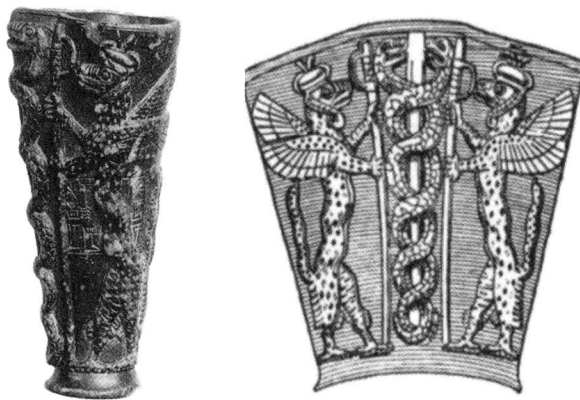

Figure 2: The libation cup (or vase) of Gudea on the left, also drawn as if it was unrolled, on the right. It shows two serpents entwined around a central staff. They are symbols of Gudea's personal god, Ningiszida, a fertility god. To the sides are two dragon figures, the mushussu,[20] which translates into "furious snake."

blade at the top of the neck and make a swift slice across the upper neck, severing the carotid artery and jugular vein. Quickly, they would position the urn to catch the spurting blood. The first priest would squeeze the lamb tightly to resist its attempts to escape, until, as the flow of blood slowed, the lamb fell still. Life is in the blood.

The urns filled with the sacred blood were brought by the butcher-priests to Gudea for blessing and then emptied into the basin. With this ultimate offering, Gudea asked Ningiszida to honor them, come back to them, and choose this temple to be his home.

Thankfully, the ray of sunlight at its lowest point was below the line Nanse had drawn, which meant the sun was higher in the sky. Nanse exhaled softly: Ningiszida had begun his northern return. She passed the seven gold rings to Gudea, who offered them to Ningiszida in thanks and placed them on the altar.

The final offerings were the choicest cuts of the cooked lambs. All the offerings would remain on the altar for several hours to allow Ningiszida time to ingest the food's spirit, its vitality. Close to sunset, all that was offered, the meat, fish, and grain, were given to those in attendance, who had been fasting all day. The first who'd arrived were the first to be served. The various liquid libations poured into the basin were never consumed; that would be unthinkable. Instead, they were poured upon the soil of the temple gardens, to return as new life, new crops.

The Symbols of Life

The above fictional vignette takes place around 2100 BCE in the ancient land of Sumer, located between two fertile rivers, the Tigris and the Euphrates, in what is now called southern Iraq. Over thousands of years, a new way of life arose—the way of agriculture. The settled life, built around crops and irrigation, transformed not only the economy but also the very conception of life itself. In the older, shamanic world, life was breath: to breathe was to live. But in temple societies, life required more than air. Life now flowed in liquids—sacred water, milk, wine, blood—offered back to the gods in rituals of renewal. Prana, in this new context, began to mean more than breath. It came to include the fluids that sustained the land, the people, and even the gods.

So many gods![21] Hundreds of them. Where the primal shaman only had to be familiar with the local spirits, those of the beasts and the land around him, priests catering to larger social groups had to contend with the heavenly hosts of gods above and gods below. It is from the earth that plants sprout, so the earth powers must be coerced into providing their bounty. It is from the sun that nurturing fire warms and stimulates growth. And it is the waters of sky and river that bring everything to life. Water is the blood of life. Priests had to know how to communicate with all these powers and convince them to cooperate with the city-state.

Agriculture on a large scale requires the ability to mark the passing of the days, the cycles of the seasons, to know when to sow and when to reap. The only way to create such a calendar and measure the passing of days, months, and seasons was by becoming intimately familiar with the stars and their changes. "As in heaven, so on earth" became the template for the social order. There were as many stars in the night sky as people in the cities: humans were a mirror below, reflecting what was happening above. And the stars were constant, always in the same relative positions to each other, rolling slowly across the night sky with the moving year. Since the stars were fixed in their place, so too should the citizens of a state be fixed in their roles in society. There was no thought of what you would like to do; your duty, your *dharma*, was defined for you by the powers above, and there was no point in questioning that. It was simply the inexorable order of the universe. The north star was always in the north, and a laborer would always be a laborer.

But there were those seven lights in the sky that were different;[22] they did change. Their behavior governed the events below them and had to be studied and known. The brightest object, the sun, was mirrored on earth by the king, who wore a crown that symbolized the sun's halo. The king ruled on earth as the sun ruled in the heavens. The sun's court of wandering planets who encircled him were matched by the king's ministers. The moon, who ruled the night and was variously described as the home of life itself, was a god of a different order entirely.

The Moon, Rebirth, and the Feminine Cycle

The moon waxes and wanes. It grows out of darkness, then becomes brighter and full over a two-week period. Then, once it has reached its prime of life, full of potency, it begins to decay and finally dies. It is gone for three nights, but then, miraculously, it is reborn and grows again. It is not a great leap to see in the moon's cycle a mirror of earthly rhythms: crops grow and die, animals reproduce and perish, and humans, too, follow this waxing and waning path. The moon became associated with life on earth. Indeed, in many cultures, the moon is a greater god than the sun because the moon is the source of life; the sun merely provides the energy for life. Ur was the city of Nanna, the moon god.[23] In India, the great god Shiva is the moon god, as denoted by the crescent moon found in his hair and by the horns of his great bull, Nandi.

Why a bull? The first sliver of a new moon and the last sliver of the dying moon form the horns of the moon. What creatures on earth have such horns? Cows! Thus, the cow is symbolically linked to the moon and is an equivalent symbol of life. Notice that in Figures 1, 3 and 4, all the gods are wearing horns, again symbolic of the power of life. The kings who represented the moon god also wore crowns of horns, unlike the kings who represented the sun god and wore the sun's circular halo as crowns.

The serpent also became a positive symbol of the moon.[24] Each year, a snake sheds its skin and grows a new one. It is not hard to see how some cultures made an intuitive leap from the rebirth of crops, the rebirth of the moon, and the rebirth of snakes to the idea that souls also come and go, through the process of *transmigration*, better known as *reincarnation*.

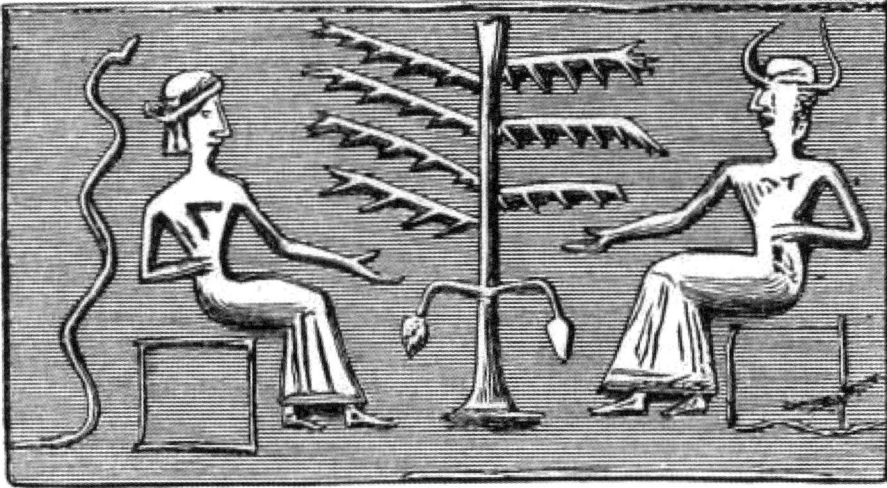

Figure 3: Drawing from a Sumerian cylinder seal impression, circa 22nd century BCE. The modern interpretation suggests it is a scene of worship, with a horned god on the right, a worshiper on the left, and a symbolic date palm and snake.[25]

Close to the snake is the goddess. Animal life comes from the female. The first woman of the Bible was given the name Eve, meaning life; she was the giver of life, the first goddess. The mother goddess and the serpent are often depicted close to the tree of life, as in the Garden of Eden. But this association predates the Bible by millennia. Figure 3 shows an imprint from a cylindrical seal from Sumer around the time of Gudea, circa 2200 BCE. The symbols powerfully suggest fertility: the horns of a god, representing the moon, the serpent, and the tree.

From Shamans to Priests: Institutionalizing the Sacred

The earliest priests were astronomers: they keenly watched the sky, where they found portents and auguries. Priests were required to predict not only one person's fate but the fate of the whole society. A shaman was an independent contractor with his own unique visions, power, and relationship to the spirits. Priests were part of a college and a caste, with its hierarchy and commitment to a shared understanding and process. When priests arise, shamans go underground. In some cases, the king fulfilled the role of the shaman, and he was used by the priests as a specific link to special knowledge and spiritual power. But, and this is important, the priests were the ones telling the king what to do: he was their talisman and, when needed, scapegoat.[26]

All ancient religions were based on the barter system. To convince a god to do you a favor, you had to return the favor—in advance. The principle of sacrifice required the priest to feed the gods and hope that in return, the gods would be pleased and grant the priest's request. Big requests required big payments. Of course, anyone could throw some butter or meat into a fire and make a wish, but a major sacrifice required special training. Rituals were developed with sacred scripts known only to the priests. This was power—the power to invoke and move the gods. This power was not shared with commoners. It was the secret possession of the priestly caste, passed down privately through the generations. Like the shamans, priests were different from ordinary people. They dressed differently, they ate differently, and they spoke a secret language of the gods.

King Gudea achieved the rank of priest-king. He married into the job, and his sisters-in-law were also in the priestly business. They knew the proper rituals to invoke and inspire the gods. While the above vignette is fictional, as we have no records of what exactly went on the day Gudea dedicated his new temple to Ningiszida, we do know Ningiszida was a new god that Gudea wanted to place into the pantheon, we know that one of Ningiszida's symbol was the double snake entwined around a central staff, and we know that Ningiszida was a fertility god, a bringer of life. But the key substance for us in this story is water, for it is water that brings life. In our search for the roots of prana, this story takes us beyond the primal shamanic tools of fire and wind, to the role of water and earth.

Water is the lifeblood of any society living in a dry land. It is the water from the river and the sky that brings life to the plants, which in turn give life to the animals, people, and gods. Water in this context is much broader than our view today: water is not simply H_2O. It is any precious liquid. The Sumerian word for water is "a" (pronounced "ah" as in "ma" and "fa la la la la"). You cannot get much more basic than that! But "a" has multiple meanings; it also refers to semen, to seed, to offspring, and to a riverway. And clearly, water is the main component of our blood.[27] The importance of water to Sumerians is found in their creation story, which is recounted in the endnotes.[28]

Water, the First Element

A key theme in many creation stories is the role of water. In the beginning, there was only water. The waters were separated and in between, land appeared. This is found in the creation story in Genesis, but there, it was not Enlil but God who did the separating. For the Hebrews, the original waters ("the deep")[29] were not a goddess, but inert and lifeless, for in that tradition, there can only be one god. But in each tradition, life came from the waters. In the Bible, God brings forth from the waters the moving creatures and the fowl that fly.[30] Over a thousand years earlier, in the Sumerian tale, it was Enki bringing forth life from the waters.

As in the heavens, so in the body: just as rivers nourish the land, the inner waters nourish the soul. In this view, prana is not just the breath that animates but the sacred flow that sustains.

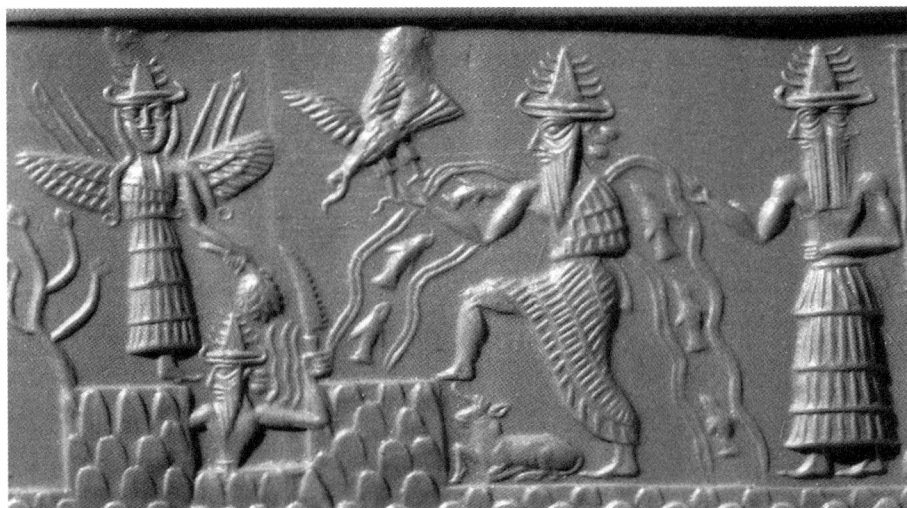

Figure 4: Detail of the Adda Seal.[31] Four gods wear pointed hats with multiple horns. Enki in the center, god of waters and wisdom, is identifiable by the streams of water and fish flowing from his shoulders. To the far right is Usimu, Enki's two-faced chief minister. Utu, the rising sun, is shown on the bottom left, digging his way up from his night's rest in the mountains. Notice the rays of light coming off his shoulders. Finally, on the far left is Inanna, who in Babylonian times would be called Ishtar, the winged goddess of war and love, with weapons sprouting from her shoulders. Originally, she may have been purely a fertility figure.

Sumerian Summary

Seen through the lens of these stories and symbols, we begin to understand how the spirit world of the shamans gave way to the divine order of the priests. A small tribal community of 100 people is concerned with their local conditions: the comings and goings of animals, the weather, events within the tribe and within the neighboring tribes. The world is small and close at hand. The shaman's role is to help coordinate the tribe's needs with the spirits that surround them. Life is equated with breath. In the larger societies of the planned agriculture world, there are tens of thousands of people. Roles are defined, hierarchies are formed, and castes are created. The sky and its stars hold the key to foretelling the future. The local spirits that worried a small tribe have evolved into the gods that live in the sky, on the tops of high mountains, in the waters, and under the earth. Where earlier, each tree, bubbling brook, and kind of animal had a spirit that needed to be accommodated, now the gods governed, directed, and commanded us. The interface between the gods and people became the priests. As priests assumed this role of intermediaries, they also subsumed the earlier shamanic roles of healer, fortune teller, and life planner.

The stories told by society and confirmed as truth by the priests also evolved. The little stories of spirits were not abandoned; they were overwritten by the grander mythologies of the gods. In these stories are found the rules of the universe and the rules of society. These tales are etiologies of life, explaining why life is the way it is, why society is the way it is, why one must obey and fulfill one's role in society.

In tribal life, prana was wind and fire. In temple culture, it flowed in water, blood, and sacred libations—vital fluids that nourished both gods and people.[32] As myths evolved, so too did the concept of prana.

Far from being merely of historical interest, I would soon come to feel these ancient echoes in my own body, in my own breath—at a yoga teacher training in the forests of British Columbia. There, amid early mornings, quiet meditations, and the teachings of Shakti, the ancient and the modern would meet. Prana would no longer be a story from the past. It would inform my daily practice.

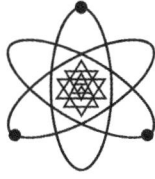

CHAPTER 6:

The Inner Ear

"Don't teach kumbhaka with empty lungs to beginners," warned Shakti. "Tell them to sip in a little air, then hold, but only until they feel the pressure to breathe again. Never force it." She was introducing us to the practice of pranayama as well as prana's intention and power.

Shakti had changed out of her morning attire of tight black yoga clothes. While mornings in the forest were cool, it was already warming up. She let her turquoise pashmina shawl slip from her shoulders to the floor. It was 11 a.m. We had done our morning asana and meditation practice, had breakfast, and completed our karma yoga chores of cleaning the various rooms, preparing meals, and washing the dishes. It was lecture time for the next two hours.

Before Shakti could carry on, the whole class was distracted by the door opening to reveal Grant and Rhonda sneaking in, with a giggle, a shush, and a hush. The teacher training retreat had only started three days ago, but it was obvious to everyone that these two had really hit it off. In the coming year, they would become a very tight couple and open the Wandering Yogi studio in Vancouver.

The retreat had begun on August 1st, a bright, blue-sky Saturday. Sixteen of us had gathered under the gaze of Shakti at the Inner Ear Retreat Centre on the Sunshine Coast of British Columbia, a short journey from Vancouver. Of the 16 students, Grant and I were the only men. Shakti designated me the "eager stiffy"—ready, willing, and unable to do every pose, regardless of the folly. My counterpoints were the "sexy flexies," like Momoko, a Japanese-Canadian yoga teacher who could bend her body into impossible shapes. Good teachers had to teach all students, from the eager but stiff to the casually hypermobile and all bodies in between.

The retreat center was in the middle of a West Coast rainforest. Meals were taken in a two-story lodge. Nearby in the woods were several rustic cabins, meaning the toilet facilities were outside. I was sleeping in a pup tent set up near a pond in front of the lodge.

Between the cabins and the pond was the Quonset hut—a half-cylinder-shaped structure that housed a recording studio. Our 6:45 a.m. yoga practices were done upstairs in its loft. Our 6 a.m. and 9 p.m. meditation sessions were held downstairs in an open area. This is where we were all sitting for our morning lecture when Shakti began to teach us about the contraindications for pranayama practice.

On the wall behind Shakti was a rendition of the rising sun made of flat strips of wood, fashioned into a semi-circle with large rays radiating outward and upward. From my vantage point, she was the source of the radiance.

Arranged on the floor in front of Shakti, on a large, red Persian rug, we sat on cushions. A few tired students were lying down on their bellies, looking up at Shakti. To my right sat Louise, sitting very proper and upright, with her constant smile and short brown hair. She looked like a pixie. To my left was Momoko, poised and serene. Though compact in stature, she could move like liquid silk. Shakti began to teach us about the breath.

Breath as a Path to Stillness

In Sanskrit, *kumbha* means pot or vessel. *Kumbhaka* is the retention of breath—held in "the pot of your belly." There are only four basic things you can do with breath: inhale, hold, exhale, and hold again. Each of these has a name:

- *Puraka*: inhalation
- *Antara kumbhaka*: holding after inhaling
- *Rechaka*: exhalation
- *Bahya* (or *bahir*) *kumbhaka*: holding after exhaling

Simple and straightforward. What else is there to do with breath? Well, later I would learn of a fifth state: *kevala kumbhaka*—an effortless, spontaneous pause in breathing that arises without trying. But at this stage, I was like a child learning the basics of reading and arithmetic. This was my first yoga teacher training, although I hadn't planned on teaching yoga; I just wanted to understand it more deeply.

From Sivananda to Shakti

Shakti's teachings drew from her own explorations, layered atop her training in the Sivananda tradition and life in several ashrams. Born in Israel, she discovered yoga at age 14, worked briefly as an actor, married, and moved to Montreal. There, she left both her husband and former life behind and met Swami Vishnudevananda, a disciple of Swami Sivananda of Rishikesh.

Vishnudevananda had opened the Sivananda Yoga Vedanta Centre in Montreal in 1959—the first of many he would establish worldwide. He pioneered the model of offering yoga teacher training certifications in the West. While Maharishi Mahesh Yogi introduced the Beatles to meditation, it was Vishnudevananda who introduced them to yoga. Shakti traveled with him and lived in Sivananda centers in San Francisco, the Bahamas, and India. Immersed in a full yogic lifestyle—posture, kriya, diet, philosophy, pranayama, and meditation—she eventually formed her own path. What we received during the retreat was a blend of classical Sivananda methods and Shakti's personal insight.

"Kumbhaka is pranayama," writes Swami Niranjanananda Saraswati, referring to a line from the Yoga Sutras of Patanjali that he translates as: "Pranayama is the pause in the movement of inhalation and exhalation."[33] Patanjali, the fourth-century compiler of yogic practice, described yoga as the stilling of the mind's fluctuations: *yoga citta vritti nirodha*. When do thoughts stop? When the breath stops.

I later heard the ashtanga teacher Richard Freeman put it like this: "The mind and the breath are like two fish in a school. When one moves, the other moves." Stilling the mind through sheer will is difficult, but the yogis found a backdoor: the breath. The tantric teacher Rod Stryker echoed this: "The moment between breaths is the moment between thoughts."

Experiencing kevala kumbhaka, the effortless suspension of breath, is the aim of pranayama—to prepare the body and mind for that spontaneous stillness. When breath ceases, mental chatter dissolves, and one may enter *samadhi*—a deep state of inner absorption. All the other forms of pranayama techniques and practices are in the service of kumbhaka.

Safe Breathing: Guidelines and Cautions

Shakti was meticulous about student safety and instilled this vigilance in future teachers. Every posture had contraindications. "Before teaching anything to anybody," she warned, "make sure it's safe to do so." Pranayama was no different. She stressed that breath control must develop gradually and never be forced or coerced.

The Hatha Yoga Pradipika, a fifteenth-century text, offers a stark caution: "Just as lions, elephants, and tigers are controlled slowly, so too must the breath be tamed gradually. Otherwise, it can kill the practitioner."[34] One of Shakti's most memorable cautions stayed with me: "Pranayama practice will make you more of what you already are. If you're neurotic, it may make you psychotic. If you're calm, it may make you blissful."

Her list of guidelines was clear: "Don't hold your breath if you're pregnant, have been using drugs, have high blood pressure or heart issues, or if you're suffering from eye, ear, or throat infections, headaches, or indigestion. If a cramp or side stitch arises—stop. Ideally, pranayama requires a clean diet, no intoxicants, and moderation in sexual activity. And above all—teachers, *watch your students.*"

To help train us in this awareness, she had us partner up and observe one another's breath. Louise and I paired off. She lay on her back with one hand on her belly. "Watch the stomach," reminded Shakti. "Do not stare at a woman's chest. You are looking at the wrong place!" As she said this, her gaze went from me to Grant, who was hovering over Rhonda.

These were foundational teachings—simple, but not easy. In theory, breath observation is straightforward, but in the classroom, it's challenging to monitor each student. Louise's belly rose on the inhale and fell on the exhale—classic *abdominal breathing*, also called *diaphragmatic breathing* (though the diaphragm is involved in all breath).

When the opposite happens—when the belly sinks on the inhale and rises on the exhale—it's called *paradoxical breathing*. We were taught to retrain the movement by placing a palm lightly on the belly and say, "As you breathe in, push my hand away. As you breathe out, allow my hand to fall."

We then repeated the exercise with the student seated. It's harder to observe belly movement this way, but a soft gaze helps. Peripheral vision can detect subtle torso shifts. In still sitting, even the breath grows quiet, but you might notice gentle belly or clavicle movements. Tiny waves—each one a mirror of the mind.

The Three-Part Yogic Breath

The focus that morning was on a foundational Sivananda technique: the *three-part yogic breath*. Sitting comfortably, we placed one hand on the belly and the other on the lower side ribs. "Begin with an exhalation," said Shakti. "Then inhale by filling the lower lungs first—feel your belly expand beneath your hand. Next, draw breath into the mid-lungs, sensing the ribs move outward into your fingers. Finally, bring the breath into the upper lungs, placing your lower hand now on the clavicles to feel their gentle lift." To complete the cycle, we exhaled in reverse—top, middle, then bottom.

After five rounds, we paused to reflect. I felt grounded, calm, and unusually present—and we had practiced for barely a minute.

Shakti then introduced a variation combining breath and movement. We began with arms resting at our sides. As we inhaled—belly, ribs, and chest expanding—we raised our arms in sync. When our arms reached shoulder height, we were breathing into the mid-lungs. As they floated overhead, we filled the upper chest. After a brief pause, we reversed the motion with a smooth, full exhalation: arms lowering as awareness descended from clavicles to ribs to belly. We repeated this sequence five times.

This simple practice, she explained, trains a deeper, slower breathing pattern. It's said to utilize the full capacity of the lungs, enhance oxygen saturation, and develop conscious control of the breath. Years later, when I delved into the physiology more deeply, I came to understand why that claim isn't entirely accurate—but I'll return to that question in Chapter 21, "The Life of Breath."

Patanjali on Pranayama

While parts of our training touched on yoga philosophy, Shakti didn't dive deeply into any one school. She did mention Patanjali's Yoga Sutras, though his treatment of pranayama is brief—just five sutras (2.49–2.53). Unlike Shakti, who offered practical techniques, Patanjali gave no how-to guidance. Still, he clearly valued pranayama as an essential limb of practice, preparing the aspirant for the deeper inner stages that culminate in samadhi.

Like a methodical engineer, Patanjali defined key aspects of pranayama. He outlined its stages: inhalation, exhalation, the intentional pauses between them, and the spontaneous stillness of kevala kumbhaka. He also listed its components: *placement* (directing awareness and energy to specific regions), *number* (repetitions), *duration* (how long each cycle lasts),[35] and *intensity* (the degree of effort or subtlety employed).

In the Sivananda tradition, the essence of pranayama lies in lengthening the breath without force. It is a practice of gentle refinement. As Swami Sivananda of Rishikesh put it, "A yogi measures the span of life by the number of breaths, not by the number of years."[36] The slower you breathe, the longer you will live.

Swami Niranjanananda claims that advanced yogis can reduce their breathing to one breath a minute, then one an hour, and eventually one a *week!* He even cites a case of a 102-year-old yogi who reportedly stopped breathing for nine days.[37] It sounded to me like something out of shamanic lore—remarkable, perhaps, but difficult to accept without a trace of skepticism.

Pranayama in the Woods

The forest surrounding the Inner Ear Retreat Centre wasn't old growth. Like much of the Sunshine Coast, it had been logged long ago, and fire had taken its toll in places. The trees I walked among were replanted decades earlier—tall and dense, but less diverse than an untouched forest. Still, there was beauty: western red cedar, Douglas fir, and hemlock, alongside deer and sword ferns, birch, and salal bushes.

I'd found a quiet meadow where I liked to rehearse. I sat atop a fallen giant of a fir tree, its bark softened by pale green moss. Mushrooms and salal sprouted from the trunk, and at the far end, a young hemlock had taken root, already reaching nearly ten feet tall. The old fir had become a "nursery tree." As planting cultures have long known, before new life arrives and thrives, old life decays and fades away.

The teacher training had progressed. Each afternoon, students took turns being the teacher, leading part of the class. Today, I would be teaching *anuloma viloma*, also called *nadi shodhana*. Shakti simply called it "alternate nostril breathing." I sat on my tree, held up my right hand with a wide "V" between the middle and ring finger, then folded my forefinger and middle finger to the palm, leaving the thumb, ring and little fingers extended.

I sang out the instructions, mimicking Shakti's tone and accent: "Exhale completely. With your thumb, press against your right nostril, blocking it, through your left nostril, inhale...two...three...four." With each count, I loudly patted my thigh with my left hand, keeping the rhythm.

"With your ring finger and thumb, pinch both nostrils closed and hold...two...three...four. Open your right nostril, keep your left nostril closed with your ring finger, and exhale...two...three...four. Now, through your right nostril, inhale...two...three...four. Again, pinch both nostrils closed and hold...two...three...four. Open your left nostril and exhale...two...three...four." Each count was one second.

With each cycle, I simplified the instructions:

Left, inhale...two...three...four.

Hold...two...three...four.

Right, exhale...two...three...four.

Right, inhale...two...three...four.

Hold...two...three...four.

Left, exhale...two...three...four.

Again, more succinctly:

Left, inhale (pat, pat, pat went my hand on my thigh).

Hold (pat, pat, pat).

Right, exhale (pat, pat, pat).

Right, inhale (pat, pat, pat).

Hold (pat, pat, pat).

Left, exhale (pat, pat, pat).

Nadi shodhana means "cleaning of the nadis". The *nadis* are the channels for prana found in the subtle body, a tantric teaching that was adopted by hatha yogis. *Anuloma viloma* means "against the grain" and refers to the practice being a counter-intuitive way to breathe.[38]

Beginners start with a 1:1:1 ratio—equal counts for inhale, hold, and exhale. As capacity grows, the exhalation is extended (1:1:2), then the hold (1:2:2), and eventually the classic 1:4:2 pattern, with a 16-count retention. Since the purpose of pranayama is to slow the breath and extend the pauses, kumbhakas gradually lengthen over time.

Advanced practitioners may add bahir kumbhaka—a hold after exhaling—creating four-part cycles like 1:1:1:1 or even 1:16:4:8. The advanced cycle translates to just two full breaths a minute. Shakti considered this too advanced for most students.

Shakti did not teach holding the breath when the lungs were empty. That was too challenging. She also mentioned that this technique of counting time was only for teaching students: when doing your own personal practice, she told us to forgo counting and hold for as long as comfortable. Three minutes of practice was the maximum for almost all students, which would be about 12 cycles of 1:1:1. Ancient yogis apparently worked up to 42 cycles or even more, while doing the most challenging ratios. That could take up to 30 minutes or longer.

As always, Shakti taught us the contraindications: nadi shodhana should not be done by anyone with high blood pressure or heart conditions, but it is okay for pregnant students as long as they omit the kumbhakas. Studies showed that for hypertensive adults, nadi shodhana without the kumbhakas can reduce blood pressure significantly (by about 10/4 points).[39] But the primary benefit, Shakti emphasized, was increased breath-holding capacity—an essential preparation for more advanced breathwork.[40]

Kapalabhati and Bhastrika: Fire Breaths

While nadi shodhana brought balance and calm, other pranayama practices were designed to energize and invigorate.[41] Of the five pranayamas Shakti taught us, my favorite was *kapalabhati*, which she said meant "shining skull." As I'd been steadily losing hair through my 30s, I joked that I already had a head start. Shakti corrected me: "Kapala means skull. Bhati means shining. After practicing kapalabhati, you'll be so cleansed that your scalp will shine!" It had nothing to do with hair loss.

Swami Niranjanananda offered a more nuanced interpretation: *kapala* as cranium or forehead, and *bhati* as light, clarity, even knowledge. "Kapalabhati," he said, "brings clarity to the frontal brain."[42] Whatever the meaning, I found it invigorating.

Shakti was meticulous about posture. She reminded us to scan students' posture: were they slouching? If so, give them a cushion to level the pelvis. Still hunched? Place a hand lightly on the lower back and another between the clavicles. "Touch," she warned, "is just to bring awareness, not to move the body." The spine should be upright, the head neutral, the shoulders and jaw relaxed. For students struggling, she recommended practicing in front of a mirror.

Kapalabhati is counterintuitive: the exhale is active, the inhale passive—the opposite of normal breathing. Students often contort their whole bodies rather than isolate the belly. Placing a hand on my abdomen, I took a small inhale. Then, contracting my abdominal muscles, I sharply drew in my belly and exhaled through the nose. "Hummpff." The belly pulled in. Then I relaxed, allowing a passive, silent inhale. My hand rose with the belly. I repeated this 30 times, then rested.[43]

Bhastrika is similar, but I didn't enjoy it as much. Used in kundalini yoga—where it's called "breath of fire"—it's more forceful.[44] Unlike kapalabhati, where the inhale is passive, in bhastrika both inhale and exhale are sharp and active, like the bellows used by blacksmiths. Some legends say mountain monks would use it to warm themselves on freezing nights.

Each inhalation is short, sharp, and fast, followed quickly by an equally short, sharp exhalation. There is a constant noise from the nose, like the noise of a bellows fanning the flames. Beginners will naturally have to learn this slowly, but experienced students will eventually cycle faster and faster. This is quite unlike kapalabhati, where, with advancing practice, the breath actually gets slower.[45] Bhastrika is deliberate hyperventilation—with its physiological consequences: elevated heart rate, high blood pressure, and dangerously low carbon dioxide levels.

It often surprises yoga students that carbon dioxide isn't just a waste product but is also essential to healthy function. While excess CO_2 is harmful, too little is also risky. That's why kumbhakas are so important after energizing techniques. They give CO_2 a chance to rebuild and stabilize the system. Skipping the pause can lead to dizziness, anxiety, or worse—a crash course in respiratory physiology. Yogis use hyperventilation deliberately: to reduce CO_2 and allow longer kumbhakas. The Hatha Yoga Pradipika even claims bhastrika awakens kundalini.[46] I would come to understand these links—especially the role of carbon dioxide—in much greater detail later (see Chapter 21, "The Life of Breath").

As always, there were cautions. Kapalabhati and bhastrika were off-limits for pregnant students ("too bouncy for the baby," said Shakti), as well as anyone who had recently eaten or who had high blood pressure, infections, or headaches. Iyengar took it even further, claiming these practices should not be taught to women at all, lest they cause sagging breasts or uterine prolapse![47] Shakti disagreed and taught them to all genders. The claimed benefits were impressive: toned abdominal muscles, cleared lungs, improved asthma, strengthened diaphragm, and stimulated heart.

One practice not found in any Sivananda text I'd seen, but beloved by Shakti, was *chakra breathing*. She often used it to warm up a class. Sitting cross-legged on a cushion, we'd slowly exhale and collapse forward, rounding the spine and bringing the head toward the navel. Elbows were bent, hands beside the hips. On the inhale, we'd lift our arms in front, arch the back, and roll the chest and pelvis forward. Then we'd exhale and collapse again. We'd do ten fast repetitions, then sit tall for three deep breaths. No kumbhaka here—"too much energy in the body," said Shakti. A variation involved raising the arms to the sides instead of the front.[48]

Coffee Enemas and Peanut Butter Sandwiches

The hardest part of the retreat for many students wasn't the yoga or the silence—it was the lack of coffee. For me, that wasn't a problem. I'd tried coffee once at age 10, hated it, and never touched it again. Our mornings always began with oatmeal and decaf tea. Lunches and dinners were equally plain: salads, rice, vegetables, and some kind of protein—usually tofu or beans. Deliberately dull. We were cleansing the body and, by extension, the mind. But by mid-August, the blackberry bushes lining the gravel road began to ripen. Each morning, angels and heroes would gather the berries, and suddenly oatmeal included a touch of sweetness. Those berries lifted everyone's mood.

Still, the diet wore on me. At 180 cm (5'11") and always on the lean side, I'd started the training at 68 kilos (150 lbs.). Two weeks in, I'd lost over four kilos and was looking gaunt. Shakti grew concerned. I tried to eat more but couldn't keep up. So one sunny afternoon, while the others napped or studied, we snuck away. Driving north along Highway 101 toward Sechelt—a name meaning "land between two waters" in the Coast Salish language—we moved between inlet and strait, past evergreens and driftwood beaches, until we reached Clayton's Market.

Inside, the artificial lighting, cold air, and buzzing sounds hit hard. Two weeks of retreat serenity dissolved instantly. We grabbed a loaf of bread and a jar of peanut butter and headed back. Shakti thought the bread might help me regain weight. After lunch and dinner, I would sneak back to my tent and enjoy my private dessert. I did not regain any weight, but at least I stopped losing more.

Meanwhile, many students were suffering caffeine withdrawal. Shakti's remedy? Enemas. It was my first—and last—experience with them. For those especially desperate, she suggested coffee enemas, which she said could "cleanse the liver." Whether any scientific basis supported that claim didn't matter—for some, desperation won out. The process was simple: first a standard enema, then one with coffee, which was to be held for fifteen minutes. Whether the caffeine was absorbed through the lower bowel or the aroma was simply comforting, the procedure seemed to work, and coffee enemas became surprisingly popular.

Bandhas: Containing the Current

As the days slid by, a steady routine took hold: early rising, 6:00 a.m. meditation and yoga, a 9:00 a.m. breakfast, karma yoga chores, lectures, a 1:30 lunch, study time or siesta, student-led asana classes, another yoga session, dinner around 8:00 p.m., and a final hour of meditation. We fell into the rhythm of retreat life. Old topics recurred in our classes, while new ones kept us alert.

After exploring the fundamentals of pranayama, Shakti introduced us to the *bandhas*. In tantra, people who are rigid or overly controlling are said to be "stuck" at the first chakra. Joseph Campbell jokingly referred to them as "creeps," though in modern parlance we might say "tight asses." In hatha yoga, however, tightening the anus is not a personality flaw—it's a technique. The repetitive contraction of the anal sphincter is called *ashvini mudra*, while a sustained lift of the perineum is known as *mula bandha*.[49]

"Bandhas," explained Shakti, "lock in the energy stimulated during your practice." They're best applied at the end of pranayama sessions—except after energizing practices like chakra breathing. Though mula bandha was the first one she taught, she called it advanced. "If you're having money problems," she quipped, "it might be because your root chakra is too tight. Mula bandha can help you control your anus—and your wallet."

To teach the technique, she led us through what, to me at least, felt like a slightly surreal exercise. Maybe I was still traumatized from the coffee enema class. We sat on our heels with knees slightly apart in a pose known as *vajrasana*. "Picture your anus as a beautiful flower," she said. "Now open the petals... and contract the flower. Pull it up—all the way to your throat. Then relax the flower. Let it sink down again." We repeated the imagery several times. She encouraged us to add this to breathwork: inhale gently, then during the kumbhaka, lift the pelvic floor. No forcing. When the breath wanted to move, we'd exhale and release the contraction.

I couldn't help wondering—why were yoga teachers so fixated on the anus? But I came to realize that hatha yoga places great emphasis on internal cleansing, the *shat kriyas*—six purificatory actions.[50] Yogic enemas were just one of them. Shakti also taught us *neti*, the nasal rinse. While many used a proper neti pot, she demonstrated how to do it with a coffee mug. All these practices, she insisted, support optimal health—prerequisites for advanced pranayama and meditation. If your system isn't clean, she warned, breath practices could make things worse.

Promoting "anal health" was part of this regimen. One morning she declared, "When you shower, cover your finger in soap and insert it into your anus. Swirl it around to clear any stuck stools." This, she claimed, enhanced mula bandha. Benefits included stimulating the area, improving blood flow, and increasing control. Personally, I wasn't sure why more control was necessary—I'd had things under control since I was two years old. Still, I was learning to suspend judgment.

Mudras: Rewiring the Circuits

Mudra means a seal or lock, according to B.K.S. Iyengar.[51] It usually involves closing the body's apertures or placing the limbs or fingers in specific positions to redirect energy. Recall that a bandha refers to specific muscular contractions, which contain and direct prana. The two terms are sometimes used interchangeably: a bandha can be a mudra, and vice versa.

David Swenson, an ashtanga teacher I would later study with, likens a bandha to a valve—allowing energy to move in one direction while preventing it from leaking backwards.[52] Iyengar compared bandhas to electrical transformers that control the voltage of prana before it flows into our "wiring." Without such control, the force could be overwhelming.

Swami Niranjanananda Saraswati uses a similar analogy.[53] He describes nadis as wires, and the circuits formed by their intersections as the subtle infrastructure of the energetic body. Mudras "rewire" the circuits; bandhas store and regulate the energy generated through pranayama. Prana is the current. The aim is to redirect apana (downward energy) upward and prana (upward energy) downward, so they meet in the core and awaken kundalini in the sushumna, the central spinal channel. Without bandhas, this energy could surge wildly, like an electrical storm, potentially harming the nadis or nervous system.

Iyengar claimed that the first bandha to master is *jalandhara bandha*, the chin lock. Shakti disagreed—she felt it was the most advanced and told us not to teach it in classes. We were to explore it privately, ideally after practices like kapalabhati. It could be combined with mula bandha, but only with a small amount of air in the lungs. Done with completely empty lungs, it's much more challenging. For some, simply bowing the head is sufficient, as anatomical variation prevents full chin-to-chest contact in many students. Paul Grilley suggested no neck movement at all—just retain the breath without tensing the throat.[54]

The third bandha, *uddiyana bandha*, involves hollowing the belly after a full exhalation. It can only be practiced on an empty stomach.[55] Drawing the abdomen inward and upward massages the organs and lifts energy up. If your digestion isn't clean, that energy may bring unwelcome revisitations and regurgitations. Iyengar poetically claimed this bandha could "make you young again" and was "the lion that kills the elephant named death."[56] Niranjanananda Saraswati warned it's not suitable for pregnant practitioners or those with heart or stomach issues, though it may be beneficial postpartum to tone abdominal and uterine muscles.[57]

With these three bandhas—mula, jalandhara, and uddiyana—Shakti introduced us to the fourth: *maha bandha*, the "great lock," which combines all three. When practiced in a specific seated posture, with one heel pressing the perineum and the opposite leg straight and that foot held by both hands, it becomes *maha mudra*.[58] These were powerful techniques—tools to safely harness and redirect the vital energy that pranayama awakens.

From the Pier to the Office

The month was ending. On the last evening, Shakti organized a gala feast and allowed us to have wine. It was a surprising luxury, and soon everyone was tipsy—although the next morning, she admitted the wine had been non-alcoholic! The evening air was filled with laughter, feeding perfectly into a talent contest held in the Quonset hut. Fittingly for a yoga gathering, the party ended early, and by 10 p.m., I was in my tent, falling asleep to memories of a month spent in the woods.

The next morning, we rose at 5:30 a.m. in darkness and made our way to the Roberts Creek pier. Over the past century, this wharf had worn many faces. It was originally built to welcome day visitors from Vancouver to the wilderness of what was once called the Sunshine Belt. Settled in the 1880s, the area had become home to pulp mills and logging camps. During the day, the wharf bustled with activity, surrounded by shops and anchored by the well-known Gumboot Restaurant. At this early hour, though, it was quiet—emptied of both busyness and business.

Shakti was nowhere in sight when we arrived. The gravel path beckoning us along the pier splitting the ocean was lined with shrubs and lit by two rows of glowing paper bags, each containing a single tea light. In the pre-dawn dark, the flickering orange lights felt magical. We were transitioning: from the forest's scent of cedar and the hush of wind through trees to the salty tang of the sea and the whisper of lapping waves. From a canopy of green to a vast, star-strewn sky. From earth and air to water and space.

We reached the wooden platform at the end of the pier in silence. Shakti was already there, seated in meditation, facing east. A faint glow to the east announced the coming day. We joined her, sitting together in stillness. The sky gradually brightened. The sun remained hidden behind the coastal hills and forest, but the day had begun. Shakti initiated the final ceremony—our graduation.

Later that afternoon, on the ferry back to Vancouver, I thought about the ceremony. One month of simple food, forest air, daily yoga, and twice-daily meditation had changed me. I felt clear. Centered. Lighter. In the early days of the retreat, I'd doubted the decision to come—my business challenges tugged at my thoughts. But now, I questioned why I was going back.

The next morning was Monday. My calendar was full: meetings, memos, phone calls, telexes, faxes—and these new things called emails. By noon, I was shaking. The adrenaline that had drained away during the retreat came rushing back. It felt like I'd drunk ten cups of coffee. I was jittery, anxious, and by dinner, exhausted. I was back in the world.

But the breath I carried with me from the forest helped. Nadi shodhana calmed the surge. Asana gave me balance. The teacher training had been a beginning, not just a break. I was returning not as the same man who had left, but as someone with tools to steady himself.

This was my life now: yoga and business. And that included more travel to faraway lands where other lessons would be learned.

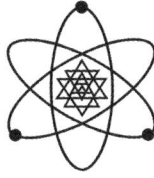

CHAPTER 7:

Mad Dogs and Englishmen

The whole week had been hot and humid. During the day, the thermometers were stuck in the high 30s Celsius (100 Fahrenheit), and the humidity was fluctuating between oppressive and miserable. Dan Friedmann and I were looking forward to our trip to Dehradun. We were promised that the weather would be cooler. On Friday morning, we hired a car to take us from our hotel in New Delhi. It was an old Hindustan Ambassador, basically a copy of the 1950s British Morris Oxford, black in color, which seemed a strange choice given how hot it always was in India, but the driver assured us it had air conditioning. A/C was the magic mantra, and he was hired. To avoid the heat of the day, we left well before dawn. Sunrise in Delhi in July is around 5:45 a.m., so we were on the road by 4:30. I was surprised how many people were up already, working in the fields and repairing roads, despite the darkness. I guessed that they too wanted to beat the heat.

We were in India to meet with the Surveyor General, the National Remote Sensing Agency (NRSA), and other government agencies to present our technology for creating maps from satellite imagery. Our company, MacDonald Dettwiler and Associates (MDA), had done business with the NRSA in the past. I had joined MDA in 1984 after working as a salesman at Xerox for seven years. I had also just completed an undergraduate degree in science, which helped me understand the technology behind MDA's offerings.

Dan, technically brilliant and personally driven, was three years younger than I but had been with MDA five years longer. When I joined, MDA was small, with only 240 employees. By the time I left MDA, in 2014, there were thousands, and the dramatic growth was mostly due to Dan. His career progression was remarkable, and my career followed in his wake, like a water skier being pulled by a fast boat. Come 1993, he was president, and I was the vice president of sales. By 1995, he was the CEO; he then made me an executive vice president in charge of the space division and, later, the larger systems division. MDA grew to be a multibillion-dollar company. But during this trip to India in 1987, Dan was marketing and I was sales.

Delhi to Dehradun was 160 miles, which by my reckoning would take us three hours. But this was India, and I should have known better. Dehradun is in the foothills of the Himalayas. Our driver hadn't lied: his Ambassador did have air conditioning, but what he didn't tell us was that he could not run the A/C while the car was driving uphill; there was not enough power in the little 1.5 liter engine to do both. Being in the foothills of the Himalayas meant that we were climbing most of the time, which also meant the A/C was off most of the time. Despite that, the driver still had to stop several times to refill the radiator, and the journey took over six hours. It was a long, hot day, and by the time we made it back to our hotel, we were cooked. I slept poorly that night and was very tired as we headed to the airport the next morning to fly to our next stop: Bangalore, a burgeoning high-tech mecca in the middle of India. I'd heard that Bangalore, situated on the Deccan plateau and sitting about 900 meters above sea level, was also cooler than New Delhi. I needed cooler.

The flight was uneventful, by Indian standards. By Western standards, it was crowded, noisy, warm, and humid. After landing and collecting our luggage, we took a taxi, which drove along an old airport road towards our hotel. Along the way, I noticed a scruffy golf course with nobody on it. There was more brown than green, but it was the first golf course I had seen in India. Our next meeting was not until Monday. We had Sunday off with nothing in particular to do. Neither Dan nor I were much for sightseeing, but I made the brilliant suggestion to go golfing. The hotel staff arranged to have a car take us. I have no idea where exactly the golf course was or even its name, but I recall it was owned or run by or affiliated with the military in some way. I had taken up golfing a few years earlier, but Dan had not golfed since he was a young teen in Chile.

We rented a half set of clubs each, which a young boy carried for us. A forecaddie ran out ahead to hunt down any stray shots. The fairways were more dirt than grass, but the forecaddie was good: by the time I got to my ball, it was always miraculously sitting on the only tuft of grass around. On a hot, sunny Sunday in July, we were alone on the course. Noel Coward's song "Mad Dogs and Englishmen" was repeating in my head.

Dan's swing was rusty. He kept topping the ball, which would hop a few feet forward, stop quickly, and mock him in its stillness. After a few holes of watching Dan miss the ball, the forecaddie got bored and distracted. Then Dan finally connected: his ball shot off like a cruise missile, never getting more than four feet off the ground—about the height of the caddy's upper back. With an alarming thud, the ball struck and the boy fell. In concern, Dan and I rushed up to him, while the other caddy lagged behind, unable to suppress his laughter. The forecaddie then popped up, one hand rubbing his back and the other pointing down to the ball, showing Dan where he would be playing his next shot.

I was 33 years old, with hair already thinning, and what remained was fair in color. Dan had a luxurious crop of black hair protecting his skull. Neither of us had thought about wearing a hat that day. Fortunately, the course was short and we finished playing in under three hours and headed back to our hotel. The next morning, I could not get out of bed. Heat stroke. Dan was not feeling great either, but at least he was vertical. I stayed in bed while he took the scheduled meetings without me. I was extremely dizzy, tired, sometimes nauseous, and sometimes hot. I had no appetite but did drink several bottles of Limca, a lemon- and lime-flavored soda pop. By the next morning, I was feeling a little better, enough to get up and catch our next flight and continue our Indian tour. The memory of what heat stroke felt like, the extreme dizziness, was vivid and unforgettable. I was later told by an Indian Ayurvedic doctor that I suffered an extreme excess of pitta, which is an Ayurvedic term for heat energy. I translated this to mean, "You fried your brains." Ever since that day, I have always worn a hat whenever venturing out of doors. Once burned, twice shy.

This trip to India was one of the first times I truly understood that the body speaks its own language—and sometimes it shouts. That lesson, delivered under a blazing sun, would echo later in my practice of yoga and pranayama: pay attention, or pay the price.

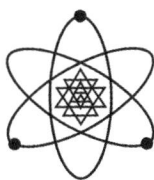

CHAPTER 8:

The Kindness of Strangers

It wasn't the end of the world. I still had my passport, wallet, and tickets, which were all in my suit pockets. But my notes of all the meetings we'd had over the past two weeks in India, and confidential copies of proposals to clients, were gone. Dan and Jayaraman—the agent our representing company, Malhar, had assigned to us for this trip—could help reconstruct some of my notes. We were leaving Lucknow to fly to Madras soon, and there wasn't much time left before the flight to find my missing briefcase.

In 1996, Madras would be renamed Chennai as part of an ongoing government directive to change the names of cities and states to reflect local pronunciation and history. Bombay became Mumbai in 1995. The spelling of Calcutta was changed to Kolkata in 2001. Mysore became Mysuru in 2007. Today, we were flying to Madras, and from there, we would board an aircraft to Hong Kong and then fly back home to Vancouver.

I had been mindless. In the taxi to the Lucknow airport, I'd placed my briefcase on the ledge under the back window. When we arrived at the airport, we got our luggage out of the trunk of the car and hustled towards the throng of people crowding the ticket agent. It was always a mad crush of humanity at every airport, a loud, colorful collection of potential passengers trying to get the agent's attention so they could claim their boarding pass. Jayaraman was a magician at getting us through the crowd and obtaining our passes. We still had an hour before the flight, so we sat down on one of the benches in the airport waiting area. Only then did I realize I had left my briefcase in the taxi. My heart sank and the pit of my belly felt hollow. Shit!

The old airport in Lucknow was small, dark, and warm. It would be replaced over the following years and modernized, but right then, I sat near an electric fan that was trying its best to keep me calm and cool. It was failing.

Lucknow is the capital of Uttar Pradesh, located in the north of India. It is India's most populous state, officially formed in 1950, following Indian independence. The region's history, however, is ancient. Archaeological evidence suggests that Stone Age humans were here as far back as 85,000 years ago. Domesticated animals and farming practices likely began here around 8,000 years ago. This is the ancient land of the Kurus and the Kosala kingdom. Many events described in the great Indian epics, the *Mahabharata* and *Ramayana*, are believed to have taken place in this region.

This history was completely unknown to me while I was sitting and brooding over my lost valise. My mood instantly improved when I saw our taxi driver walking towards me. He had my briefcase. He said it took him a while to realize that I had left it in his car but as soon as he noticed it, he came back to the airport and sought us out. It was fortunate that I had not yet boarded the plane. Through the kindness of a stranger, weeks of work were salvaged.

Decades later, I discovered that the roads the taxi driver followed en route to the airport were the same that mystics, monks, and yogis had traveled. Knowledge and kindness had been shared among strangers here in the north of India for millennia, as the following story illustrates.

That art thou!

Winter was cool, delightfully so. It had rained the day before, and Kapila's gourd was now full of fresh water. But his mind was troubled by a recent conversation. A monk had greeted him yesterday with the standard greeting, "Who are you? Where are you from? Who is your teacher? And what does he teach?" When Kapila had asked the same questions of the monk, he received the reply, "I am Mankha, from Savatthi. My teacher is Gosala and he teaches heresy!" Mankha shared his teacher's heresy, leaving Kapila confused and unsettled. While the day was pleasant and the walking easy, his mind could not dislodge the seeds of doubt that Mankha had sown.

All of Kapila's teachers had trained him in the four Vedas. He had memorized them in childhood and could recite each verse by heart. He knew all the limbs of the Vedas—the Vedangas: pronunciation and phonetics, grammar and meter, etymology and semantics. He had studied the sky and the movement of stars. He understood rituals, ethics, and duty. Yet he understood life poorly and knew nothing of how to avoid grief. He had set out to find new teachers to complete his education. Instead, he found only confusion.

Kapila was tall, with long, unbound hair cascading down his back. He was naked, save for a strip of cloth around his loins and a necklace of wooden beads. He was clean, despite being covered in ash. He carried only a cloth bag tied to the end of his walking stick, along with a gourd and a begging bowl. This was standard attire for mendicants who lived off whatever alms they could obtain.

There was no hurry. Kapila was walking east, with no particular destination in mind. He had begun in Kuru, where he'd been born and raised, then wandered through Pancala and now Kosala. He supposed he would eventually reach Magadha. In the distance he spied a solitary figure, struggling to walk with a long wooden staff. When he was close enough, he could see the old man was an ascetic, thin as a spoke and bent from years of harsh living. He too was nearly naked, wearing only a worn, tawny rag around his loins. "Grandfather," said Kapila, "How do you fare? Are you in need? May I help you?"

The ascetic paused, smiled, and replied, "Thank you, son. What is your name? Where are you from? And… do you have any water? I have not yet broken my fast today, nor have I drunk anything."

Kapila gave the old man his water, answered his questions, and suggested they rest beneath a banyan tree he had passed earlier. It was beside a brook that gurgled into a small, bright green lake. The ascetic agreed, took Kapila's hand, and was led to the tree. Children were playing in the green water while their mothers washed clothes.

The wide branches of the banyan tree served as drying rods for the women's laundry. Baby monkeys plucked the last of the dried figs from the branches and tossed them at the women below. As he sat down, the old man picked off a piece of bark and began to chew it slowly. He didn't swallow—just chewed.

Once they were seated, Kapila felt emboldened and dared to ask the old man some questions. "Grandfather, what is your name? Where are you from? In all your years, you must have had many teachers. What have you learned of the source of life and the causes of pain? Please be so kind as to teach me while we sit and rest."

"I am Svetaketu from far to the west, past the land of Kuru. My family now lives in the city of Taxila. My father was a great sage, as was his father before him. I have spent my life learning the secrets of kings and brahmins. I have heard much and deliberately forgotten even more—useless teachings that lead only to confusion.

"And I have taught many. My *shishyas*, my students, earned their privilege through serving me over months and years. I have never taught the unworthy or those who were not ready. You ask me to teach, but you have not earned that right! I am old, though, and my remaining days are few, so I will not live long enough for you to earn my trust. And yet—should I share with you?

"Grandfather," said Kapila, "I am young, and much remains hidden from me. You are old, and your eyes are open. Please, dispel my darkness."

Svetaketu nodded, then looked around the small lake. "I have not eaten today. Take my bowl and ask for alms among the women. If you succeed, I will answer seven questions." Kapila took the old man's bowl and approached the women, but they had no food to offer. He followed their directions to the village and an hour later returned with a dried chapati and a lump of stale dahl. While Svetaketu ate, Kapila waited by the water, pondering what to ask. He didn't want to waste a single question.

When Svetaketu had finished eating, Kapila cleaned his bowl and then sat beside him. Svetaketu waited until the women and children were gone before signaling for Kapila to begin. It would not be proper for others to overhear the knowledge to be shared this day. They had to be alone. A few monkeys sat in the branches above, but they too could not be allowed to listen. Svetaketu instructed Kapila to chase them away.

Alone in the midday sun but shaded by the branches of the banyan tree, Kapila began with his most perplexing concern: "Grandfather, what is the source of suffering?"

Svetaketu seemed annoyed by the question, and his answer was brief: "Ignorance of Sat is the source of all suffering."

Kapila did not understand. "Grandfather, what is Sat?"

"Sat is the source of self."

"What is self?"

"The self is the one who is listening to you ask this question."

Kapila discovered that asking questions was tricky. He had already used three. He decided on a different approach. Remembering yesterday's conversation with the monk Mankha, he said, "I was recently told that the gods are dried-up shit-sticks, and that rituals are pointless. Priests are pointless too. They do not understand the cause of suffering, nor how to escape it. As a brahmin, these words cut me. I was confused and angry."

Svetaketu softened and looked directly at Kapila. "That is not a question—but there is some truth in it. The gods are symbols, reflections of aspects of Sat. Those who worship gods give Sat the name of gods: Sat is called *Prajapati, Purusha, Hiranyagarbha, Prana, Vayu, Rudra*. All these are aspects of Sat. Just as the arm, the leg, the mouth, the ears, the eyes, memory, and mind are aspects of the body, so too are the gods aspects of Sat. Rituals have their place—but they will not reveal Sat."

Svetaketu paused for a moment, but Kapila dared not speak. He hoped there was more to be revealed and felt silence was the best question now. He was rewarded when Svetaketu continued. "Around us is the world of endless forms. Look—and all you see stretches on and on. This is the world of names and forms: *namarupa*. This is the world of gods and men, of animals and plants. It seems so vast, so real—but it is illusion. This entire universe you see... is within you." At that, Svetaketu poked his finger at Kapila's heart and continued, "All the heavens, all the hells, all the gods... they are within you!" Svetaketu's finger tapped Kapila's chest again and again. "You must follow their signs, like a farmer tracking the footprints of a lost cow.

"This is the truth of truths: it is ignorance of Sat that leads us to identify with the body—and to suffer its frailties. When we realize we are not the impermanent physical form, but we are Sat, what can we suffer? A drop of water is not truly a drop—that is only its name and form, its namarupa. It is water. That is its nature. If it believes itself to be a drop, it suffers: fearing loss, longing for permanence, caught in desire and aversion. But in truth, it is water. When it falls into the ocean, a drop dissolves into its true nature and there is no drop to experience suffering. Salt in water dissolves and becomes one with the water. In its separateness, it is subject to suffering. When it realizes it is one with all, there is no separateness and there is no suffering.

"This world of names and forms is made of *prakriti*—matter, memory, thoughts, and feelings. But the self is pure awareness—*purusha*, or consciousness, which remains unattached to the physical world. Like two birds perched on the same branch: one, prakriti, eats the fruit of the tree, while the other, purusha, merely watches. That second bird is the self."

Svetaketu noticed the confusion remaining on Kapila's face, sighed, and said, "You don't understand. That's all right. Pick up that fig on the ground. Good. Now break it open. What do you see?"

Kapila complied and said, "I see small seeds."

"Good, now break open one of the seeds and tell me what you see."

"I see nothing, sir."

"You perceive nothing—yet from that seeming nothing at the center of the seed arises the great banyan tree." Svetaketu raised his arms, indicating the breadth of the tree they sat beneath. "All that exists has that invisible essence, including you, Kapila. *Tat tvam asi!* You are that![59] That is the self."

Happy that his approach was working, Kapila risked one of his four remaining questions. "Please teach me more. How does the drop of water return to the ocean?"

"Ah," answered Svetaketu, "that is a big question. Do you know of the five fires? No? It is a secret teaching of the caste of kings, the *Kshatriyas*.[60] We *Brahmins*, being of the priestly caste, learn the secret rituals of the Vedas and know the power of sacrifice, of *yajna*, but kings and warriors preserve their own branches of knowledge—wisdom they do not share lightly. This teaching was revealed to me and my father, Uddalaka, by King Pravahana, son of Jibala, and it explains the cycle of becoming and leaving."

Svetaketu adjusted his seat, sat tall, and began the lesson. "The heavens are the first fire. To them, the gods offer faith, and from this offering, the moon is born. The god of rain, *Parjanya*, is the second fire. To him, the gods offer the moon—and from this, rain is born. The earth is the third fire. To it, the gods offer rain, and food is born. Man is the fourth fire. To him, the gods offer food, and semen is formed. Woman is the fifth fire. To her, the gods offer semen, and a man is born. At life's end, that man is carried to the funeral pyre and consumed by fire—returning to that from which he came."

Svetaketu turned his head to look at Kapila and explained, "This is the path of the moon, the path of smoke, young Kapila. When a man dies, the smoke from the funeral pyre rises into the sky and reaches the moon. There, the self abides for a time, nourished by the light of the ancestors. Then the moon releases water back to the earth—as rain, as dew. That water feeds the plants. The plants are eaten by animals and by man. Within man, this essence becomes semen. When the seed is planted in the garden of a woman, new life arises. And so the cycle turns again. Those who live have lived before. If they follow the path of the moon, they will return. But those who, at the moment of death, know that the self is Sat—those rare ones follow the path of the sun, the path of fire. They go through the sun-door and do not return. The self is Sat. When this is known, there is no more need to come back and live again. Do you understand, Kapila?"

Kapila nodded, though not with confidence. He had heard such teachings. *We return. The self comes back again and again.* "I understand the teaching, and it feels right to me… but how can I know if it is true? I have heard many stories from many sages along the road—some say we are born once, others say many times. How can I know what is true?"

Svetaketu looked into the distance, as if listening to his own teacher from years ago.

"You can know the truth in two ways: through *sruti*—what has been heard in the ancient teachings—and through *yukti*—reason, reflection, and observation. If I tell you that water comes from fire, how will you know that is true? See for yourself. What happens when the fire within you is too strong? You sweat. Where does the water come from, if not from fire? Pour water upon the earth—what happens? Plants grow. A man eats plants—his body grows. He generates semen. When that seed is planted in a woman, a baby grows. Everything I have told you can be known—not only by scripture, but by seeing, thinking, and reasoning."

Kapila nodded again, this time more thoughtfully. "I understand now—it is a series of transformations. From fire comes water; from water, plants; from plants, men, and so on. But all of these are physical things. Is the self also physical?"

"The self is not physical like the body, the mind, the moon, or the earth," said Svetaketu. "The self is a drop from the ocean that is Sat. All things—whether physical or not—are aspects of Sat."

Kapila paused for a long time. He knew he had only one question left, yet so many remained. What was most important to learn—was it better to dispel confusion or seek new understanding? To clarify a hidden point, or pursue something entirely new?

In the end, he gave up trying to plan his final inquiry and blurted out, "It doesn't make sense! How can the immaterial self bring life to a material form?"

"Prana!" came the swift reply. Kapila's shoulders sagged with disappointment.

Seeing this, Svetaketu smiled softly and began to explain. "Remember the two birds I spoke of earlier? The bird that eats the fruit is prakriti—the material world, with all its suffering, memories, and thoughts. The second bird, purusha, is the self—the observer, the witness, consciousness itself. Now, the branch they sit on is like a thread connecting them. That branch, that thread, is prana. Prana is the activity that binds the self to prakriti. When prana weakens—through old age, illness, or injury—the self's tether to the body begins to loosen. And when prana leaves the body, the self leaves as well."

Kapila showed a glimmer of understanding, but Svetaketu could see he had not yet fully grasped it. He continued: "There is the physical aspect of Sat—what we call nature, or prakriti. But without prana, nature is senseless, inert, dead. Nature is part of Sat, and so is the self. The self—some call it purusha, some say soul or *atman*, some say consciousness—is not the mind. It is not the intellect. It is not the ego. These are all aspects of nature. Sat is the material body. Sat is also the immaterial self. Prana flows through both. When prana departs, the body fails and decays. The self then takes one of two paths: it may pass through the moon door, follow the path of smoke, and be born again, or it may pass through the sun door, follow the path of fire, and never be reborn.

"Now, just as Sat has many aspects, so too does prana. There are five aspects of prana. Each has its role and location, but all are *vayus*—the winds, the breaths of life.

"Vayu is the breath of Sat, and it is also found within each of us. Air, a form of vayu, is more powerful than any other substance. When fire goes out, it is swallowed by air. When the sun sets, it is swallowed by air. When water dries up, it is swallowed by air.

"Vayu is the swallower. In man, prana is the swallower. When you sleep, your eyes, your ears, your thoughts are all swallowed up by prana, and you are aware of nothing.

"Understand? Prana is both a cosmic principle of life and also the personal life-activity within you. The self does not animate the body—prana does. It is the thread that ties the self to life, to prakriti.

"Prana moves within the body, but that is a longer telling. I grow tired now, Kapila. If you were my student, I would tell you to return tomorrow for further instruction. And there is still much for you to learn. One day, you will be told about the secret channel that runs from the heart to the head—the path through which the self, no larger than your thumb and dwelling in the heart, is driven upward by prana to the crown of the head. When that happens, you will depart through the sun door—or the moon.

"Please remember—nothing I have told you must be taken on faith. By one's own wit, one knows the truth. Studying the Vedas and relying on ritual will lead to the moon. Heaven may be attained, but it is neither free from pain nor permanent. All who reach it must one day return here. To follow the path of the sun, rely on reason and observation. They will reveal the truth to you. You can work this all out for yourself.

"And now that your seven questions have been answered—and I am weary—I ask you to leave me. Continue your journey, young Kapila, and ponder my answers well."

Kapila was filled with gratitude. His mind overflowed with what he had received. He honored the knowledge by prostrating before the sage. Touching Svetaketu's feet and then his own head seven times—once for each question—he rose, bade the yogi farewell, and resumed his eastward journey.

Samkhya

Kapila walked for hours. His pace was slow, unhurried—but his mind was far from calm. Thoughts swirled: of Sat and self; purusha and prakriti; smoke and fire; moon and sun; the power of prana. But one idea rose above the rest: reason! His whole life, he had been taught that true knowledge came only through *shruti*, the revealed wisdom of the Vedas. Now, he realized that through logic and observation, he could find answers to the questions that had long plagued him. Many of the teachings Svetaketu had shared didn't fully make sense. But if he applied his mind, if he reasoned carefully, they might yet be made reasonable. It was not just permitted—it was necessary to question what he had once been told to accept without doubt. Even Svetaketu's revelations could be explored, tested, and perhaps improved upon.

He struggled to understand how his own self could be part of Sat, and Svetaketu's self also part of Sat. If Svetaketu became free from illusion, then wouldn't Kapila, who shared the same essence, also be free? When one self passes through the sun door, why do others still pass through the moon door? If one drop of water realizes it is the ocean, and the ocean is present in all drops—why are not all drops liberated at once?

There is a time when the curious mind seeks new information, eager to expand. And then comes a time when the cup is full—when no more can be poured in until the contents are digested. Kapila had reached that point. When he saw another monk walking toward him, he slipped away. He did not want more teachings—not now. The time for divergent thinking, for gathering, had passed. It was now time for convergence—for synthesis. He needed to digest what he had learned and make sense of it.

The logic of Svetaketu seemed sweet and compelling. Fire devolves into water, water into plants. Plants grow in the earth. But perhaps, Kapila thought, this could be looked at in reverse. Earth evolves from water; water evolves from fire. But whence fire? Svetaketu had said it comes from air. And air? Air must evolve from a subtler substance—space. Akasa. Thus, there must be five basic evolutes from which the visible world is made manifest. Kapila named these *bhuta*—not mere "elements," for they themselves evolved out of something subtler. They are formed from the higher forces of nature, from prakriti itself.

"Think deeper!" he told himself. "How do I know these *bhutas*, these evolutes? I sense them. I can smell the earth. I can taste water. I see fire. I feel the wind. And space? I hear sound. Each of the five evolutes has a sense through which it is perceived." These five cognitive senses Kapila called *jnanendriya*—the organs of knowledge.

Deeper still. "In order for me to see fire, something must link the flame to my eyes. To hear a bird's song, something must carry its sound to my ears. Logically, there must be subtle flows from the objects I perceive to the sense organs. Since there are five evolutes and five cognitive senses, there must be five subtle potentials, the essences of these perceptions. These," Kapila reasoned, "are the *tanmatras*—the subtle elements."

And deeper still. "The senses receive—that is one kind of action. But the body also performs outward acts. I defecate. I grasp. I walk. I speak. I procreate." These active faculties Kapila named *karmendriya*—the organs of action.

"I think. But what is this 'I'? I sense, I act, I desire—but who is this I who claims these actions? Is it purusha? No—Svetaketu was clear: purusha does not act. Purusha is the silent witness, like the bird who watches from the branch. The other bird—the one who eats, who engages with the world—that is this *I*. This acting *I* must lie above the body, the senses, even the mind. It is subtler." Kapila called it *ahamkara*—the ego, the maker of "I". But where does *ahamkara* come from? From intelligence, from *buddhi*—the faculty of discernment, of reason. And what gives rise to *buddhi*? The first principle to evolve from nature itself: prakriti.

Thus, Kapila reasoned his way to understanding.

He thought through all this as he walked over the next few days. In time, he arrived at a village, where kind people offered him a small hut to rest in. As he sat, his thoughts returned to prakriti. Was it elemental—or was prakriti itself made of something more fundamental?

Outside the hut, he saw a young woman weaving a basket, intertwining thin strips of bark. At her side, her mother spun coarse fibers of hemp into rope. His mind leapt: perhaps prakriti, like the basket and rope, was woven from basic threads. He called these threads *gunas*. They could not be fire, or water, or plants—those were effects. These threads had to be more basic, more subtle—made only of themselves. But how many threads? The women used three. Two would not hold; more seemed unnecessary. Three were enough. Kapila had his inspiration: gunas—three in number, each with a different quality—might be the underlying substance of all prakriti. And not just of matter. Could these threads also weave the mind?

Kapila continued wandering eastward, slowly. By the time the rains returned, he found himself in another small village, where he was again offered a humble hut to pass the wet weeks. Though small, it was dry and warm, its walls well lined with cow dung. During this time of stillness, he completed his reflections and compiled the teachings he had received—now tempered and clarified through reason.

What Svetaketu had taught, he now fully grasped. Nature—prakriti—was the manifest form of the universe. In its quiescent, unmanifest state—*mulaprakriti*—it was space and time itself, a latent potential. From this root evolved intelligence (*buddhi*), which others called *mahat*—the great principle, source of discernment and will. From *buddhi* emerged the ego (*ahamkara*), the sense of individuality. From ahamkara came *manas*, the coordinating mind; the ten *indriyas*, or sense faculties—five for perception, five for action; and the five tanmatras, the subtle essences. From these tanmatras, the five bhutas—the gross elements—finally took shape.

The universe, Kapila realized, was an evolution from the subtlest forms of nature to the grossest particles of matter. At the summit of subtlety stood only two principles: prakriti, the material substratum, and purusha, pure consciousness. Or rather—*purushas* in the plural. Svetaketu had spoken of Sat, a single unitary principle from which all emerged. Others called it *brahman*—not a god, but the ground of all gods.[61] But was such a notion necessary? Kapila reasoned, "I have no need of that principle. The existence of one aware being—a purusha—suffices to explain consciousness. Since my awareness does not encompass what Svetaketu perceives, each of us must possess our own purusha, separate, singular, yet all tethered to the same world of prakriti. To posit Sat only complicates what can be made simple.

"If the universe is an outward unfolding from the root of prakriti, then freedom must be an inward return. Liberation is an *involution*—a reversal through the layers of existence, until mulaprakriti is reconstituted, still and untouched. At that point, purusha can detach. It enters the sun door—and is never again reborn into this world."

When the rains had passed, Kapila saw no need to travel farther. He had arrived. He began to teach, just as Svetaketu had taught him. But unlike Svetaketu, he would teach anyone who asked, regardless of caste or learning. He laid out the nature of existence, calling his teaching *Samkhya*—to reason, to deliberate, to enumerate. It was an ontology, a map of how things came to be. To those weary of the endless cycles of life—rebirth through the moon door again and again—he offered release through two means: an ascetic way of life, to shed attachment to the pleasures of prakriti; and *viveka*—discernment—an understanding of Samkhya, the way of the world. His way was a yoga, but one of separation: purusha must scrape itself free from the clutches of prakriti so it is never tempted to return to this physical world.

In the beginning, his students were few. But in time, his nephew Asuri came and became his disciple. Asuri's student was Pancashikha. Together, they carried the teachings forward—some say expanding, some say transforming them. The village where Kapila had settled grew into a small city, its fame rising alongside his own. After his passing, his disciples renamed it Kapilavastu. And there, a few generations later, two great sages are said to have been born: Mahavira, the Jain teacher; and Siddhartha Gautama of the Sakya clan, who would come to be known as the Buddha.[62]

The Axial Age East

To understand a story, context is required. To understand the import of the above story, some history is required. Most historians agree that a group called the proto-Indo-Europeans lived on the steppes between the Caspian and Black seas 5,000–6,000 years ago. Over millennia, they migrated into Europe and South Asia. One group, the Indo-Aryans, entered the Indus Valley and Gangetic plains between 2000 and 1500 BCE, during a time of climatic upheaval. Their sacred texts, the Vedas—from the same root as "video," meaning "to see" or "to know"—were passed down orally through priestly lineages.

The Rig Veda, oldest of the four, tells of Purusha, the cosmic being with a thousand heads, eyes, and feet, whose body became the world. From his mouth came priests, from his arms kings, from his thighs the commoners, and from his feet the servants. His breath became vayu, or prana.[63] Prana combines *"pra"* (forth) and *"an"* (to breathe or move), signifying the source of all movement—especially breath. But it is more than breath. In the Atharva Veda, prana is exalted as a god—ruler over all forms, the vital breath at the heart of existence. "Reverence to Prana, to whom all this (universe) is subject, who has become the lord of the all, on whom the all is supported!... O Prana, be not turned away from me, thou shalt not be other than myself.... O Prana, do bind to me, that I may live."[64] Prana was not just wind or life-force—it was thunder, rain, sun, moon, death, power. The gods worshipped prana. It ruled all.

After the Vedas, new teachings emerged. Some were called the Brahmanas and Aranyakas and elaborated on priestly rituals. A different set of texts—the Upanishads—took a more philosophical turn. Often interpreted as "learning by sitting near a teacher," *upanishad* also means "secret doctrine."[65] These texts explored the nature of reality. They often disagreed with each other but shared one idea: brahman, the essence of the universe, is atman, your personal essence. *Tat tvam asi*—you are that.

Between 800 and 200 BCE, a profound shift occurred across China, India, the Middle East, and Greece—a period the German Philosopher Karl Jaspers called the Axial Age.[66] Independently, these regions began to question inherited religious traditions and explore the nature of knowledge, existence, and reality. Philosophy emerged—not just in Greece. It was the time of Daoism, Confucianism, and many other schools of thought in China, the time of the prophets of the Old Testament in the Levant, the time of philosophers in Greece, and the time of the Upanishads, Jainism, and Buddhism in South Asia.

It was also a time of wandering sages—hermits in China, ascetics in India, philosophers in Greece, and prophets in Israel. Many of these seekers founded schools to share their insights. In India, *shramanas* roamed the Ganges and Indus valleys, rejecting priestly authority and societal norms in pursuit of spiritual liberation.

Early shamanic cultures linked life to breath. As societies grew, so did their understanding—life also needed water, fire, and earth. These elements were personified as deities, but later thinkers sought deeper explanations. If life is breath, what causes that first breath? What draws the soul into the body—or causes it to leave at death? Is breath enough for life? Can a soulless body live? Are breathing animals soulless? Such questions chipped away at the old stories, calling for new narratives.

The old priestly model—intervening with gods on behalf of humans—was giving way. The divine was no longer "out there" but "in here," within each person. As the Upanishads taught, "All the heavens, all the hells, all the gods... are within you." If so, who needs priests? This was the radical heresy of the Axial Age.

This revolution birthed enduring ideas: reincarnation in both India and Greece; theories of elemental matter; debates on dualism and non-dualism; and the concept of a prime mover behind all existence—unknowable and without qualities (*nirguna*), yet often described with qualities (*saguna*) for the sake of language. In India, it was called Sat, brahman, Purusha, or Prana. In Greece, Zeus or apeiron. The same mystery, just different names.

The fictional meeting between Svetaketu and Kapila above draws from two early Upanishads: the Brihadaranyaka, where the sage Yajnavalkya debates profound questions, and the Chandogya, where Uddalaka teaches his son, Svetaketu, what he hadn't learned in school.[67] During this time, a new philosophy called Samkhya emerged, attributed to the mysterious Kapila. Was he real? We don't know. Many bore that name, and there's no evidence that Kapila met Svetaketu. The imagined story explores what might have happened if he had.

In the Upanishads, prana evolved into more than mere breath. It was cosmic and personal—linked to wind, fire, and space, akasha.[68] In the Kaushitaki Upanishad, prana is volition, the cause of effort. The wind is merely its external manifestation.[69] Indra, highest of the gods in the Vedic pantheon, announces that he is prana, life is prana, prana is life, and by prana, a man obtains immortality! Indra equates prana with *prajna*—consciousness itself.[70] In this particular Upanishad, prana is equated with the consciousness of brahman.[71]

Samkhya was a departure from the Vedas and the Upanishads. It proposed dual realities: purusha (soul) and prakriti (matter), rejecting the need for a single, unifying source like Sat. Unlike the Vedas and Upanishads, Samkhya did not include prana in its cosmology.[72] Kapila had no use for this concept—nor, it seems, did Patanjali. The collection we call his Yoga Sutras was profoundly shaped by Samkhya's metaphysics. He adopted its dualism of purusha and prakriti but said little about prana—mentioning it only in the context of breath control (pranayama), not as a cosmic life-force.

Unlike the later yoga systems we will explore—such as hatha or tantric yoga—Patanjali emphasized mental discipline over energetic manipulation. In these later schools, prana became central: as breath, as life force, and even as consciousness itself. As McEvilley writes, prana became "the substance on which the yogi works... to know and manipulate the force of life."[73] Prana, as brahman, was seen as the underlying current of all things.

While for Patanjali, pranayama was a preparatory practice—a method to calm the mind, not a primary path to transformation—for later yogis, prana was central to their philosophy. The practice of pranayama became entwined with asana. This I discovered during my venture into ashtanga practice with David Swenson in Vancouver and Costa Rica.

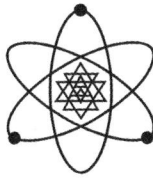

CHAPTER 9:

Pura Vida

Louise told me that it literally means "pure life." She would know; Louise spoke Spanish fluently, and her partner was Chilean. I spoke no Spanish and only a tiny amount of French. Here in Costa Rica, though, "pura vida" meant more than a pure life. It referred to the simple life—a way of living. Louise and I were staying for a couple of days 5,000 feet above sea level at the Pura Vida Resort, nestled in the mountains above the capital of Costa Rica, San Jose, amid hills filled with coffee bushes. It was January of 2001, winter in the northern hemisphere, but the weather in Costa Rica was warm and a bit humid. It reached 27°C (81°F) on the day we arrived. Quite the change from the 8°C (46°F) we had left in Vancouver.

We were in Costa Rica to meet up with David Swenson, who was conducting revolving, 11-day ashtanga teacher training sessions in the jungle at the Bosque Del Cabo Resort, on the Pacific coast of Costa Rica. Ashtanga is a particularly challenging form of flowing yoga postures, with lots of sweating, compiled and taught by K. Pattabhi Jois. I had met David, one of the leading purveyors of the practice, the previous summer when he led a teacher training in Vancouver, hosted by Mike Dennison, the founder of City Yoga. For about six months, I had been taking ashtanga classes given by Mike and Fiona Stang in a space they rented across from the Vancouver General Hospital on West 12th Avenue. It was basically a gymnasium. Mike eventually moved to better locations. His second space was the upstairs storage room of the first Lululemon store. Like Greenpeace twenty years earlier, Lululemon began on Vancouver's West 4th Avenue. We would do our sweaty ashtanga flows between racks of clothing that we pushed aside to create space. Eventually, Lululemon moved across the street, giving us solo access to the whole floor. It was spacious and almost perfect but a bit dark and cool. We needed a while to warm up in the early mornings.

By 2005, Mike was able to acquire a space on West Broadway and kitted it out with furnaces to keep the room toasty. While Mike looked after the business aspects of City Yoga and taught from time to time, Fiona was the main teacher. Originally from the American East Coast, she had chucked a job on Wall Street for the delight of yoga teaching and landed in Vancouver when her husband relocated here to study for his master's degree. At the time, she was one of only two teachers in Canada accredited by Pattabhi Jois. Over the years, Mike invited many of the famous ashtangis to come and teach workshops and trainings, including David Williams, Tim Miller, and Nancy Gilgoff. But the first was David Swenson. It was in City Yoga in the summer of 2000 that I first trained with David, and I needed more.

From San Jose, we boarded a small plane that took us to the tiny town of Puerto Jimenez. There was not much to see. This little town, named after the first Costa Rican president to visit the area, in 1910, had two moments of fame. The first was in the late 1930s, when a small gold rush brought hopefuls to the Osa Peninsula, a hook of land jutting out into the Pacific and pointing its finger south, towards Panama. The bay corralled by the finger of land was called Golfo Dulce, the sweet gulf. The gold panners stayed on even as their dreams died, becoming farmers and squatters. By the end of the 1970s, the peninsula became the Corcovado National Park. The farmers were bought out and relocated, but in the 1980s, a new gold rush ensued, thanks to the rising price of gold internationally. It took a while to get these new miners out, but eventually, the peninsular park was preserved. Ecotourism became a leading source of revenue for the region and the country.

At the very tip of the finger was Bosque del Cabo, a tropical "forest at the cape." It was, in a word, gorgeous. Like the rain forests of British Columbia, everything was green, but a different green. Brighter. The smells were more humid. The grass was broadleaf, and the trees were not quite as high. This was a second-growth forest; all the original trees had been felled generations ago. Where the cabins in the Inner Ear Retreat center in British Columbia were roughly made of cedar and hemlock, the bungalows here were elegant, fashioned of tropical hardwood and topped with peaked thatched roofs. The king-sized beds had mosquito netting, which draped from a centered circle high over the bed to the four corners. Being a hundred feet or so above the coast, there was almost always a cooling breeze. There was no need for an alarm clock to wake us in the morning; the howler monkeys did that. As soon as the sky lightened, they started checking in with the rest of the troop with hoots and hollers, just as they did each night before going to sleep, curled up in the trees. I knew Louise was awake each morning when I heard her howl in harmony with the monkeys.

Since it was the middle of the dry season, our lessons were outdoors, on a long veranda attached to a rectangular, single-story building. There were 16 of us, including David, which seemed to be the limit the veranda could hold. David repeated the same training that I had taken the previous summer at City Yoga. In the mornings, he led us through a set sequence of postures, called the primary series.[74] After breakfast, he would walk us through each posture of the series, showing several variations to accommodate students of different abilities. He would demonstrate on volunteers how to "adjust" the students to fit the postures. Adjustments were a big part of the ashtanga practice. They involved arranging the student to fit the ideals of the pose. Often, these adjustments would entail significant force, so positioning the teacher's body to acquire appropriate leverage was part of the art.

The Five Tools of Ashtanga

"There are five main elements of ashtanga yoga," David explained, "asanas, bandhas, vinyasa, drishti, and breath."

Asanas, of course, are the physical postures, which David recommended we practice at about 85% of maximum intensity, to ensure we did not injure ourselves or push too hard.

Vinyasa is the flow, the movement from one posture to the next. It is the movement that generates the heat of the practice. In ashtanga yoga, the heat comes from inside the student, but at City Yoga in Vancouver, the room was also heated. Fortunately, the furnace never pushed the ambient temperature above 30°C (85°F).

Bandhas, in David's view, as mentioned earlier, are less the locks that Shakti taught and more like valves. They help to regulate and direct the flow of prana. Unlike a lock, which blocks all movement, a valve allows things to move in one direction but not in the opposite direction. A locked door cannot be moved at all; the valve of your bicycle tire allows air to enter the tire but prevents it from leaving.

Only two bandhas are lightly engaged during the ashtanga practice: the root valve, mula bandha, and a softer version of uddiyana bandha. David Williams, who was David Swenson's first teacher of ashtanga, told me that mula bandha must be done consciously—when the mind is gone, the bandha is gone.[75]

Normally, a full uddiyana bandha is only engaged during a held breath, a kumbhaka, as part of a formal pranayama practice. However, in ashtanga, a subtle engagement of the lower belly is preferred during asana practice. This is a slight lifting action deep in the central core that, when activated, creates stillness in the outer body. In the ashtanga tradition, all movement caused by the breath occurs above this level, but below this level, the lower abdomen is still.

The third valve, jalandhara bandha, is normally reserved for formal pranayama practice and only during a kumbhaka, but there are some postures where it can arise spontaneously, such as shoulder stand (salambasarvangasana) or plow pose (halasana), where the chest is pressed against the chin.[76] These are very temporary throat bandhas.

Drishti is a Sanskrit word with a number of meanings. According to Georg Feuerstein, a noted yoga scholar and writer, it can mean a view or an opinion. David was using the term in its context of a gaze. During meditation, there are three drishti options: eyes closed, eyes half-opened, or eyes fully opened. When the eyes are open, the gaze can be directed towards the middle of the eyebrows, which always makes me feel tired, or to the tip of the nose, which causes me to be cross-eyed and is also tiring.[77] During asana practice, there are seven places the gaze can be directed: the navel, a hand, a thumb, the toes, far to the right, far to the left, or up to the sky. These are external foci; with a deepening level of practice, the foci are inward. These inward drishtis may include focusing on the breath, or sensations in particular areas of the body that are undergoing a stretch, or any place tension may be gathering. The intention is to build awareness and then, like viewing an object under a microscope, zoom in on it, observing more and more detail.[78] David Swenson quoted David Williams, "What's important is what's invisible." The outer physical shapes we assume during asanas are the outer form of the practice; the real yoga is being aware of what is happening inside. This thought made me wonder whether the shape of the postures we were being adjusted into were the real point after all.

In the manual given to each student at the start of the course, David had written that "the essence of the subtle internal science of yoga is present in the breath. Without knowledge of breathing, the yoga can become nothing more than an arena for contortionists. When we apply the specialized techniques for breath control, we move from the mundane into the divine. The simple act of breathing holds the key to life and death." Ashtanga is the dance between breath and movement.[79] And the name of the breath employed in ashtanga is *ujjayi*.

Ujjayi Pranayama

Ujjayi means victorious. Victorious over what? No one ever says. If you are feeling poetic, come up with something: victorious over sloth (finish your practice!); victorious over death (gain immortality! Sure, why not?); victorious over *samsara* (overcome the need to be reborn); victorious over *avidya* (dispel your ignorance about the world). Richard Freeman defines ujjayi pranayama as "victorious stretching of the Prana."[80] It seems you get to choose what you want to conquer.

The practice of ujjayi sounds simple: make a sound while you exhale. David taught it by having us stand up or sit up tall and whisper, with our mouths open, "Hhhaaa." You should feel the air swirling in the back of the mouth and throat. We did this a few times, breathing in through the nose and out through the mouth, and then in mid-exhale, he told us to close the mouth but still create the sound "hhhaaa." Almost done. Now, do the same thing with the soft sound but add the smile. Once we had mastered this simple breath, we employed it throughout our practice. The volume of our ujjayi was loud enough so our neighbors could hear us, but not so loud that we couldn't hear them. Darth Vader jokes abound around the sound of ujjayi, but it should be neither harsh nor overly loud.

Ujjayi is ubiquitous in ashtanga practice, and it was carried over into most of the derivative forms such as power yoga, flow yoga, or vinyasa yoga. It was not, however, practiced during asanas in all traditions. I don't recall Shakti using it, for example. Where it was used, it was promoted as a tool to build inner heat and to help focus the mind. It was also a barometer of the practice. If you stopped doing it, your attention was undoubtedly wandering. If it became uneven or too loud, you were straining too much. Ujjayi should have a smooth even rhythm and a grace to it.

In the early texts of hatha yoga, ujjayi meant something different. There, ujjayi referred to a form of inhalation with the mouth closed, and a holding of the breath while employing jalandhara bandha. While a soft, snoring sound accompanied the inhalation, that did not seem to be its primary characteristic.[81] In the Hatha Yoga Pradipika, ujjayi involved inhalation through both nostrils, a kumbhaka, and exhalation only through the left nostril.[82] Even up to the 1930s, teachers like Sivananda and Kuvalayananda were still teaching ujjayi as breath retention followed by exhalation through the left nostril, although they were using more modern terminology, such as "constrict the glottis," which produces the hissing sound.[83] In his 1961 book *Yoga Mala*, Pattabhi Jois mentions ujjayi but does not describe it.[84] By 1966, B.K.S. Iyengar wrote about the practice in his book *Light on Yoga*, but the requirement to exhale through the left nostril was dropped. He advised holding the breath, but only for a second or two. He did mention that while the syllable "*jaya*" can mean victorious, conquest, triumph, or success, it can also mean to curb or restrain. Ujjayi can be done while sitting but also while walking. He said it is the only form of pranayama that can be done at any time of the day.[85]

Over the next few years, other teachers I studied with gave different views on ujjayi. Some differences were subtle, some significant. A teacher City Yoga hosted was David Williams, one of the first Americans to study ashtanga in Mysore, India under Pattabhi Jois. David Williams said that he eventually realized yoga had less to do with the poses, forms, or shapes the body can take and more to do with the breath. In his teaching, while we held a posture, only the ribs were to move while we breathed. He said, "It is the movement of the ribs that causes the stretch." While normally jalandhara bandha is used only in pranayama practices, David said that in all forward bending postures, we should engage jalandhara bandha: the chin lock. One way to do that was to gaze towards the navel in every forward fold; that would require the chin to come to the chest. He said that even in a straight-legged seated forward fold, like paschimottanasana, bring your chin to your chest and do not look towards the toes. Keep jalandhara bandha engaged. One of his statements resonated with me so much that I had to write it down: "To deepen the breath, don't inhale more, exhale more!"[86]

In the early days of Western students coming to Mysore to learn ashtanga from Pattabhi Jois, he would offer pranayama practice for 20 to 30 minutes every day after completing the primary series of asanas. He always employed the chin lock on kumbhakas and would cool down at the end with *sitali* pranayama, breathing in through a curled tongue. Another breath practice was to take five full inhalations and exhalations through both nostrils, followed by inhalations and exhalations through just one nostril, then the same through the other nostril. Eventually, the exhalations would last longer: a 12-count inhalation and an 18-count exhalation. As the number of students coming to Mysore grew, Pattabhi Jois offered pranayama less, eventually only to students who had completed the third series.[87] Part of the reason for this was that he didn't have time with so many students now requiring his attention, but another part of the reason was the dangers inherent in practicing pranayama. David Williams's teaching of pranayama evolved as well. He taught only gentle versions, eschewing the long-held retentions commonly advocated by other teachers.

Bandhas continued to be an important part of the yoga practice. David Williams thought that pranayama should be done with *jnana mudra* (the wisdom seal formed by touching the tip of the thumb to the tip of the index finger, forming a circle)[88] and mula bandha. David admitted that it took him 10 years to really get mula bandha, another 10 years to really understand it, and another 10 years to realize that yoga *is* mula bandha. The release of the stretch is the source from which we draw energy. Yoga redirects that energy, that prana. Above all, one must not waste the prana by skipping the end of practice relaxation and restoration called *shavasana*! If you skip shavasana, the energy you release will go into your next activity. During shavasana, that energy will go into healing the body.

Unlike Pattabhi Jois, David Williams abandoned doing physical adjustments on his students. He felt they were too strong, and would eventually be damaging, especially if done the way Pattabhi Jois did them.[89] Another important point was to avoid fatigue! When you are tired, stop for the day. You are done. I know that I heard him say this, because I wrote it in my notebook. But hearing something and understanding something is not the same thing.

In 2003, I took a vinyasa teacher training with Shiva Rea in Los Angeles. I had been doing Shiva's power yoga videos at home for a few years and wanted to learn from her directly. She was fated to be a yoga teacher, as her father named her Shiva at birth. What a start! She was a leading light in Western yoga, with a long, lean, lithe dancer's body and a presence that captivated students. At one point during the training, she quoted Ken Wilbur: "Most of us have not lost our minds, we have lost our bodies. But," she promised, "as soon as we connect our breath to movement, we cultivate embodiment."

This was what David Swenson taught. Which breath were they referring to? Ujjayi! Shiva had done ashtanga yoga for seven years, and then had a baby. After delivering her son, Jai, she went back to the practice, but it wasn't the same. A year later, she'd quit. She said she had lost the "spark" and it now left a bad taste in her mouth. Instead, she had developed her own flowing style of yoga movement, breath, and practice. Her way of teaching ujjayi was similar to David's but slightly different. She suggested touching the collarbones to bring awareness there. Like David recommended,

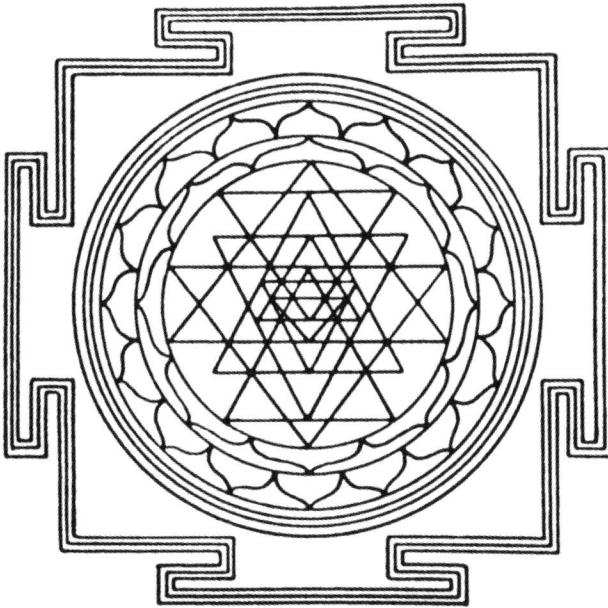

Figure 5: The Sri Yantra. To find the nine main triangles, look for the four tips of the ascending triangles, which represent Shiva, and the five tips of the descending ones, which represent Shakti.[91]

it was best to learn the practice with mouth open, say "hhhaaa," then close the mouth midway through the exhalation so you were noisily breathing through the nose. But somewhat differently, she suggested opening the mouth again and still making the breath come out the nose. She claimed this was more advanced, which of course made me want to try it. To my unadvanced ears, it sounded the same.

Shiva had guests give talks. One guest teacher was Mark Whitwell. Mark had lived for several years with Krishnamacharya and his son Desikachar. He said that he co-wrote Desikachar's book, *The Heart of Yoga.* He looked like a guru: slender, with long, blonde hair flowing over his shoulders. He was a few years older than I and spoke with a charming New Zealand accent. During his talk, Mark noted that in New York, too many ashtangis were burning out. The reason, he suggested, was because their ujjayi breathing was all exhale focused! There was too much masculine energy, the "*tha*" of ha-tha yoga, the sun's fire, and not enough feminine energy, the "*ha*," the moon's coolness.[90] The feminine part of the breath is the inhalation. Yoga, in Mark's mind, was the surrender of the male to the female. Yoga is the union of in and out, of up and down.

Mark described the *Shri Yantra*, a geometric drawing or device with five large triangles representing Shakti pointing down and four large triangles representing Shiva pointing up. Shiva, Mark explained, is coming up! Shakti is pouring down. The feminine descends and is stimulated by the inhalation. If a man learns to inhale in his yoga, he will receive love. Mark was very poetic.

Sarah Powers had a different take on ujjayi. During my training with her and Paul Grilley, she asked us to place a finger under our nostrils while we breathed normally, and feel the air. Then, we added the ujjayi.

"Whisper RRRR as you exhale," she said, "with the mouth open. Try it again. And again, but this time, close your lips. Once you have the sound on the exhalation, make the same sound during inhalation." So far, very familiar. "Now, place the finger under the nose again and feel the breath. Slow your breath down to four-second inhalations and exhalations." I tried that for a while. It was pretty easy to feel the wind on the finger. The practice helped me focus on the breath.

Next, Sarah applied this technique while we lingered in a posture. "Now, breathe like this into the edge." We were sitting cross-legged on the floor. She asked us to lean forward, our hands crawling out in front of us, until we felt a distinct sensation. That was our edge. "Where your attention goes, the prana flows." That was not the first or last time she mentioned that.

"Move to the edge," she said, "until it grows from mildly interesting to strongly interesting. If it becomes exceptionally interesting, you have gone too far. Play with the edge, staying in the middle of the range of interesting sensation."

Unlike the ashtanga and vinyasa forms of yoga, where ujjayi married movement to the breath and breath to the movement, Sarah employed ujjayi as a tool to direct the breath to the sensations within the postures. In all cases, the breath was in service to prana.

Overheated Again

The days with David Swenson flowed like a well-choreographed vinyasa class. The practices were warm and lovely, but I was starting to feel tired and a bit light-headed. Towards the end of the stay, I went for a hike. On my own, I set off down one of the paths from the lodge to the beach. The downhill walk was refreshing, with a breeze off the ocean and birds' songs. I lingered on the sands, talked to several of the students who had been there for a while, and then headed back up the path. That is when I realized that I was not as strong as I'd thought. The walk uphill exhausted me. By the time I got back to my cabin, I had to lie down and rest for the remainder of the day. I was pushing myself too much. I had to take it easier.

At the end of the training, we piled into the open-aired taxis and drove back en masse to Puerto Jimenez's airport. As we said our goodbyes, a plane landed with another group of 15. David greeted his next group of students while our group departed.

Back in San Jose, Louise and I returned to Pura Vida for a short holiday and some sightseeing. We decided to visit a cloud forest. The Braulio Carrillo National Park lived up to its promise of green treasure. On the well-groomed trails of smooth surfaces and wooden walkways overlooking deep ravines, we moved into and through the clouds. The Barva volcano rises almost 3,000 meters above sea level, but we could not see the peak, as it was wreathed in mists. Our trail intersected many streams and waterfalls, which contributed to the damp air. On one occasion, while we overlooked a long waterfall, the clouds briefly parted, allowing a ray of light to create radiant rainbows. Other tourists quickly got out their cameras. Those who were too slow missed it, for the clouds came together again quickly and the vista changed. Due to the mists and shade, the air was cool, which was perfect for a long hike. I felt tired at the end, but it was a normal tired, a good tired, not a light-headed, disabling fatigue.

On our last full day in Pura Vida, we joined a yoga class. There was one small, heated room set aside at the resort as their hot yoga studio. Neither Louise nor I had done any form of hot yoga. I lasted about 30 minutes. The heat, combined with the strenuous practice, made me faint, and I left to lie down in my room; Louise carried on and finished the class. By the time she checked in on me, I was no better. I felt just like I had in India, the day after golfing without a hat under the noon-day sun. I had been experiencing some minor versions of these symptoms over the previous year, but nothing like this. I couldn't stand; I couldn't even sit up. I had to remain horizontal and motionless.

Louise was worried but felt helpless. There was nothing she could do. I slept fitfully that night. Fortunately, I had recovered enough by the next morning to get to the airport and fly home. On the flight home, I resolved to figure this out and started to plan my investigations into the reasons for these symptoms. I had studied physics in university, but all sciences fascinated me, and I knew some of the basics of chemistry and biology.

It was time to start diving deeper into human physiology and the medical sciences. While I had always been a student of science, I was equally fascinated by the history of science as well—a history that stretched back to the time of the ancient Greeks, whom we will visit next. What did the Greeks believe to be the essence and vitality of life? What was their "prana"?

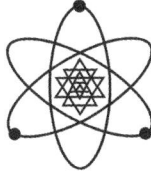

CHAPTER 10:

The Lyceum

The view from the Acropolis looked nothing like the postcard I'd sent my children. The air was thick with smog, and the heat was stifling. I'd hoped to see the hills around Athens or the Aegean Sea in the distance, but a gray haze obscured everything. Apparently, this was the norm. Fortunately, the view of the ruins made up for the disappointing vista.

The ancient columns still soared, but broken marbles and fragments of friezes lay scattered on the ground—a reminder of a seventeenth-century explosion during a war with the Ottoman Empire, when gunpowder stored in the central chamber was ignited by a cannonball. The statue of Athena, once nearly 12 meters tall and overlaid with gold and ivory, had disappeared over a thousand years earlier. All that remains is her base. Once, Athena had held a small statue of Nike, the goddess of victory, and a spear around which a sacred snake looped.

Wandering the ruins with me were John MacDonald, co-founder of our company, and his wife, Alfredette. It was the spring of 1988. We had been attending a remote sensing conference, listening to presentations on the latest approaches for analyzing the digital pictures satellites were taking of the earth's surface. From Athens, John and Alfredette were heading to the holy land for a vacation, and then Alfredette would stay for a couple of months, volunteering at an archaeological dig near Jerusalem. I was heading to Islamabad, in Pakistan.

Before we left, I gazed to the east, overlooking the Lyceum, an ancient grove where once had stood a gymnasium, lecture halls, dormitories, and a famous collection of philosophers: the Peripatetic school, founded by Aristotle in 334 BCE.

The Ionian Philosophers

"Plato wrote books," said Theophrastus, "Aristotle wrote notes. Books are easy enough to copy, but my task is to organize Aristotle's mass of lectures into something coherent—before Ptolemy sends his agents to take them. Better to be generous than to be plundered."

"Your job," continued Theophrastus, looking directly at Neleus, his old friend and former student, "is to copy the works of the Ionian teachers: Thales, Anaximander, and Anaximenes."

Together, they wandered down a path between olive trees and the occasional carob tree within the Lyceum. Named after Apollo Lyceus, the god of light and music, the Lyceum had been used for hundreds of years—for military training, exercise, sports, and public debates. It was a region rather than a building, an area just outside the walls of Athens. Fifteen years ago, Aristotle had purchased one of the buildings and founded a school. He had structured it similarly to Plato's Academy, where he had long been a student. Thanks to the patronage of Alexander of Macedonia, the Lyceum had grown into a renowned institution for learning and thinking. It became one of the first organized centers of study in Europe, with a significant library and a collection of botanical specimens—plants Alexander had sent from across his empire.

Though once protected by his most famous student, Aristotle found Athens hostile after Alexander's death. Anti-Macedonian sentiment was rising, and he wisely fled, entrusting the Lyceum to Theophrastus. Meanwhile, Alexander's generals divided his empire. Ptolemy claimed Egypt and set out to create the greatest library the world had ever known. His agents scoured Greece for manuscripts, and the Lyceum's trove of knowledge was a prime target.

Theophrastus, tall, slender, and as yet unbowed by his years, although there was more gray than black in his short hair and trimmed beard, walked upright without a cane, proud in his bearing. The himation covering his left shoulder and tucked under the right was white, always white. Neleus, younger by a generation, with a fine, full beard, was shorter and broader of shoulder. His himation was a dark navy blue, a bold choice among the subtler tones favored at the Lyceum. These were busy times, and the two friends rarely got to walk together in the woods surrounding the school. It was their habit of walking while discussing philosophy that gave Aristotle's followers their name: the Peripatetics—from *peripatein*, to walk about. Theophrastus and Neleus were enjoying just such a walk as they headed south along the shaded paths toward the river Ilisos.

"All right," replied Neleus. "I have studied the Ionians in depth. We are all in their debt. I would be happy to arrange the copying of the manuscripts we have. They are almost 200 years old and fragile, and we will have to be very careful with them."

"Good. I didn't realize we had an expert available for the task," said Theophrastus with a mischievous twinkle, "and since you are a self-proclaimed expert, tell me, then, about the greatest gift they gave us. Based upon your answer, I will either confirm or deny your expertise."

"A test?" responded Neleus with surprise. "Am I once again your student? Let us instead enter into a debate worthy of the philosophy of Thales, Anaximander, and Anaximenes, who never took the words of their forebears to be truth unless the truth could be ascertained without recourse to authority."

"A discourse, then, Neleus! State your first position and then convince me of its validity."

"Very well. Here is my first statement: Anaximander was the greatest *physiologos* of them all, a natural inquirer, surpassing even Thales. And, before you ask, here is what I base this claim upon. It was Anaximander who reasoned that the earth hangs free in the center of the cosmos, unsupported, because it has no reason to move in any particular direction. There is space above us and space below us, but against the critique that if there was no support under the earth, it would surely fall, he plainly stated that the earth would not fall because there is no particular direction for it to fall. Nothing dominates the earth, as it is already in the center of all things, so it remains in its place."

"A bold statement, Neleus, and one that many would dispute, but let me leave my thoughts until later, for I fear you have missed the essential point of Anaximander's view. Continue, for surely one proclamation would not give rise to your generous appointment of his primacy among the early physicians."

"Indeed, several were Anaximander's views of the way the natural world unfolded. Unlike Thales, who thought the primary source of the world was water, from which emanated the earth and upon which the entire earth floats, Anaximander went further and proposed the *apeiron* to be the ultimate source of all. The apeiron is neither one of the elements (like water or air) nor describable in terms of qualities. It is eternal, ageless, and divine in some sense. From the apeiron emerged the fundamental opposites—hot and cold, wet and dry—through which the cosmos was ordered. The earth did not arise out of water. However, in the beginning, water undoubtedly covered the earth. In time, due to the heat of the sun, the waters evaporated, revealing the surface of the earth. Anaximander proposed that rain, thunder, and lightning arose from natural interactions of heat and moisture—clouds crashing together and releasing sparks of fire—creating the thunder and lightning that frighten both the young and the superstitious."

"What you relate is what I have heard as well, but again, you are missing the key stroke of genius. It is not the particulars of Anaximander's musing that are remarkable but something you have not mentioned. If we stick to the particulars, some say Anaximenes returned to a more tangible principle—air—as the *arche*. But in doing so, he gave us the ideas of rarefaction and compression: through condensation, air becomes water and then earth; through rarefaction, air becomes fire. All things, he claimed, are transformations of primal air. But let's stick to Anaximander. Please try one more time. Whence did Anaximander claim life arose?"

Neleus gave a small smile. "Life, said Anaximander, began in the waters. From those primordial forms emerged creatures who, driven by necessity, took to land and changed their nature. Over time, these creatures became us—walking, talking, pondering under olive trees. It is this—*necessity*—that I believe is Anaximander's greatest gift."

"Well argued, Neleus. Necessity is indeed a wondrous notion… but still, not quite the key I had in mind."

"What have I forgotten, then? Please go on, my instructor," requested Neleus with a bow of respect.

"In all you have relayed, in all that Anaximander wrote and taught, not once does he invoke the gods to explain the workings of nature!" Theophrastus' hands began to gesticulate, as was his habit whenever he was teaching. "This is the greatest gift of Anaximander's philosophy. The gods are not needed! You spoke of necessity: when I release a pebble from my hand, it falls to the earth, not because a god causes it to fall, but of necessity! The earth dominates the pebble. The thunder heard from the clouds is not caused by the anger of gods but arises out of necessity. The earth occasionally quakes, not because gods are warring but because the sun dries it and, out of necessity, it cracks. Water rises into vapor out of necessity due to the heat of the sun; the vapor turns back into water to fall as rain, not due to some action of gods but out of necessity due to the cold. This is the beginning of *physis*! This is the beginning of a purely natural-ist approach to understanding the world, and this is why I called Anaximander the first *physician*. Not even Thales could bring himself to ignore the gods so fully."

"Yes, you are correct, my teacher. Thales believed the gods to inhabit everything that had the power to act or react, to move, to change or grow. Even the magnetic lodestone that moves when placed near iron, and all plants and animals, are full of god."

Theophrastus nodded. "And you can see how Anaximander went further than Thales. To truly honor one's teacher, one must study his wisdom deeply, but then one must seek his errors and fix them. Anaximander saw the flaws in Thales' view and set about to com-pletely ignore the gods. Not deny them, mind you, for that will always cause chaos in society; people need their gods. But there was no need to invoke their presence in natu-ral events. At the heart of it is this ability to refuse to bow down to someone's authority simply because they claim authority or because someone claims they must be believed. Authority can be questioned."

"Thus was Socrates condemned to drink his poison," murmured Neleus.[92] He was growing worried about his old friend. It was all very well for philosophers to play the game of questioning authority while in the sheltered walkways of their schools, but this was dangerous in the world at large. Aristotle had questioned Alexander and been cut off from the king's grace. He had been luckier than Socrates and escaped execution, but luck usually runs out.

The Source of Life

"Yes, yes… you are right, Neleus," sighed Theophrastus. "I am getting old and must remember there is a world of men who only see what is right in front of them and must follow the obvious. Let us change the subject. Tell me more about life and its causes. We know what Anaximander thought—the gods are not required—but what is the view of today's philosophers? If the view before Anaximander is discarded, that the gods dictate when and where life begins in the womb of a woman, what has replaced it?"

"So many views!" started Neleus. "Let's start with the poets of old. Homer spoke only vaguely of life and death; his heroes were animated by breath or spirit. But later thinkers sought to locate life within the body. Some suggested that semen came from the brain, flowing through the spine and out into the world—a soul-bearing essence. Democritus agreed, offering a more refined, atomic view: life was composed of tiny elements carried in the seed. In this 'one-seed view,' the man provides the soul-bearing substance, and the woman bears the soil in which it takes root."

"I like this summation," said Theophrastus, "and your characterization of this being a pre-Socratic view. But how did Plato, Socrates' greatest student, accommodate this idea?"

"Plato made everything more complex," Neleus smiled. "He gave us not one soul but three: the rational soul in the brain, the spirited soul in the heart, and the appetitive soul in the belly. Reason seeks truth; spirit seeks honor; appetite seeks pleasure. And the seed, Plato claimed, draws its power from that lower soul—from desire.

"According to Plato, each human soul begins as a celestial being, assigned to a star. When the time for incarnation comes, the soul descends from its star and enters the body, taking up residence in the head—specifically, the brain, which houses the rational part of the soul. True *eros*, true longing, is the soul's desire to return to its divine origin in the heavens. But the lower souls—centered in the heart and belly—can distort that longing. When desire overwhelms reason, it stirs the vital forces of the body, directing a soul-infused substance down the spine, through the marrow, and into the reproductive organs. This, Plato says, is how semen is formed: not as mere fluid, but as a carrier of life, infused with the soul's animating power.

"While Plato agrees with the one-seed view of generation, he says that the woman does have a role to play. In his book the *Timaeus*, he likens the womb of a woman to a wild creature with its own independence. Plato saw women as less perfect reincarnations of men and believed a womb unoccupied by pregnancy could wander and obstruct the breath, cause choking, suffocation, and many diseases."

"You summarize Plato well, Neleus," said Theophrastus, "but many philosophers today believe Plato was speaking metaphorically. Did he really believe that a uterus wandered, or was this merely his way to explain the varieties of female sensations, the craving for children, and the desire for intercourse that moves throughout a woman's body?"

"I take Plato at his word and feel he meant what he said," replied Neleus. "Why else would he say it? But his views do raise questions he never addressed. For example, if the higher soul resides in the brain, arriving there before birth, what is it that flows from the brain into the womb? He calls it soul-stuff, but is the father's soul somehow partitioned, and part travels to the new child? If so, what role do the stars play? If not, why is semen soul-stuff? And if the woman has no role in the generation of the new life other than providing the soil in which it grows, how can children look like their mothers? There must be something of the mother in the child."

"Good points," replied Theophrastus, "and the wandering of the womb would fit with the sayings of the followers of Hippocrates, who also believe that the uterus can move around the body unless it is tied down in a proper location by pregnancy or the moisture of constant intercourse. For this reason, doctors say that young girls and old women are more likely to suffer the distress of a wild uterus, for they neither have intercourse nor bear children, and so the uterus, untethered, may roam. But Hippocratic doctors differ from Plato and Aristotle in that they propose a two-seed model: both man and woman contribute generative seed, with the woman also offering her womb and blood. This, they claim, explains why children may resemble their mothers as well as their fathers."

"They do hold this view, but Aristotle does not," said Neleus. "He rejected earlier theories that both sexes contributed generative seed. In his view, only the male produces true seed—semen—which is created by the transformation of blood through the action of vital heat in the testicles. Women, being naturally cooler, lack the heat necessary for this transformation. Instead, they contribute menstrual blood, which acts as the raw material for the new being. During intercourse, the male's semen, carrying both vital heat and form, acts upon the female's menstrual blood, shaping it into a developing body. Generation, then, is the result of form acting on matter: man provides the initiating force and structure; woman provides the substance."

"So neither Homer nor Hesiod, Plato nor Aristotle think that women contribute much to the generation of life. And yet a child can look a lot like its mother. So please," urged Theophrastus, "explain how a woman can affect the fetus as it grows."

"Well, again, many views!" said Neleus. "Aristotle thought that if the seed is deposited into the right side of the womb, a boy will be born; if it falls to the left, a girl. The Hippocratic physicians believed that a woman possesses two wombs, just as a pig has many—boys from the right, girls from the left. Others claim it is the seed itself that determines sex: semen from the right testicle creates a boy; from the left, a girl. But Empedocles, the Sicilian, said that left or right is irrelevant—it is heat that dictates the outcome. A womb with sufficient heat will produce a boy; if it lacks heat, a girl will be born."

"But there are yet other views, are there not Neleus?"

"Yes. The first view I spoke of, that of Plato and some earlier thinkers, might be called *preformation*: the belief that semen contains a miniature, complete being, needing only nourishment to grow. In this one-seed model, the male alone provides the seed. Where exactly this seed is produced varies—Plato suggests the brain; others, the marrow; still others say it forms through the foaming or concoction of blood, as Aristotle claimed. A second view, *pangenesis*, holds that semen is drawn from all parts of the body, flowing through the blood to the testicles. And then there is the *two-seed theory*, held by Empedocles and the Hippocratic school, in which both male and female contribute seed, which, when mixed and anchored in the womb by *pneuma*—vital air—can result in new life."

"In the two-seed view, if two strong seeds merge, a boy will result. If two weak seeds merge, a girl. If a strong seed merges with a weak seed, the result will be driven by the total number of male seeds or female seeds. The most abundant seeds will determine the sex of the baby."

"Let us return to your comments about the soul, for surely life is only possible when the body hosts a soul!" said Theophrastus, changing the topic slightly. "You mentioned Plato's view that we have three souls: one higher and two lower. I have just finished organizing Aristotle's various talks and lectures on this topic and compiled a single manuscript called *On The Soul*. In this work, he compares many views, explains where they all miss the mark, and offers his own understanding, along with his rationale. Do you recall his teachings?"

"Yes, I paid close attention to those talks," said Neleus. "Aristotle taught that we have three types of soul. The first, the nutritive soul, is the most basic—it governs growth, nourishment, and reproduction. Plants have only this kind of soul, but it is also present in animals and humans. Animals possess a second kind: the sensitive soul, which enables perception, desire, and voluntary movement. And humans, in addition to these, have the rational soul—the power of thought, reason, and understanding. This, Aristotle believed, is what sets us apart from other living things."

"So," said Theophrastus, "both Aristotle and Plato believed we have three souls, but the natures of these souls are quite different. However, there is one key difference you have not yet described. For Plato, our higher soul is immortal; it exists before and after the body and can be ensouled over and over. And Aristotle—what does he believe?"

"That is what I hope your studies will answer!" exclaimed Neleus. "As far as I can recall, Aristotle kept avoiding this question. Does the rational soul or any of the souls pre-exist the body? He seems to disagree with Plato, because he claims that soul and body are inseparable, like form and matter. This yew tree before us has matter, substance, but its nutritive soul is what gives it form. When the tree is gone, cut down and burned in the hearth, the form is gone; its soul is gone. Soul does not have an independent existence, so how can it survive the body? Soul is a capacity or a potential for the body to take a specific form, but that capacity cannot exist without the body. He does hint, in one cryptic talk, that the intellect may be separable—but he never says this plainly, and his overall argument suggests he viewed the soul as perishable, like the body it animates."

Theophrastus nodded. "Exactly. He avoids proclaiming the soul's end but also refuses to claim its persistence. Unlike Plato or the Pythagoreans, Aristotle did not believe in the soul's pre-existence or its postmortem survival. Soul is the actuality of a living body, nothing more."

The two Peripatetics fell silent, contemplating the weight of their discussion. Theophrastus, visibly tired, finally smiled. "Thank you for proving my original proposition."

"Your proposition?" asked Neleus.

"Why, that Anaximander's greatest gift was his refusal to invoke the gods. In all your explanations—from Plato to Empedocles, from Hippocrates to Aristotle—none of them needed gods to explain life. They sought natural causes. You may lament that the final answer still eludes us—but you must admit, these are *natural* explanations, not theological ones."

Neleus softly chuckled, which prompted Theophrastus to raise an enquiring eyebrow. Neleus explained, "I was just thinking of three new students yesterday who expressed a great deal of frustration over such matters. They said that while all these dead philosophers spouted handsome words and would seem to be wise, not one of them offered any form of evidence to prove their contentions. Where is the proof?"

"Yes," laughed Theophrastus, "the folly of youth. I hope you set them straight. I would have turned to Pythagoras. He put the power of necessity into the language of numbers and shapes to prove ideas to be true."

Neleus smiled and nodded. "I did cite Pythagoras, but they were not impressed. They found it all too abstract. But I reminded them: the senses deceive; only the mind grasps truth. In the realm of forms, circles and lines are perfect—here, they are flawed. If observation contradicts a clear idea, perhaps it is the observation, not the idea, that is mistaken."

"Well done, Neleus," replied Theophrastus. "We owe a great debt to the Ionians, and perhaps the greatest debt is to Pythagoras. Most of what Plato describes is a restating of Pythagorean thought, and even Aristotle acknowledged Pythagoras' influence.

"Sadly, my dear Neleus, I must take my leave now. I fear I will need a nap before attending to the rest of my duties today, but please remember my request to oversee the copying of the Ionian manuscripts. I still fear for the future of our library, and I will leave it in your hands to make sure it is safe."

Neleus nodded and placed both hands on Theophrastus's shoulders in a gesture of parting respect. He watched his friend walk off to his afternoon siesta and then turned his attention to the Ionian texts.

In time, Theophrastus retired, bequeathing the entire collection of manuscripts to Neleus. As the political mood in Athens soured, becoming less tolerant of the Lyceum's questioning spirit, Neleus gathered the works and returned to his family estate in Scepsis. There, he protected the library—though later generations would neglect it. Some of the texts were eventually sold to agents of the Ptolemies, who preserved them in the Library of Alexandria. Others decayed in obscurity until, centuries later, fragments of Aristotle's library were brought to Rome.[93] Much of Aristotle's philosophy remained unknown in Western Europe until the Middle Ages, when Muslim scholars, having preserved and elaborated upon the ancient Greek knowledge, reintroduced Aristotle and the Ionian thinkers through Latin translations of Arabic texts.

The Axial Age West

"Even a bean has a soul," Pythagoras was purported to have claimed. "Everything is full of god," insisted Thales. Pythagoras was claiming that all living things have a soul and that life requires a soul. Souls can pass from one living thing to another and another, the theory we today call reincarnation and that he called *metempsychosis*. Thales used the term "god" in a specific way, as he felt that everything was full of an animating divine essence. He saw a unity in nature, an underlying order to the natural world, and this divine essence was the source of all life. Thales and Anaximenes called it *arche*. Anaximander called it the *apeiron*. Svetaketu would have called this *brahman*.

Ionia was a strip of land along the west coast of modern Turkey. While it was small, its colonies ranged as far north as the Black Sea and to the west to Sicily and southern France. Along the coast of Asia Minor, 12 cities banded together, creating the Ionian League. The greatest of these independent cities was Miletus, the home of Thales, Anaximander, and Anaximenes.

Thales of Miletus, 625–545 BCE, is known as the "Father of Philosophy." Anaximander, younger by about 15 years, has been called the first scientist, but it has to be pointed out that this is not referring to science as we know it today. Missing in Anaximander's writings were any hint of mathematical models, experimentation, or proof. It would be more accurate to call his study *physis*, which is the explanation of natural events.[94] Physis means "nature," and its adherents were called *physicians*—not necessarily doctors, but philosophers who sought explanations for events in the natural world without recourse to supernatural agencies like gods and demons.

In no other center of high learning and civilized culture had such an emphasis on seeking knowledge from the natural world arisen. Although Babylon and Egypt were renowned for their priests and scribes, their writing and mathematics, they never made the leap to understanding the world through natural causes. The conservative and structured hierarchy of the courts of these kings worked against new understanding. The knowledge of the ancients was sufficient to explain everything. Authority was vested in the priests and the kings and arose from ancient, transmitted teachings.

Why was Ionia so different? What allowed philosophy and physis to arise there and not in the other great centers of civilization? Well, firstly, there were no kings in Ionia. And there were no priests. Each city was fiercely independent and would tolerate no foreign rulers. Ionia was born out of a dark age, which began with the fall of the earlier Mycenaean civilization. Ionia had no unquestioned heritage from ancestors and no hereditary caste to be threatened. Secondly, the people were cosmopolitan. They were seafaring and traveled widely, learning many languages and customs. This was a young civilization without the weight of past traditions, knowledge, and rituals.

Thirdly, and perhaps most importantly, the Ionians could read and write and knew mathematics. In all other civilizations, only priests and clerics could write and work with numbers. Rarely, a king might learn to read or write, but never was this a practice of the aristocracy, let alone the lower classes. The Ionians, however, took the alphabet of their mercantile neighbors, the Phoenicians, and made it their own. Reading became so easy that the general population and the aristocracy could become literate, write manuscripts, and share ideas. A similar revolution occurred with mathematics: symbols representing numbers in a base 10 format with columns assigned for each digit allowed everyone to understand how to add, subtract, multiply, and even divide! In Ionia, information was not restricted to clerics and clergy. Anyone could learn and add to a growing body of knowledge.

In Ionia, ideas could be challenged. New thoughts were encouraged and celebrated. The old ideas served as a baseline upon which new concepts could arise. Nothing was fixed. For example, the idea that life comes through the male, and specifically through his semen or water, could also be reprised and revised. The baseline belief that life comes through the male goes way back in time. Sumer had tales of the god Enki, the god of fertility, ejaculating semen, generating great rivers that begat all forms of life. In Egypt, the connection between gods and fertility was mediated by seminal liquid. Hieroglyphic symbols of an erect or ejaculating penis formed the base for words like "man," "husband," "semen," as well as "offspring," "fetus," and even "mother." It was also the base sign for verbs like "to beget" and "to impregnate."[95] The womb received little credit for bringing forth new life. This idea, common in the stories of early Greek poets and teachers, implied that the role of women in generating new life was minimal; they were simply the hosts.

The Greeks took these base ideas and expanded upon them. They believed that life—or even soul—originated in the seminal fluid, often considered the vital "water" of men. Plato described a semi-mystical process in which the vital substances of the body—including marrow and brain—were linked to reproduction. Some interpretations suggest he believed semen carried elements of soul, though the process is more symbolic than biological.[96] Where the semen was stored varied according to the school describing the process, but both Aristotle and Plato believed it resided in the brain or the marrow. Marrow in this case was not what we think of today, the tissues found within bones, but a broader, grander substance. Marrow, according to Plato, was the generative force of the soul-stuff. He never provided a good biological description of it: Plato was no scientist. Aristotle, on the other hand, believed marrow to be the soft tissues of the body, which were responsible for generating vital heat. Blood took up this vital heat and distributed it to all the other tissues and organs. When the seed was implanted into the womb, it was fixed in place by pneuma, the elemental air, which joined the soul to the new body.

A distinction must be made between soul—and the Greek word used here is "*psyche*"—and spirit, "*pneuma*." In all references made to soul above, the Greek word used was psyche. Just as the Upanishads drew a distinction between soul, in this case "*atman*," and the breath of life, "*prana*," so too did the Greeks. Soul, psyche, is an essence required for all life. It is an animating principle that causes growth, movement, and development, which are the basic life processes, but soul also causes rational thoughts, emotions, reason, and self-awareness in humans. Spirit, pneuma, on the other hand, is breath, air, or the wind residing within the body, mainly as respiration, without which life cannot continue. Plato uses the word pneuma to describe the material substance used to shape the human soul and body.[97] It is a divine breath infused into the mortal mixture of soul and body. Aristotle uses pneuma more biologically, regarding it as respiration and the vital activity associated with breathing and the circulatory system in living beings.[98] We can consider psyche or soul to be psychological and pneuma or spirit to be physiological. Both are essential for life.

Thales and Anaximander lived about the same time as Svetaketu and Kapila, near the beginning of the Axial Age. There are many surprising similarities between the emerging world views in the East and West. To be clear, however, psyche is not equivalent to atman, although both terms can be interpreted as soul. While both Plato and Kapila posit a dualism between soul and matter, they draw the line between them in different places. In the Samkhya philosophy of Kapila, atman is pure purusha. It is consciousness distinct from mind, memories, intelligence, or reason. Those attributes are prakriti. For Plato, and especially for Aristotle, psyche includes attributes such as logic, reason, and memory, which Kapila says are part of the physical realm.

Channels of Life and Ensoulment

Plato said there was a soul channel, a "holy tube," down the center of the spine. Today, we call this conduit the spinal cord, and yogis call it the *sushumna nadi*. For Plato, this sacred channel was a pathway for semen, the source of life, flowing from the brain to the genitals. Similar ideas appear in the teachings of the Pythagoreans, in the Orphic tradition, and in Heraclitus' writings. Heraclitus, a sixth- to fifth-century BCE philosopher, pointing to the reality of impermanence and constant change, recommended a lifestyle of sexual abstinence and semen retention—echoing teachings that would later appear among tantrikas in India.[99] If semen is composed of soul-stuff, then diminishing one's supply will deplete vitality and shorten life. Plato also described two side channels paralleling the holy tube, foreshadowing the ida and pingala nadis of tantric anatomy. Greek philosophers associated the right side of the body—including the womb and testicles—with masculinity and heat. The left side was considered feminine and cooler. This dualistic framework echoes the later tantric models of energy flow and polarity.

When was the soul joined to the body? This process, called *ensoulment*, has confounded philosophers, theologians, and scholars for millennia. Aristotle's views became canonical in Europe for over a thousand years. Aristotle proposed that the nutritive (or vegetative) soul was affixed first, followed by the sensitive (or animal) soul. For male fetuses, the rational soul was believed to arrive on the 40th day after conception; for females, on the 90th. (This delay was attributed to the belief that females possessed less innate heat, so they developed more slowly.) The ensoulment of the rational soul turned the fetus into a person, and it was marked by a quickening: the first movement of the fetus in the womb. (It was believed that when a woman first felt her baby kick, the soul had arrived—and she was now carrying a person.) This philosophy is known as "delayed ensoulment."[100] The contrasting view, called "immediate ensoulment," held that the soul entered the body at the very moment the two seeds fused.

In either case, the question of what constitutes life remains far from clear. According to Aristotle, there are levels of life: a human life is not the same as plant life, because humans have three souls: the nutritive, the sensitive, and the rational. A plant is still alive, despite possessing only the nutritive (vegetative) soul. While the soul appears to be the carrier of life, it cannot generate life on its own. Other processes must also be involved. Pneuma, air, is required to fix the soul to the body. If we attempt to map the concept of prana onto these ancient models, we quickly find complications. Life is a complex process with many requirements. It is not merely psyche or pneuma. As Aristotle emphasized: the soul requires a body—and the body, a soul.

Physis Is Not Yet Science

In our imagined dialogue between Neleus and Theophrastus, they concluded their walk by pondering how we come to know the truth. Observation is helpful—but it is inferior to reason, logic, and imagination. Their conclusion reveals something fundamental about the ancient Greek worldview: knowledge was shaped more by abstract principles than by sensory experience. While the early Greeks took bold steps toward understanding life through nature—through physis—their approach had not yet become what we now call science. Theories were rarely tested through experiments. If an observation seemed to contradict a cherished idea, the observation was often dismissed, ignored, or reinterpreted to fit the prevailing worldview. Even the quest to understand the soul, breath, and life itself was shaped more by philosophy than by physiology.

One example, drawn from the early medical tradition of Alexandria, illustrates how powerful ideas could obscure the evidence before one's eyes. Herophilus was a contemporary of Neleus and Theophrastus, living in Ptolemy's Alexandria. Ptolemy wanted Alexandria to be the world's greatest center for knowledge and allowed certain explorations that would have been prohibited in other cultures. Herophilus was allowed to dissect human bodies. Through their anatomical explorations, Herophilus and his teacher differentiated the roles of arteries and veins.

Herophilus was the first to discover ovaries, which he equated with the testicles of men.[101] Like most ancient civilizations, the Hellenic world was fiercely patriarchal. In the prevailing Greek view, the female body was an imperfect copy of the male body—malformed, weaker, and improperly built. Female bodies had many similarities to men, but their differences attested to their inferiority. For Herophilus, it was well known that the seed of the male carried the important formative template or soul, which guided the growth of a newborn (the one-seed view), and that women were simply the vessels nourishing the new life. Women were not the progenitors of life but the keepers of it. Herophilus discovered that women had testicles just like men, but due to their imperfection, a woman's testicles were undescended. They remained inside the body.[102]

Herophilus' conclusions were filtered through the lens of prevailing gender ideologies. Since Herophilus believed that female seed played no role in reproduction, he missed the fact that the female semen flowed through tubes to the uterus. Instead, he believed he saw channels from the ovaries to the bladder. Thus, he concluded, female semen, being imperfect, did not enter the uterus but was discarded from the body, proving again that women contribute nothing to the newborn except nourishment. Despite the evidence to the contrary being right before his eyes, Herophilus' confirmation bias caused him to miss the obvious, and instead, he imagined that he saw something that did not actually exist.

The ideas of Greek philosophers held sway over European thinking for centuries. New evidence could not dislodge them. The revolution begun by Anaximander and the other Ionian philosophers, of questioning and doubting received wisdom, ground to a halt as the new authoritative views supplanted the old and became equally petrified. It took until the time of Giordano Bruno, Galileo, and Newton before physis would rise again and become modern science. What Anaximander called "necessity" Newton would call a "law." No god or angels were involved in the description of nature. In 1663, the newly established Royal Society of London coined a Latin motto: *Nullius in verba*, "Take no one's word for it." Centuries then elapsed before the methods of repeatable experimentation and falsifiability—hallmarks of modern science—finally emerged.

While East and West offered differing answers to the question of what animates life—whether it be purusha or psyche, prana or pneuma—both traditions agreed that something more than matter was needed. Breath was not just a physiological act but a bridge between body and soul. In India, this became prana, in Greece, pneuma. These concepts did not remain confined to philosophy. They began to influence medicine, healing practices, and theories of disease. If breath is life, what happens when it is obstructed? If prana is the thread that links the self to the body, can that thread be manipulated to restore health?

It is to these questions that we soon will turn, looking at how prana can be understood not only as a metaphysical force but as a vital function within the living body—central to both diagnosis and cure. But before we alight there, allow me to share with you an important lesson about respecting the body, which has little to do with prana and a lot to do with listening.

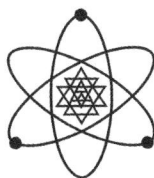

CHAPTER 11:

Bhakti and Broken Knees

The Hatha Yoga Pradipika says that padmasana, or lotus pose, is the "destroyer of all disease." Apparently, this power is available only to the very wise.[103] As I was to discover, for the not-so-wise, padmasana is the destroyer of knees.

I remember exactly when they broke and what I was doing. It was the fall of 1999. I had been practicing yoga for two years and was now a certified teacher. But what kind of teacher couldn't do lotus pose? I was determined to master it—quickly. I had heard Rodney Yee suggest it might take Westerners 10 years to achieve full Lotus. I didn't want to wait. I could almost get into lotus without using my hands, but the last bit required pulling.

As I pulled my feet into place, I felt sharp burning inside both knees. I ignored it. "No pain, no gain," as they say. I stayed for two minutes, even trying tolasana, lifting my body up by pressing my hands to the floor. But when I came out, the pain didn't end. It lingered through the rest of my practice. After shavasana, it was still there. A month later? Still there. Years later? Yes. I had crushed the medial menisci in both knees. That pain was not going away.

The problem wasn't my knees—it was my hips. When the femur lacks sufficient external rotation, the only way to get the foot onto the opposite thigh in lotus is by twisting the tibia around the femur. The knee ligaments, relaxed when the knee is bent, allow a bit of twist—but for me, not enough. Forcing the foot compresses the meniscus between the medial femoral condyle and the tibial plateau. I was lucky not to have torn the lateral collateral ligament as well. The solution, I thought, was clear: open the hips.[104] For months, I worked at it: pigeon pose, lunges, seated twists—anything that might improve external rotation, flexion, and abduction. In late 2000, I even moved closer to Prana Yoga Studio so I'd have more time to practice. I was convinced my hips would open any day now. The pain, though? Still constant.

I hadn't yet met Paul Grilley or heard his teaching on skeletal variation. I didn't know that my femur's shape and the orientation of my hip sockets meant I would never comfortably do lotus pose. Stretching could bring me to my personal limit—but not past it. My bones said no. But this realization still lay ahead of me.

Eventually, I saw my doctor, who referred me to Dr. Horlick, a surgeon at St. Paul's Hospital. The X-rays ruled out arthritis or fractures, but they showed thinning of the meniscus. Horlick said I could live with the pain—as he did—or have arthroscopic surgery to trim the torn bits. But that would reduce cushioning and accelerate wear. He warned that osteoarthritis was inevitable—maybe in five or ten years. To slow the damage, he advised me to stop activities that stressed the knees: no running, no tennis. He didn't mention yoga—I exhaled with relief. I gave up tennis, hockey, and even golf. Yoga would be my path.

The Canadian health system covered the cost, but the wait for elective surgery was long—about 18 months. My surgery would be in late 2001. In the meantime, I studied all I could. With aching knees, I went to Costa Rica to study with David Swenson. The pain remained—but by then, I had bigger things to deal with.

Seeking Support

Flying back to Canada always felt like coming home. As the plane descended into Vancouver on my return from Costa Rica, the mountains were dusted with snow. I was weak, dizzy, and exhausted—but relieved to be back. While I did go to work that week, I was highly unproductive.

In the previous June, I'd had a mild experience of this tired, dizzy feeling. Then, the lightheadedness occurred while driving. I'd had to pull over, recline my driver seat, and rest there for over half an hour before I could continue. A co-worker at MDA, Wendy Keyser, suggested I go see her husband, Jack, a physician specializing in naturopathy. He ran the requisite tests, which showed low blood pressure, elevated white blood cells, and a bit of overactivity in the thyroid. My lightheadedness was not due to any inner ear problems. My blood pressure being low was normal for me. Jack prescribed supplements—and made one major recommendation. I had been a vegetarian for about 15 years at that point. He suggested I add small amounts of chicken and fish. Adding some meat to my diet did seem to help, until it didn't.

Throughout the rest of 2001, I was mostly okay, but there were days when I did have to leave work early to go home and lie down. None of the episodes that year were severe. But Costa Rica took my condition to a whole new level. To figure out what was happening, I added a few new health advisors to my team.

Shakti Mhi suggested I visit an Ayurvedic physician she trusted: Dr. Shiva Varma. Shiva had set up his offices right beside a Vancouver landmark on the westernmost end of West 4th Avenue, called Banyen Books. Banyen Books was a mecca of New Age and alternative books, music, yoga props, incense, and delightfully colorful clothing. Shiva's office was next door, on the bottom floor of a two-story, old wooden building. He and his partner, Dr. Susan Barr, lived upstairs. They looked me over, listened to my story, took my pulse (in both wrists), and quickly concluded that I was suffering from an overdose of pitta and *Candida*. *Candida* is a genus of fungi commonly found in the mouth, gut, and skin. Usually benign, various *Candida* species can grow unchecked when the immune system is compromised, causing issues like thrush or yeast infections. Susan was sure I had a *Candida* overgrowth.

Pitta is one of the three Ayurvedic constitutions, the other two being kapha and vata. These three doshas are formed from Samkhya's five evolutes of space, air, fire, water, and earth. Pitta, made of fire and water, oversees our basic metabolism and is characterized by heat and fluidity. According to Shiva and Susan, my inner heat was out of control. This observation made me think of golfing in India and doing hot yoga in Costa Rica. It seemed plausible that this pitta stuff was contributing in some manner to my problem. Kapha, made of earth and water, governs our inner structure and manifests as heaviness, slowness, and steadiness. I had very little kapha. Vata, made of space and air, governs the breath and movements inside and outside the body. It manifests as dryness, coldness, and lightness. While I had a considerable amount of vata, it did not seem to be the cause of my problems. All three doshas contribute in varying degrees to our basic constitution, but when these basal levels are disrupted, ill health arises. In my case, the suspect was overactive pitta. I needed to cool it and foster more kapha.

Shiva put me on *Candida* killers and a liver-strengthening supplement. No more sugar, spice, or sweet lassis. My new diet was mostly kitchari, dahl, rice, and beans. Bland but, apparently, healing. Over the next year and a half, I slowly felt better. I can't say for sure whether the treatments helped—or whether time did. But even as I improved, I wasn't fully back to normal. Perhaps that was because I was still doing my very active yoga and pranayama practices.

One of the first yoga videos I owned was *Yoga Mind and Body*, hosted by Ali McGraw—but it was Erich Schiffmann's voice and teaching that hooked me.[105] When I saw he would be leading a retreat at Silver Bay in New York, alongside teachers like Richard Freeman and Donna Farhi, I knew I had to go. I was mostly better—aside from the knees.

Lines of Energy

The land beneath Silver Bay had been rising for over a billion years. Formed by a geologic dome, the Adirondack Mountains are a quiet testament to time. It is still slowly rising to this day. The dome stretches from the St. Lawrence Seaway to the Mohawk Valley, from Lake Champlain to the Black River. Worn by time and ice, its peaks and valleys cradle a long glacial lake called Lake George. On its western shore, near the northern end, lies the Silver Bay Conference Center, a YMCA facility nestled among the forests and slopes. The facility dates back to the first years of the 1900s. The center comprises numerous cottages, buildings, and halls, surrounded by trails and beaches. In the auditorium tower hangs a 500-pound bell, cast in 1909. I don't recall ever hearing it ring. Each morning, I would walk through the fields to attend my first yoga class of the day.

The conference ran on a tight, generous schedule: a two-hour asana class with a different teacher each morning; a midday lecture on yoga philosophy or practice; and a three-hour afternoon session with our chosen lead teacher. We were guaranteed time with every instructor, but for our deep dive, we had to choose one. For me, it was no contest: I chose Erich Schiffmann.

Erich was a large, warm presence—part teddy bear, part laughing sage. His graying hair fell in waves down to his shoulders. His personality was bright and his energy eager, reminding me of a large, jovial leprechaun. I felt lucky to be among the 50 students accepted into his group. On the first day, he described his approach to teaching yoga: begin simply, like opening a chess match with known moves, and then allow the flow to emerge naturally. He shared his habit of sketching classes with stick figures, a shorthand that soon became mine too. He assigned only one piece of homework: pause. Pause whenever you remember. In the pause, you might find yourself.

Erich preferred spontaneity. At home, he practiced to music, surrounded by notebooks and a tape recorder. He would document a sequence, then drop back into the flow. This became the template I used for designing my classes. While Erich loved using music for his own practice, he no longer used it in a class setting. I love music with classes, so when I pressed him on why he no longer used it, he demurred and said, "No real reason... there are always sounds around anyway."

Unlike many teachers, Erich didn't teach pranayama. When asked about it, he smiled and offered his own version: "smelling a flower." That was his pranayama— a breath of enjoyment. "Pause," he said, "and breathe like you're smelling flowers." Personally, he had gotten away from pranayama because he found he could "get there" faster by relaxing. He did not clarify where "there" was. He did admit that mantras were good—great, even. But he suggested we make one up and use that, and then, sooner or later, let it go and return to pausing. I eventually figured out that for Erich, the pause was the "there."

Erich often talked about energy. He told us how Iyengar could look at him in a pose, touch his arm, and say, "Move this to here." A subtle shift, a line of energy redirected, and suddenly, everything aligned. Years later, Erich read Joel Kramer's article "Yoga as Self-Transformation," which described energy flowing through the body and guiding practice.[106] Erich realized: he could move not from instruction but from sensation. "Send a line of energy through your arm," he told us, "and see what happens." From Joel, Erich came to understand that all the yoga he had practiced was someone else's yoga: that of B.K.S. Iyengar, Jiddhu Krishnamurti, T.K.V. Desikachar, but not his own yoga. At last, he knew how to do Erich yoga.

Erich gave us an assignment: hold your arm out, feel a current of energy from shoulder to fingertip, then turn it up—30 miles per hour, 40, 50, more—until you almost tremble. Then shift the angle, explore the direction, feel where the energy wants to go. Let the line move you. This is an organic form of yoga. You feel more alive. It is more fun. This wasn't a metaphor, either. For Erich, energy was palpable, experiential, and directive.

We experimented with star pose: feet wide, arms stretched, heart lifted. Five clear lines of energy radiated outward from the hara—the Zen name for the center of the body situated below the navel.[107] The goal wasn't to perfect the pose but to feel the flow. Look for blockages. Follow the energy. Adjust until you felt alive again. When a posture became stale, you sought the next movement. "Yoga," he said, "was a dance with awareness."

"Start from something easy," he said, "and then turn up the current. See what happens." It was less about alignment, more about aliveness. It wasn't about getting it right. It was about getting it real.

The Knee-dy Student

One of my intentions for the week was to ask each teacher for their advice on tortured knees. Erich was open about his own knee troubles. In fact, many yoga teachers I've studied with have admitted to joint injuries caused by their practice. Erich claimed he "popped both knees, twice!"[108] His recovery involved strengthening, not stretching—starting with mini-squats while holding ten-pound weights, and eventually building up to one-legged squats. It took a year, but he resolved it. This theme came up repeatedly: if something is too loose, don't stretch it—strengthen it.[109]

After one afternoon session, I joined a queue of students waiting to speak with David Life. He had completed an impassioned lecture on veganism and ahimsa, the practice of non-harming. He'd made the point that simply being alive creates harm—eating a carrot is, after all, bad for the carrot.

David was kind to each student, listening without a trace of impatience. Like many yoga teachers, he had a long, lean frame—almost gaunt—with serpent tattoos coiling up both forearms. When my turn came, I stepped forward and asked him about torn menisci. He was sympathetic—he'd torn both of his. He'd declined surgery and instead spent four years healing his knees through two practices: sitting daily in Vajrasana and riding an exercise bike. Like Erich, his message was clear—strengthen the knees.

The next morning, I saw Richard Freeman walking across the field to his first class. He moved slowly, mindfully—like a monk. I hesitated only a second before falling into step beside him. He gave a small nod, acknowledging my presence. We walked in silence for a few paces before I asked about knee injuries and meniscal tears. To my surprise, he stopped. I took one more step before turning to face him. He gave me his full attention.

He explained that the cartilage between the femur and tibia—the meniscus—has no direct blood supply. There are no arteries feeding it, and thus, healing is slow, if it happens at all. If pain persisted and healing didn't occur, surgery might be the only effective option.

I thanked him, realizing I shouldn't delay him further. His presence was luminous—calm, clear, fully there. I knew he had lived for years as an ascetic renunciate in India, studying Sanskrit, Sufism, yoga, and philosophy. Just those few minutes with him felt like a blessing. I took his advice seriously. I would continue strengthening practices, as suggested by Erich and David—but if the pain remained, I would also proceed with surgery. I was already on the waitlist. When the time came, I'd be ready.

Bhakti on the Beach

Earlier in the week, I met some fellow Canadians from the Santosa Yoga Studio in Ottawa. I also met Nancy (her last name is now lost to me), who was offering massage to soothe the sore bodies of students doing hours of yoga each day. My neck had grown particularly stiff, so on Wednesday night, I took her up on the offer.

Her style was called Thai Yoga Therapy. It was amazing, like having yoga done *to* you while remaining completely passive. Nancy bent and folded me into various postures, mobilizing every joint. Not only did my neck feel better—my whole body melted into ease. After that blissful session, I went to meet the Santosa teachers, gathered on the deck of their cabin overlooking the beach. Just as I arrived, someone pulled out a guitar—and another instrument I had never seen before: a harmonium.

I knew the word, but only from Kurt Vonnegut's *The Sirens of Titan*. In his novel, harmoniums were thin, blue, pancake-like creatures clinging to cave walls on Mercury. They ate sound and adored music, especially the haunting voices of the Sirens—beings of pure harmony, never fully explained. The real-life harmonium that night was something quite different.

It looked like an accordion had mated with an apple crate. Tipped on its side, with a keyboard in front and bellows behind, it produced both melody and a sustained drone, like a bagpipe—but far more pleasing. Someone explained that the harmonium had been invented in France in the mid-1800s as a poor man's pipe organ. It caught on in Europe and North America before making its way to India, where it evolved to suit Indian classical and devotional music. By the early 1900s, it had died out in the West—replaced by electric organs—but in India, it became a staple of kirtan.

Kirtan. I only had a vague notion of what it was, but it would become a major part of my yoga journey in the years ahead. Kirtan—also spelled *kirtana* or *keertan*—means to narrate, praise, or tell a story. It's often practiced in a call-and-response format, where a leader sings a phrase and the group repeats it. Or, as that night unfolded, it can be a simple circle of friends singing devotional songs, full of divine names.

Kirtan is common within bhakti yoga—the yoga of devotion and ecstatic joy, of tears and dancing, worship and surrender. This was the yoga of gospel singers and church choirs all over the world, not just in South Asia. Kirtan taps into the power of "Hallelujah!" The words were simple, easy to learn, and we sang and sang. After 40 minutes, I felt mellow and wide open. I thanked my new friends and left to walk home alone along the beach.

The air that night was charged with something still and holy. I don't know whether the peace I felt came from inside or from the shimmering moonlight on the water. Maybe it was the warm night breeze, the quiet lake, the drifting clouds, the just-past-full moon casting silver paths on the rippling waves. Maybe it was everything.

I'd felt something like this before—often on long flights, gazing out a window at the stars, high above the earth. I used to think it was due to the thin air at high altitudes, a kind of hypoxic high. But now, after massage and chanting, I realized it was something else—an altered state of stillness, of presence. It was beautiful. That moment stayed with me.

My return from Lake George required an overnight stay at a hotel in New York City. I arrived late on Sunday, September 2. With little time and fewer options, I decided—without knowing why—to visit the World Trade Center. It was late, and the towers were closed. I wandered the empty food court in the basement. Nothing was open. The whole place was silent, save for a single man slowly mopping the floor.

The next morning, I flew home to Vancouver.

Nine days later, on September 11, the World Trade Center ceased to be.

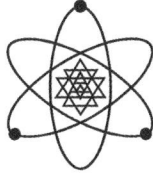

CHAPTER 12:

Taxila

The World Trade Center's memory lives on in the memorial built at Ground Zero. In my travels, I had visited many sites where great buildings had stood and great deeds been done, but little now remained. One such place was the ancient city of Taxila, in what we today call Pakistan.

I do not remember much about Pakistan. I was there only once, almost 40 years ago, and our company never did win any business. I no longer recall the name of the local agent who assisted me, nor even the name of the government official we visited. But I do remember a river, a mosque, and a large, empty room.

The flight from Athens to Islamabad was on a Sunday afternoon. As I gazed out the window, I saw the Indus River meandering below. Wherever it wandered, the land was green. Wherever it wasn't, the land was dry and barren. I've flown over many great rivers—from the Amazon to the Mississippi—but few match the historical significance of the Indus. This river halted Alexander the Great; his army never crossed it. Civilizations have risen and fallen with the floods and droughts of this river, including the Indus Valley civilization, which thrived long before Babylon existed.

Islamabad, Pakistan's capital, lies nestled in one of the middle bends of the Indus. The river winds between the hills of Rawalpindi and Peshawar. To the north rise the westernmost hills of the Himalayas—the mighty Margalla range. As we landed, I could see their forested slopes forming a green wall behind the city. I was due to visit Rawalpindi the next day to learn what the government needed. The twin cities of Islamabad and Rawalpindi sit on the Pothohar Plateau, and very close by are the ruins of ancient Taxila.

I met with the director of the Pakistan Remote Sensing Agency. He outlined their goals and proudly gave me a tour of their new facility. We stopped in a long hallway before a glass-walled room. Behind the glass was their newly-constructed computer center, empty for now, but equipped with raised flooring for cable management and a high ceiling to accommodate the future air conditioning demands of high-powered machines.

One of my company's advantages was the simplicity of our software and the sophistication of the hardware we used. I explained how our system would spare them from needing upgrades for many years. I showed photos of the equipment. The director nodded and murmured politely. He did not seem impressed.

After our meeting, my agent suggested I take the afternoon off and visit the Faisal Mosque. I had never been to a mosque, and this one, he told me, was the largest in the world. It had just been completed and was open to the public. I went—and I was amazed.

In the early 1970s, I had backpacked through Europe. One of the highlights of that trip was visiting Vatican City and St. Peter's Basilica. There, I stood transfixed by Michelangelo's *Pietà*—its grace, sorrow, and beauty turned the tragedy of Jesus' death into a sublime, eternal moment. That masterpiece carved itself into my heart. I can describe what I saw, but I cannot fully describe what I felt. Awe is the closest word.

Faisal Mosque was entirely different from St. Peter's. Although austere and devoid of images, it was just as arresting. It too was immense. Like St. Peter's, it could hold 300,000 worshippers, but that day, I seemed to be the only one there. Its folded roofs slanted like the canvas of a great Bedouin tent. Four sharply pointed minarets stood like sentinels at each corner, twice the height of the main roof.

I wasn't sure whether I was allowed to enter the prayer hall, so I stayed outside and wandered the spacious grounds, nestled against the Margalla Hills. Everything I saw was in balance—geometrically ordered, serenely beautiful. It left an impression I've never forgotten.

A few weeks after we submitted our bid, our agent told us, as expected, that we'd lost. I asked him why. His answer surprised me: the director was horrified by our proposal. Our computer was too small! He imagined his superiors touring the shiny new facility, only to find one tiny machine hiding in a vast, empty room. He feared being accused of incompetence for overbuilding.

I had misread the client completely. I assumed he wanted what *I* would want: the latest, most powerful system available. But he wanted something that fit *his* existing structure, that projected the scale and seriousness of his effort. He wasn't seeking progress for its own sake—he was seeking harmony with what he already had.

That experience taught me a lasting lesson about international sales. More importantly, it taught me something about cultural perspective. We can't see the world clearly if we assume others see it as we do. Cultures differ. People differ. Time itself differs. The knowledge we take for granted today didn't exist in earlier eras. Every culture, every era, has to work with what it knows. Ideas that now seem fantastical or naïve were once the best tools available. No one begins from nothing—we all build on what came before. To understand the past, we must forget the present. We must learn to see with the eyes they had, and through the world they inhabited.

Crossroads: West Meets East at Taxila

In the twenty-fifth year of the reign of Chandragupta II, a saffron-robed monk entered the ancient city of Taxila. According to the Western calendar, the year was 400 CE. The monk had traveled by foot from his home in Shanxi, in the land known then as Qin—the Middle Kingdom—in search of manuscripts. He was a Buddhist. His family name was Gong, but his dharma name, given at ordination, was Sehi, meaning "seeker."

Despite his smooth, bald head and long, gray beard testifying to his 63 years, the journey had strengthened him. Sehi had traveled with merchant caravans and fellow pilgrims for safety. Though Buddhist monks were expected to live aloof from worldly concerns, Sehi relished conversation and camaraderie. His goal was to visit the places where the Buddha had walked and taught, to find the oldest and most authentic scriptures, and to translate them from Sanskrit and Pali into classical Chinese.

Buddhism had long flourished in Gandhara, the westernmost province of the Gupta Empire, which included Peshawar and ancient Taxila. Sehi was pleased to find shelter at the Jaulian monastery, perched on a hill overlooking the city. Its great central stupa and dozens of smaller ones depicted scenes from the Buddha's life. The monastery was a serene place of study, silence—and, surprisingly, mystery.

It was there that Sehi met the young courtesan named Lalita. In most monasteries, a woman of her station would have been shunned. But here, in Taxila, Sehi encountered a form of Buddhism utterly unfamiliar to him—one with esoteric practices and tantric influences. Lalita, like this hidden path, was both alluring and enigmatic.

He first noticed her because she spoke to one of the delivery boys in his native tongue. This was astonishing. Few in Gandhara spoke Chinese. It turned out that Lalita had been born Lin Mei, in Qin. Sold to a trader in childhood, she had journeyed west with him along the Silk Road. Eventually, the trader sold her to Kamala, the matriarch of the courtesans in Taxila. Lin Mei's musical talent, graceful dance, and skill with languages soon made her one of Kamala's favorites. Her delicate features and pale skin were considered rare and desirable, but her birth name, Lin Mei, was unfamiliar to local ears. Kamala renamed her Lalita, the playful one.

Sehi was intrigued by her—not for her beauty, though it was undeniable—but because she was a bridge between his world and this new land. When he asked about the whispered secrets of the local Buddhist traditions, Lalita agreed to teach him—on one condition: he must never speak of them to others, nor write them down.

She chose a special night to begin. While the other monks prepared the evening meal, Sehi slipped away and met her just outside the monastery gates. She was dressed in an indigo sari that shimmered with gold thread, and tiny bells at her wrists and ankles chimed with each step. She carried a tanbura, its long neck resting on her shoulder. Tonight, Lalita intended to play.

She led him down a quiet lane to the home of Vasubandhu, newly appointed physician to the Maharaja of Gandhara. Vasubandhu was famed not only for his healing skill but for hosting the gosthi—intimate gatherings of thinkers, artists, and seekers. Kamala had convinced him to invite Sehi, praising the monk's cosmopolitan knowledge and command of Sanskrit. Vasubandhu, curious to meet a Chinese scholar, had agreed—and had chosen the other guests accordingly.

A gosthi was like a Greek symposium: an evening of wine, conversation, and companionship. While some gatherings drew dozens, Vasubandhu kept his intimate—just enough to provoke deep discussion without breaking the bank. He greeted Sehi and Lalita warmly and ushered them into a low-lit hall where the first round of watered wine was already circulating, its purpose more social lubricant than intoxicant.

The air carried a heady blend of sandalwood, rose, and jasmine. Silk tapestries and carved friezes adorned the walls—dancing girls, musicians, and erotic unions between devas and devis mingled with more sober content in the form of scenes from the Buddha's life. Sehi recognized several of the latter immediately, though the setting felt jarringly sensual for a householder who wore the dharmachakra pendant of a committed Buddhist.

Six low couches encircled a polished mahogany table covered with fruits, breads, spiced meats, and honeyed confections. Men reclined on their left sides, right hands free to lift cups. Four courtesans, dressed in vibrant silks, knelt beside them, their eyes alert to laughter and opportunity. Servants moved with choreographed grace to keep dishes replenished and cups full.

To Sehi's left, two men conversed with a courtesan in a language he did not recognize—Greek, he learned later. To his right, two others spoke Prakrit, the local vernacular, familiar yet elusive. Lalita settled beside him, quietly translating where needed.

Kamala, the matriarch of the Taxilan courtesans, sat regally near Vasubandhu on a grand couch across the room. Sehi sat stiffly at first. He was not unaccustomed to philosophical discourse, but rarely had it been served with wine, incense, and sensual distractions. He leaned toward Lalita and murmured, "Is this truly the way of the dharma?"

She smiled, eyes twinkling. "There are many paths, Sehi. Some begin in silence. Others, with a song."

Vasubandhu rose briefly, scanning the room, then lifted his cup in greeting. "Welcome, friends. Let this evening be a meeting of minds—and perhaps, new insights."

As Sehi raised his own cup, uncertain but curious, he sensed that tonight, he would encounter teachings far beyond sutras and scrolls.

The Gosthi at Taxila

Vasubandhu continued, "To my new Greek friends, a special greeting, for long have I wished to discuss the Greek views on life, current affairs, and medicine. Please do introduce yourselves for our other guests."

"Thank you, Vasubandhu!" spoke the eldest of the two Greeks. "I am Menecrates, formerly of Alexandria but, alas, I had to flee that grand city nine years ago after the razing of Serapeum by Christian mobs. I was trained in the teachings of Hippocrates and Galen. When I fled the city, I managed to save a few manuscripts, treasures I now carry with me."

"And I," added the younger Greek, "am Philolaus of Delphi. After Emperor Theodosius' decrees, our sacred sites were laid to waste. I now serve as physician and astrologer to the local Greek community and travelers along the Silk Road. I arrived in Taxila five years ago and, thanks to the friendship of Menecrates, I was able to find work as a physician and astrologer."

Sehi, cross-legged on his couch beside Lalita, listened attentively as she translated. The Greeks wore simple togas, their hems stained with road dust—a sign, Sehi thought, that they were men of modest means.

Vasubandhu turned to his left. "Divodasa?"

"Greetings," said Divodasa, raising his cup. "My brother Dhanvantari and I follow the teachings of Charaka and Sushruta, physicians of Ayurveda, the ancient knowledge of life. While Sushruta wrote of surgery, we practice internal medicine, guided by the balance of the doshas."

All eyes then turned to Sehi. He hesitated. Lalita offered a reassuring smile.

"I am Gong Sehi of Zhongguo," he said quietly, as Lalita translated. "I am a Buddhist monk and seeker of texts. I have traveled here in the hope of finding manuscripts of the Dharma to bring home to the Middle Kingdom. Though I am no physician, there are many at my home monastery in Shanxi who are very skilled in this art, and I would be happy to share what little knowledge they have shared with me."

The Greek View: Humors and Pneuma

The five men and three courtesans bowed to Sehi, while Lalita looked up at him with a smile. Vasubandhu gestured with his goblet. "Then let us begin. Menecrates, Philolaus, tell us—how do the Greeks understand health and disease?"

Philolaus leaned forward. "We once believed illness came from the gods. But reason taught us that if a god caused disease, then no medicine could help. Now we know that three main factors govern illness: the disease, the patient, and the physician. Often, more important than what kind of a disease a patient has is what kind of patient the disease has! Healing lies in understanding nature. Illness may arise from food, water, air, the seasons—or imbalance within."

"We hold that the body contains four humors," continued Menecrates, "blood, phlegm, black bile, and yellow bile. Each is influenced by qualities of hot, cold, wet, or dry. As Philolaus has said, health is the balance of these fluids. Disease, an imbalance."

"These humors also shape the psyche," added Philolaus. "Blood makes a man sociable; black bile, melancholic; yellow bile, choleric. Phlegm dulls the emotions."

Vasubandhu nodded. "And how do these humors flow through the body?"

"Through vessels," said Menecrates, "but the key is pneuma—life's breath. Respiration brings raw pneuma into our lungs, where it is taken to the heart. It is within the heart that this primordial pneuma is refined by the heat of the heart and combined with blood, creating the essential life-giving fluid. From the heart, arteries carry the refined pneuma-enriched blood to other organs and tissues. It is pneuma that maintains the heat and vitality of the body. In distinction to this vital pneuma carried by the arteries, our veins carry a non-vital form of pneuma, produced by the liver. The veins carry this lesser form of pneuma away from the tissues and help to remove these waste products from the body."

Philolaus continued, "In the Hippocratic school, the nerves, originating in the brain, carry the humors. Galen, however, determined that there were three different types of nerves, which are hollow tubes that conducted different forms of pneuma. The first type is nerves that affect and control the movements of the body. Secondly, there are nerves that bring sensation to the brain, such as touch, pain, heat, and so on. And finally, there are mixed forms of nerves, which both transmit and receive pneuma."[110]

"And emotions?" asked Vasubandhu.

"Emotions arise from the organs," said Menecrates. "The liver, spleen, gallbladder—all play a part. The brain may reason, but the body feels."

Ayurveda: Doshas and Dhatus

Vasubandhu turned to Divodasa and said, "A fine overview of the Greek philosophy of medicine is laid at our feet, Divodasa. Please describe the Ayurvedic principles for our friends."

With a flourishing wave of his wine cup, Divodasa began. "Indeed. Thank you, Menecrates and Philolaus. There seem to be many similarities in our understanding. It leads me to wonder whether at some time, your Greek physicians had visited the East and learned such things here!"

Menecrates laughed and said, "Or perhaps your sages came West and learned from our teachers?"

Divodasa bowed slightly. "We share your view that healing is natural, but we do not abandon the gods. Think of the gods not as personalities, but as principles: Agni, the fire of digestion; Indra, the sense of self; Soma, the joy of being."[111]

He continued, "Like your views of the humors, we also hold that there are essential substances, called the doshas. In fact, there are three: vata, pitta, and kapha. The doshas are combinations of the five elements, or 'evolutes,' as we call them. Vatta is the combination of air and space and is responsible for motion, coolness, lightness, and other qualities within the body. Pitta is a combination of fire and water. It is responsible for our inner heat, intensity, and transformations. Kapha is the combination of earth and water and is responsible for heaviness, cold, durability, and endurance. Each dosha has the attributes of the gunas: tamas, rajas, and sattva. These gunas are the basic constituents of the whole universe. Tamas is what you call cold; it is inert, placid. Rajas is what you call hot; it is activity. Sattva is harmony."

Philolaus asked, "And what of the tissues of the body?"

Dhanvantari replied, "We call them *dhatus*. The first dhatu is called *rasa*, which is like the lifeblood of a river, the water that flows. All the juices secreted from the digestion of food are rasa, and this is the basis for all the other tissues. *Rakta* is what you call blood, and like in your view of blood, it carries vayu—wind or air—or more specifically, the *prana vayu*, of which we should speak more a bit later. The next four rasas are *mamsa* or muscle, *meda* or fat, *asthi* or bone, and *majja* or marrow. Finally, we have *shukra*, our reproductive substance. In men, this manifests as semen."

Divodasa took up the thread and said, "There is an order here. Rasa is concentrated to become rakta, this blood is concentrated to become mamsa, mamsa becomes meda, meda becomes asthi, and finally, asthi becomes semen. It takes 40 days and 40 drops of blood to make one drop of semen."[112]

"Yes," interrupted Philolaus, "this is something we agree upon. And, if the semen is strong, a boy child will be conceived. However, if the semen is weak, a girl child will be born."

Amala, one of the courtesans injected, "But this is not true! Everyone knows that a boy or girl child is determined by the day it is conceived. A son is conceived on the even days and girls on the odd."[113]

Lalita also spoke up, "I recall when I was young and lived in the Middle Kingdom, a physician told my father that the age of the mother and the lunar month of conception determines whether a son or daughter is born."

"In Ayurveda," said Dhanvantari, "the understanding is closer to what Philolaus suggested. The relative strength of the *retas*, or seed, from the father and from the mother prevails in most cases. If the father's seed is stronger than the mother's, a son is conceived; if the mother's is stronger, a daughter comes forth.

"But," he continued, "we should speak now of the *vayus* or vital airs, of which there are five:[114] *prana, apana, vyana, samana* and *udana*. The prana vayu is the most important air—responsible for our breath, our senses, and it resides in the chest and head. Apana vayu, located in the lower belly and legs, governs downward movements and eliminations, such as defecation, urination, and menstruation. Samana vayu, located in the mid region of the torso, governs digestion, assimilation, and the initial distribution of the healthy parts of foods, the nutrients. Vyana vayu pervades the body and governs the movement of blood and nutrients created by samana vayu. Udana vayu, also located in the upper body, governs the actions of speech and thought. Of the five vayus, prana vayu is paramount, for it brings the vitality of life into the body, and this vitality is transformed into the other vayus, in a similar way that your rarefied pneuma becomes the grosser form.

"The channels you called nerves, veins, and arteries may well be the ones we call nadis. Some carry physical substances—blood, air—but others carry the subtler currents of prana."

Philolaus was listening very intently. He asked, "I would like to hear more about this prana vayu you mentioned. You have likened it to our pneuma."

Divodasa replied, "The prana vayu provides the vitality of life. Due to this quality, a loss of prana can contribute to or cause illness or death. Prana's role is more than respiration; it has a role in digestion, the movement of food within and throughout the body, and contributes to the proper functioning of the tissues and organs. Prana works in harmony with the doshas and dhatus, and any imbalance in prana will manifest in sickness."

Vasubandhu now interjected, "Indeed, and prana not only is vital for life and healing but also supports atman, the soul."

Dhanvantari added, "And to understand that function of prana requires a teacher of dharma. Perhaps you, Vasubandhu, should continue?" he said with a smile.

Chinese Medicine: Qi, Shen, and the Dao

Before responding, Vasubandhu looked towards Kamala, who slightly shook her head and glanced towards Sehi. Taking her cue, Vasubandhu said, "Perhaps later. Venerable Sehi, we have not yet heard from your land."

Sehi had been leaning a bit towards Lalita, but now he sat up straight and tall, paused for a moment, and began. "There was once a grand idea carried mostly by wandering philosophers in the land of Qin. These ascetics built no temples, they had no orders, they belonged to no city or king. They lived off the land and the kindness of simple people. They followed 'the way,' which they called the *Dao*. Dao can also mean "to speak," so it is fitting for me to speak of this with you."

Sehi spoke slowly in his native tongue, which gave time for Lalita to translate. When she had finished and everyone was nodding, he continued. "In the Middle Kingdom, medicine flows from the Dao, the way of nature. From Dao comes the primal *qi*, which splits into *yin* and *yang*, which in turn give rise to all things. Qi is the spirit of all existence—not just of life.

"Yin and yang are not opposites but complements. Warmth reflects a surplus of yang; coolness, of yin. Their balance governs all things."[115] Out of yin–yang, the third, come five elements, which are not quite the same as yours. For a Daoist, the elements are water, wood, fire, earth, and metal.[116]

"As you have pointed out, air has a vitality that is essential to life. The spirit of the air, which you call prana and pneuma, we call *kong* qi. But qi is not only found in air. There are many ways qi can invest the body. The spirit of good food can be digested and turned into *gu* chi. There is a spirit we receive from the earth and a spirit from the sky. Each organ has its own spirit."

Sehi paused to allow Lalita time to translate and then continued, "The organs of the body are linked to *jing luo*, channels that guide both qi and blood. There are 14 main channels, 12 of which are tied to an organ."

Dhanvantari asked, "Are these like our nadis?"

"Perhaps," Sehi replied. "But qi is more fluid than prana. Qi can be deficient, which means we do not have enough of it; qi can be excessive, which means we have too much of it; it can be stagnant, which means we have enough, but it is unresponsive; and qi can be rebellious, which means the qi is out of control. Each imbalance of qi presents symptoms, and from these, a Daoist physician will diagnose the cause of imbalance and then suggest the appropriate diet, lifestyle, or intervention to re-establish the balance. In this manner, the physician's approach in my land seems very similar to your own: first, find the cause of the imbalance, and then, seek a cure to regain harmony."

Sehi again paused, and then with a slight smile said, "And our physicians have a unique method of restoring qi balance—*zhen*, the insertion of fine needles."[117]

Menecrates was incredulous at the idea and laughed. "You mean your physicians stick sharp needles into the body in order to heal the body? That sounds very strange!"

Kamala silenced his laughter. "Strange to us, perhaps—but would not bloodletting seem strange to others?"

"Fair enough," said Philolaus. "We bleed the body to balance the humors."

"As do we," said Divodasa.

"And as do our physicians," added Sehi. "Though we may use leeches instead of blades."

"Is there anything else to share?" asked Vasubandhu.

"Perhaps one last comment," said Sehi. "What you might consider the soul, which you call atman, we call shen, and we discern not one, nor three, but five forms of it: *shen* (spirit), *hun* (ethereal soul), *po* (corporeal soul), *zhi* (will), and *yi* (intellect).[118] Each resides in a different organ and governs aspects of the self. Though as a Buddhist, I do not believe in a soul that survives death,[119] I do believe that while we are alive, qi and shen support each other."

"In this, we agree," said Dhanvantari. "The body, mind, and spirit are one. No part can be treated in isolation."

"As a Buddhist," continued Sehi, "I know many Daoist physicians who also do not care whether or not hun continues after death. What is important to the physician is that shen represents the character of a person and his ability to understand himself and others. Shen is embodied. Let the priests worry about the patient after death. The concern of the healer is the patient before death occurs. While alive, qi and shen balance and affect each other. Qi supports the stability and clarity of shen; shen contributes to the harmonious flow of qi."

When Lalita had finished relaying these last words, the room fell silent in contemplation of their meaning. Kamala decided that this was the time to allow Vasubandhu to reveal a bit more about their inner teachings. She quietly looked at him and gave a slight nod. He understood her signal and began to share, but only to the degree that they had privately agreed upon.

The Triad: Macrocosm, Mesocosm, and Microcosm

"Venerable Gong Sehi," he began, "thank you. Your views have remarkable parallels to our own understanding of Sat, or existence. We too recognize the tripartite nature of the world. Between heaven and earth, what you have called yang and yin, there is an interface. Let us call these three realms the macrocosm, the microcosm and, in between, the mesocosm.

"There is the creator and the created—gods above, people below. What binds them together is sacrifice. This is the divine order, which we call *rta*."[120]

"This triune of the divine, sacrifice, and human is reflected in the triad of fluid, air, and fire, which is to say of rasa, vayu, and agni. This formula leads to success in any field of application. For the spiritual seeker, there is the triad of moon, wind, and sun. For the alchemist, there is the triad of mercury, air, and sulfur. For the physician, there is the triad of semen, breath, and blood. The highest principle is represented by the moon, mercury, fluid, and semen. The gross is represented by the sun, sulfur, fire, and blood. Mediating between these are the actions of air, wind, and breath. As physicians, our practice is finding the appropriate adjustment, or sacrifice, to restore harmony between the macrocosm and the microcosm. Just as sacrifices to the gods employ the fire of agni, we too employ transformations through the fires of digestion, cooking, and austerities.

"The Ayurvedic view of the body is also tripartite: there is the mind, the soul, and the body, which we can call *sattva*, *atman*, and *sarira*. The microcosmic body can become out of harmony with the macroscopic universe, and this imbalance is manifested as disease. To restore harmony, the sacrifice of digestion must be perfected.[121]

"Just as the moon waxes over 15 nights, so too can the dhatus be replenished in that time. Mercury, the alchemists say, is the vital fluid of Shiva—and thus nourishes semen, already alike in nature.[122] Semen can also be considered the rasa of the moon, which yields *soma*, the nectar of immortality. However, care must be taken, for the fiery blood of a woman's womb can neutralize the power of a man's semen. There are times when such a sacrifice is required; the loss of semen to the heat of a woman is necessary to generate a child; but in general, it is better to keep this seed in the vault of the cranium and not let it fall into the fires of the lower belly. The process of breathing in and breathing out will suffice to perfect the microcosm and harmonize it with the macrocosm,[123] but of that, I will not speak further tonight. It is more important to discuss the role of rasa and the practice of *rasayana*.

"There are many ways to understand rasa. It may refer to the six tastes, which affect the body and mind: these are sweet, salty, sour or acidic, hot or pungent, bitter, and astringent, but it is more. Rasa is the sap of trees, the water of life, the vital fluid known as *ojas*. It is amrta, the nectar of immortality, the soma of the moon. It is the offering in every sacrifice. And during sacrifice, rasa's vitality is carried by vayu—the wind—refined by agni's fire and delivered to the gods. This is the meaning of the triune *rasa–agni–vayu*. The body's rasas are refined by the inner agni of digestion and prana, and the inner vayus fan the fire. This inner fire is the tapas of the yogi and the goal of the physician for his patient.[124]

"Rasayana is the vehicle or practice of healing the body by making it whole, of returning the microcosm into a perfect reflection of the macrocosm. Once this has been achieved, the result is a long life, good memory and intelligence, freedom from disease, good complexion, a deep, powerful voice, and great bodily and sensory powers. This practice includes elixirs, which are referred to as the rasayanas. In the hands of the alchemist, these elixirs may include the homologues mercury, sulfur, and mica, which equate to the semen of Shiva, the fire of agni, and the menstrual fluids of the goddess, respectively. For this reason, alchemy is also known as rasayana."

Sehi tried to follow the layers Vasubandhu was weaving together—alchemy, anatomy, sacrifice, spirit. Like a new star blazing in the night sky that had not been there the day before, Sehi's world was being illuminated in a way he'd never known. It was as though the whole universe had been reduced to a single formula of breath, blood, and fire.

Seeing the puzzlement upon the face of Venerable Gong Sehi, Vasubandhu paused and laughed at himself. "I do get carried away and speak too much. Enough of metaphysics. Kamala! Perhaps it is time to change the mood?"

Kamala smiled and clapped her hands. The courtesans reached for their instruments. Susmita played her tabla, Lalita her strings. Amala danced while the men murmured quietly about herbs and remedies. As the wine flowed and music swelled, the night deepened.

When the Greeks had eaten all the meats and the laughter became louder, Kamala lightly touched the back of Vasubandhu's hand. This not-so-subtle signal again turned the evening. Amala led the two Greeks to a private room while the brothers remained with Susmita, Kamala, and Vasubandhu in the main hall. Lalita guided Sehi to their own room. What happened next was never revealed. As Sehi had promised, he never spoke or wrote about whatever it was Lalita revealed to him when they were alone.

That night, back at the monastery, Sehi tried to understand the layers Vasubandhu had woven together—alchemy, anatomy, sacrifice, spirit. He lit a candle and sat with brush and parchment. To bring order out of complexity, he drew a chart:

GONG SEHI'S TABLE OF TRIADS

Realm	Alchemical Symbols	Medical Analogues	Spiritual Symbols
Macrocosm	Moon / Mercury / Semen	Rasa / Ojas / Soma	Heaven / Divine / Yang
Mesocosm	Wind / Air / Breath	Vayu / Prana / Nadis	Sacrifice / Agni
Microcosm	Sun / Sulphur / Blood	Agni / Digestive Fires	Human / Earth / Yin

As he studied the chart, Sehi felt a subtle unease. Daoist cosmology resisted tidy arrangement. Yin was not always below, yang not always above. Their relationships shifted, like clouds in the wind. Still, the chart illuminated him like the full moon shining light on an unfamiliar terrain.

Two weeks after the gosthi, it was time for Sehi to continue his journey—eastward this time, toward the Ganges and the sacred sites of Lord Buddha. Sehi documented the practices and rituals of every monastery he visited. He gathered many manuscripts describing the dharma. In total, he spent 10 years in Southern Asia, visiting cities like Kapilavastu and Varanasi. He went further south and spent two years in Lanka. From there, he sailed back to his home, settling in Nanjing. He changed his name to Faxian, which means "the splendor of dharma," wrote about his travels, and translated many Buddhist sutras into Classical Chinese. He entered nirvana in 422 CE at the age of 85.

The Golden Age of Gandhara

What makes an age golden? A golden age is a time of peace, a time of economic growth, and a time of cultural advancement. From the first to the fifth centuries CE, the Gupta Empire provided an umbrella of peace. A vibrant cultural scene existed, fueled by a fusion of Roman and Greek art and sculpture with South Asian techniques, which, combined with the rich tapestry of Buddhist stories, created a very distinctive Gandharan style. There was an intellectual exchange due to the ongoing trade and movement of people along the Silk Road between the Roman, Egyptian, Greek, and Persian worlds and China and South Asia. This trade brought considerable wealth to the region.

Yet even with the advancements in art and architecture, literature and philosophy, culture and wealth, there were still great inequities, both socially and economically. Not everyone benefits during an age of gold. The blending of many religions can lead not only to cross-fertilization but also to factions and disputes, with social borders being invisibly drawn. As had happened in Ionia almost 900 years earlier, political, cultural, and economic changes brought alterations in the way people viewed the world and thought about their place in it. In Gandhara, the seeds of a radical new form of Buddhism were sown, a form that would mature into Mahayana Buddhism, which would be exported to and dominate China, Korea, and Japan. Other seeds would develop into forms of tantra yoga, which would eventually inform medieval hatha yoga.

Gandhara was a melting pot of many cultures and ideas, making it a perfect place and time to contrast and compare several medical philosophies that would have been tested against each other. A perfect place to see how the ideas of prana and the causes of life were evolving. In the above vignette, only Gong Sehi is a real historical person. The general outline provided for his life and his journey from China to South Asia and back again are true, but the details of his stay in Taxila are purely fictional, as are all the other characters in the story.[125]

Appreciating Fifth-Century Medicine with Modern Minds

Today, we have GPS in our cars, and we always know where we are. We have the history of the world in our pockets, and humans have been to the moon in rockets. Our world would be unimaginable to someone living 1,600 years ago—and it's equally difficult for us to imagine theirs. When we eavesdrop on a conversation from Gandhara in 400 CE, we must remember what they didn't have: clocks, compasses, antibiotics, any knowledge that the Americas existed.[126] Glassblowing had not yet produced lenses, so there were no microscopes or telescopes—the very tiny and very distant were invisible. Even ideas like progress or discovery were foreign. As Ecclesiastes put it, "There is no new thing under the sun."[127] In that world, qualities like hot and cold were not measurable. Galen believed the physician's hand was the perfect tool to assess such states.[128] Galileo later described a professor who dismissed evidence of nerves connecting to the brain—because Aristotle hadn't said it was so.

Scientific instruments like thermometers and barometers eventually gave us new senses. As the invisible became visible, it also became mechanical, less spiritual. Many ancient beliefs now seem mistaken. Mice were thought to arise from straw,[129] a theory known as spontaneous generation, rooted in Aristotle's view that life could emerge from non-living matter given pneuma and heat.[130] Even more difficult to spot are the omissions: glands and plexuses were unknown. Only in modern times were they incorporated into metaphysical models like the chakra system—ideas completely foreign to our fictional characters.[131]

Ancient physicians across cultures recognized internal channels. Daoist doctors, for example, described meridians (*jing luo*), but not veins, arteries, or nerves in the anatomical sense understood today.[132] Ayurveda also spoke of nadis: "There are a hundred and one nadis of the heart," says the Chandogya Upanishad.[133] In the Brihadaranyaka: "Just as the spokes of a wheel are fixed to the hub, so too are these nadis fixed in the heart."[134] These channels likely appeared self-evident. Cut a body, and blood flows—clearly, there must be inner conduits. Surgeons and butchers would have seen stringy, tubular structures. Nadis were probably considered real and gross, not subtle. But after the scientific revolution, when William Harvey discovered the circulation of blood,[135] and nerves were understood centuries later,[136] the role of traditional conduits was displaced. If arteries and nerves weren't carrying prana or qi, perhaps other, subtler pathways were. Thus, the modern concept of subtle channels may have been a response to science's demotion of older models.

Despite differences in names and views, the approach to medicine was remarkably consistent across cultures. Physicians used holistic models, sought to restore balance, and often linked illness to cosmic or divine causes. Most ancient texts focused more on treatment than on systematized anatomy. Whether Hippocratic, Ayurvedic, or Daoist, healing involved food, herbs, ritual, and sometimes prayer.

The earliest Ayurvedic texts—the Charaka and Sushruta Samhitas—mention vayus, prana, and nadis, but not in the metaphysical way found in later tantra or yoga. Nadis were functional conduits for breath, blood, and waste.[137] Prana was breath and life's vitality, not yet spiritualized. The spiritual roadmaps of tantra came later.

From the time of Aristotle to Harvey, there was little distinction between physical and energetic conduits. But as microscopes deepened our understanding of the physical body, these earlier concepts lost their footing. This created the need to redefine them as subtle—real but undetectable by physical means.

Before the scientific revolution, there was no need to separate gross and subtle. The world was unified. But once it was divided into atoms and then quarks, into seen and unseen, science staked a claim to the physical, and spirit was left to the mystical. Science is based on hard facts and empirical knowledge; spirit is metaphorical and poetic. Consider, as one example, the understanding of snakes. A zoologist will fascinate us with their anatomy and biology, but the yogi fascinates us with their homologues.

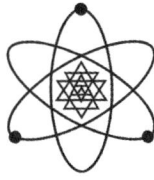

CHAPTER 13:

A Serpentine Interlude

What is a homologue? In the vignette set in Taxila around 400 CE, Vasubandhu used this term. It derives from "homologous," meaning things with a common origin or substance, though they may differ in form or function. For Vasubandhu, the moon and semen are not *symbols* of the macrocosm—they *are* the macrocosm. Similarly, sun, fire, sulfur, and blood are not metaphors for the microcosmic human; they are its expressions. This is not a simile. This is identity. The Upanishadic realization *tat tvam asi*—you are that—is not a poetic metaphor. You, the microcosmic individual *are* the macrocosm!

To grasp this, consider two examples—one secular, one sacred. First, money: coins and paper bills are different, but both are money. A gold coin is not a metaphor for wealth; it is wealth. These are homologues—different embodiments of the same reality.

Now, the sacred. In Catholic mass, the bread and wine do not merely symbolize Christ's body and blood. Through the rite of *transubstantiation,*[138] the priest converts the bread and wine into Christ's body and blood. These become homologues, not metaphors. The parishioners are actually consuming Christ's body and blood, as he commanded.[139]

Keep this in mind as we explore ancient beliefs. Semen *is* divine, the essence of life. For the alchemist, mercury *is* Shiva's semen. The snake is not a symbol or metaphor, it is a homologue—in this case, of life.

The serpent named "endless," Ananta Shesha,[140] is the embodiment of time itself and the foundation and source of each new universe. At the end of each cosmic cycle, Shiva dances the *Tandava,* consuming the universe in fire. Shesha sheds his scales— each one a memory—which are reduced to cinders. In this void, Vishnu awakens and, moved by necessity, infuses the ashes with his energy. From the remnants of Shesha, stars and galaxies are reborn. The serpent coils once more beneath Vishnu, forming the base of the new cosmos.[141]

Serpents are chthonic beings—creatures of the underworld, burrowers in dark soil.[142] They are liminal, living above and below, mediating between worlds. They are death and rebirth, wisdom and danger, guardians and destroyers. They molt and renew, bearing the secrets of transformation and immortality. In the positive light, they are beings of wisdom, fertility, transformation, and life. In the negative view, they are beings of danger, darkness, death, and decay.

In some Indian building traditions, a spike is driven into a snake's head to anchor the structure.[143] A grand naga, the snake *Mucalinda*, shelters the meditating Buddha from a fierce storm.[144] Ningiszida, the ancient Mesopotamian serpent-deity, coils around the tree of life. The serpent appears again in Eden, and again in Greece, entwined around the staff of Asclepius—son of Apollo and healer so skilled he could raise the dead. (Hades, fearing loss of souls, complained to Zeus, who struck Asclepius with a thunderbolt. Deified in death, he became the patron of physicians, his single-serpent staff the symbol of healing.[145])

To yoga students, the most familiar serpent-avatar is Patanjali. In a story related to me by T.K.S. Desikachar, Gonika, a devout woman past childbearing age, prayed for a son. Ananta Shesha, resting beneath Vishnu, heard her. With Vishnu's blessing, he fell to earth into her cupped hands, incarnating as Patanjali—*pat* meaning "to fall," *anjali* meaning "prayer" or "grace." He was the falling answer to a prayer.

In Buddhist and alchemical traditions, we also find Nagarjuna—"the Arjuna of the snakes." Myth abounds with divine pairings: the bird and the serpent, the heavens and the earth. Garuda, Vishnu's eagle, battles Ananta, Vishnu's snake. These beings are homologized as the upper and lower parts of the yogi's body. In the vault of the skull resides the bird that carries the immortal seed, semen, and at the base of the spine sleeps the serpent, Kundalini. The seed of immortality drips incessantly into Kundalini's mouth, ensuring her immortality. This is the story of a bird nesting high in the branches of the tree of life, and the serpent on the ground beneath that same tree. The serpent is a homologue for the earth and the microcosm, while the bird is a homologue of heaven and the macrocosm.

In Vedic ritual, the mesocosm—the link between gods and mortals—was sacrifice. In tantra and hatha yoga, the mesocosm is practice. The heat of the sacrificial fire becomes the tapas of the yogi. The new sacrifice is inner. The serpent rises to meet the bird. (Kundalini must be awoken and raised to the top of the head.) In that yoking, union is obtained, realization occurs, the microcosm is fused with the macrocosm.

Another homologue to the mesocosm is the practice of alchemy. This is so important to our understanding of prana that it warrants a look at how yoga is an alchemical practice.

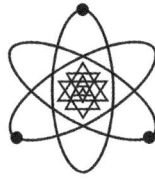

CHAPTER 14:

Yoga Alchemy

*Our true purpose in yoga is to awaken the guru within. This is what
the alchemical tradition refers to as turning lead into gold.*
– Tim Miller[146]

Tim Miller stood before the class, with short, wavy brown hair with a touch of gray and a slender, athletic build. It was a typical body shape that I noticed in all the famous ashtanga teachers. He called ashtanga "yoga alchemy."

"The word alchemy," he said, "evokes an image of a medieval conjurer murmuring incantations over a boiling cauldron, attempting to turn lead into gold." That had been my own impression: alchemy as an outdated precursor to modern chemistry, a quaint footnote in the story of science. But Tim offered something deeper.

He continued, "In a broader sense, alchemy refers to the process of transmuting one thing into another through the kindling of a vital transformative energy, known as *Mercurius*. Turning lead into gold is a metaphor for the liberation of spirit from matter, which is the primary goal of both alchemy and yoga."

It was October 5, 2001. In less than a week, I was scheduled for arthroscopic knee surgery. Dr. Horlick told me it would take six weeks—perhaps three months—before I could resume a full ashtanga practice. Fortunately, Mike Denison, the owner of City Yoga, had arranged for Tim to teach in Vancouver just before my operation.

Tim had begun yoga in the 1970s as a university student and soon discovered ashtanga.[147] Then he met Pattabhi Jois in 1978 and became one of the first ashtanga teachers in the United States. By the time of our workshop, he was well known not only for teaching physical practice but also for weaving in philosophy and therapeutic insight. For Tim, yoga was a fire—a crucible. Through breath, movement, and tapas, this inner fire could purify the practitioner and spark real transformation.

Tim began the weekend with a talk on the Yoga Sutras. "A sutra," he said, "is a few words with big meanings." He walked us through the opening lines of Patanjali's text, unpacking the Sanskrit phrase *yoga citta vritti nirodhah*. "Yoga," he said, "is the cessation of the fluctuations of the mind," pointing out that this means yoga has nothing to do with stretching your hamstrings. For Tim, yoga wasn't about acquiring skills, strength, or even flexibility. It was about letting go. "Yoga is not addition," he said. "It's subtraction."

The first line of the second chapter of the Yoga Sutras—*tapah svadhyaya ishwara-pranidhanana kriya-yogah*—can be interpreted alchemically. In Tim's translation, Patanjali offers one of many approaches to yoga: "Kriya yoga consists of three stages—tapas (heat), svadhyaya (self-study), and ishwara-pranidhana (bowing to god)."[148] The heat generated through asana and movement is the yogi's tapas, a kind of physical alchemy that purifies and transforms the body.

Svadhyaya, or self-study, is a mental alchemy. Tim explained it as the act of witnessing ourselves with attention—through posture, breath, and gaze (drishti)—which refines awareness and leads to self-knowledge.

Ishwara-pranidhana is spiritual alchemy. It's the process of releasing ego and recognizing the spark of divinity within. "Between us and the Divine sits the guru," Tim said. "But the true guru is not the teacher in front of you—it's the one within."

Prana, he taught, is "citta in motion"—the mind in movement. Ujjayi pranayama helps settle the mind by anchoring attention in the breath's sound. "Attention is not concentration," Tim reminded us, "it's interest. Be curious about your breath, but not attached to it."

When Tim first started doing pranayama, under Pattabhi Jois' direction, he worked on very long holds of the breath so much that he started having diarrhea. Jois' advice was to not worry; keep doing the practice 10 or 12 times a day, and all will be well. "It is just cleansing," Jois said.

Tim admitted that Pattabhi Jois stopped teaching pranayama. Perhaps it was because Pattabhi Jois was just too tired or too busy. But Tim continued to teach it. He believed that the breathwork was essential for balancing all the intense physical work of ashtanga. He taught what he called "baby versions"—gentle practices like alternate nostril breathing—eschewing more vigorous forms like kapalabhati and bhastrika.

Recall Swami Sivananda of Rishikesh's belief that we're born with a fixed number of breaths. Once they're used up, life ends. For that reason, slow breathing—pranayama—is a path to longevity. "A yogi's life," Tim said, "is measured in breaths." Pranayama extends life by slowing down the breath.

Tim offered an etymological insight: the common translation of pranayama as "breath control" comes from splitting the word as prana + yama. But he suggested it's more accurate to read it as prana + ayama. "Yama," he noted, is the god of death; "a-yama" means not-death, or the extension of life. Pranayama, then, becomes a means of sustaining breath, prolonging life, and ultimately entering into a stillness where the nadis are purified.[149]

One of the pranayama practices Tim gave us was viloma—segmenting the breath. During cat-cow pose, we inhaled in stages while lowering our spine deep into the body in cow pose, looking forward and then up. We started with a little breath in while lifting the tailbone; pause; breathe in a little, softening the belly; pause; a little more inhalation while lowering the spine by dropping the belly, chest, and then lifting the throat, and head; pause. We had six separate little inhalations in total, then we exhaled smoothly, arching the spine upward. We repeated this six times, then practiced the same segmenting breath while standing, knees bent, hands on thighs. Tim taught that the quality of the next breath will show whether the previous breath was held too long. If you're gasping, reduce the sips or the pauses.

As we progressed, Tim introduced variations in breath ratios and subtle engagement of the bandhas. Moola and uddiyana bandha should remain gently engaged throughout—but intensified during breath retentions after exhalation. He encouraged continuous practice, flowing one breath sequence into the next without pause.

Eventually, we combined all of this with alternate nostril breathing, and finally, with a mantra: silently chanting "Om Namah Shivaya" on the exhale. After about 30 minutes of breathwork, I felt the same quiet calm I'd experienced at Lake George, after a long kirtan session. When I stood up, I was a little lightheaded—but only for a moment.

A week later, I had my knee scoped.

A look inside

St. Paul's Hospital is one of Vancouver's oldest buildings, dating back to 1894—just eight years after the city was incorporated. On October 11, 2001, I sat inside, awaiting arthroscopic surgery on my right knee.

The admitting nurse asked whether I'd had anything to eat or drink since midnight. "Just some water," I said. She was horrified. "You weren't supposed to drink even water!" Apparently, it stimulates digestion, which complicates general anesthesia. I explained I was hoping for a local anesthetic so I could watch the procedure. She went to check whether I'd ruined everything. Thankfully, the doctor said I was fine.

They wheeled me into the operating room, where the surgical staff introduced themselves. Dr. Bob, the anesthesiologist, was preparing for a general, but I reminded him I preferred a spinal. The assistant anesthesiologist, Dr. Doug, started an IV. I curled into a fetal position, and they began a sequence of three injections in my lower spine—each one numbing the next.

Dr. Horlick arrived and outlined the procedure. He would make three incisions around my knee to insert a fiber-optic camera, a saline injector, and a surgical tool. The joint would be filled with saline for better visibility. "Don't worry," he said, "I'll suck it all out after." He expected a torn medial meniscus and signs of arthritis. He had me write his initials in pen on my right leg so everyone knew which leg they were operating on. A sterile blanket was set up to keep microbes—and my eyes—away from the incision site. I was okay with not seeing the actual cutting: I just wanted to watch the video.

The anesthetic was kicking in. I felt like my legs had just gone to the dentist's. Everything was going numb from below the belly button. It was a dissociative experience. I was out of touch with half of my body. I watched them lift my leg but couldn't feel it. I became the ultimate Zen observer.

Inside the knee, Dr. Horlick found the expected tear—more of a fold than a rip—and pockmarks in the cartilage on the tibia and femur. There was also a scratch beneath the kneecap. "This is arthritis," he said during his running tour, "but it looks much better than I'd expected." The lateral meniscus and cruciate ligaments were healthy. He trimmed about 40% of the damaged meniscus while flushing the joint. This cleansing, or lavage, helps delay arthritis by clearing old synovial fluid—like changing a car's oil.

When the screen went dark, the staff bandaged the wounds and wheeled me to recovery. It took three hours to regain sensation in my lower body. The last area to revive was, predictably, the one no man wants numb. Once I could firmly clench my butt cheeks, I was cleared to go. My daughter Jessica drove me home, bringing balloon flowers and a book. Ryan, my son, met us in case I needed help going up my stairs. But I was okay. I had no pain in the knees, just a swollen sensation. I needed neither crutches nor pain meds.

Despite the doctor's prediction of a six- to 12-week recovery, I was optimistic. In fact, I'd already registered for a Thai yoga therapy training in Santa Barbara with Saul David Raye, seven weeks away. As an ashtanga teacher who frequently adjusted students, I wanted to deepen my sensitivity. The course, held on the floor, demanded knee flexibility—but I was sure I'd be fine by then.

A White Lotus in a Sacred Land

"This land is sacred," said Saul.

We stood on the grounds of the White Lotus Foundation, perched on the slopes of the Santa Ynez mountains, just east of Santa Barbara. It was the end of November 2001. Below us, the San Jose Creek wound through the steep canyon known to the original inhabitants, the Chumash, as Taklushmon—"the gathering place." In the distance, the canyon opened toward the Pacific, and the Channel Islands shimmered on the horizon.

Saul had a grounded presence. Long and lean, with a few days of beard and dark, close-cropped hair, he seemed as if he could have lived among the Chumash centuries ago. There was something shamanic about him. He was here to teach us a healing art he called Thai yoga therapy.

Saul's father, born in Burma, occasionally practiced asana, but Saul's first teacher was a friend of his father, a Buddhist monk named Yoga Vachara Rahula.[150] Later, inspired by *Autobiography of a Yogi*, Saul traveled to India to learn yoga as therapy. A side trip to Thailand changed everything: he witnessed a small woman working on a large man, moving him into postures that looked like yoga. Her form of massage seemed both powerful and therapeutic. Saul returned again and again to study this art.

The course was full—30 students. On the first day, Saul traced Thai yoga's roots back to the Buddha's time. Its origin story featured Jivaka Kumar Bhaccha, the Buddha's personal physician. As Buddhism spread through Southeast Asia, so did Jivaka's healing methods—massage, acupressure, and herbal remedies—eventually blending Daoist energetics with Ayurveda.

In Thailand, the energetic channels were called *sen*, through which flowed *lom*, the vital wind—like prana or chi. Lom was both an external and an internal entity. Blockages in the sen lines would disrupt its flow and could affect physical health and emotional health, as well as one's spiritual state. The view in the Thai model is holistic: the physical is interconnected and inseparable from the psycho-emotional and spiritual.

Saul went over his approach to the practice and his own philosophy. For the skeptics who doubted the existence of meridians, nadis, or sen lines, he said that was okay. But he added, "Even skeptics have felt energy. So something is happening." In the Eastern view, the healer does not cure the patient; the body heals itself. The practitioner's role is to restore balance and offer space for healing.

"In the Chinese tradition," he pointed out, "each meridian corresponds to a major organ, whereas in the yoga tradition, the nadis are more esoteric and refer to sun, moon, etc. The Chinese tradition is more practical from a therapeutic standpoint."

Performing Thai Yoga Therapy

After the introduction, we were ready to begin practicing on fellow students. "Before doing anything," Saul said, "look at your partner and notice their body. Are they stiff and stressed or relaxed? Ask about their overall health. Even if you do not know the conditions they may be concerned about, that is okay. Over time, you will learn more, but don't worry about being an expert. No doctor knows everything. Listening is a magic all on its own."

Thai yoga therapy combines acupressure and assisted yoga postures. We began with "palming"—using the heel of the hand to apply broad pressure along the sen lines of the inner legs, which Saul called the Shakti or yin lines.[151] There were three:
- Line one was along the medial or inner side of the shin bone, from the ankle to the kneecap and then onto the front of the thigh, tracing the Spleen meridian.
- Line two followed the midline of the calf and inner thigh—Liver meridian.
- Line three traced the lower side of the calf and the adductor muscles—Kidney meridian.

We used our body weight to lean into the palms. The trick was to keep the arms straight and lean forward from the hips. I couldn't sit on my heels yet—my knee was still recovering from surgery. I had to stand on my knees, awkwardly, at first. Yet within an hour, something shifted. I was getting closer to being able to sit on the heels. By the end of the day, I was sitting on my heels.

Saul said, "Consider yourselves as conduits of grace. You are not healing anyone; rather, healing flows through you into your partner. If we think that we are providing healing, we will exhaust our energy stores." Perhaps as the energy of grace flowed through me, it healed me as well. Or, as my rational mind decided, motion was the lotion: stressing and moving my knees for hours every day was highly therapeutic.

We followed palming with thumbing, applying deeper, more focused pressure using our thumbs along the same lines. It took longer—our thumbs covered less surface area than our palms. We worked one leg fully before switching to the other.

Next, we moved to the outer leg lines, the yang or Shiva lines.

- The first line traced the lateral shin and top of the thigh, following the Stomach meridian.
- The second line followed the side of the legs and the iliotibial band— Gallbladder meridian.

A third, deeper line, which we did not work just yet, began between the ankle and Achilles tendon, then followed the hamstrings to the hip—Urinary Bladder meridian. We would explore that one later.

Saul encouraged us to press only as deeply as our partners could tolerate. "You don't have to wait for someone to complain," he said. "Watch their face, their breath. You will see tension before they say anything. Beginning therapists often stare at their hands, but with time, your hands will know what to do. Watch the face. Read the breath. Ahimsa is the guiding principle—no pain, no pain!"[152]

When we moved to the back body, Saul introduced two vertical lines along the spine—the first close to the spinous processes, the second about a thumb's width farther out. Both were part of the Urinary Bladder meridians.[153] Down the center of the body, front and back, he said, ran the *sen susmana*, analogous to the sushumna nadi in yoga.

Along the arms, we learned three main channels:

- The pericardium line, running from the middle of the wrist to the shoulder.
- The heart channel, running medially toward the little finger.
- The lung line, running laterally toward the thumb.[154]

After all the palming and thumbing, we began to move our partners into postures. Once we learned several shapes, we linked them into a flow, just like a yoga class. I could feel differences in the ranges of motion of the students' bodies. One student easily folded into *karnapidasana*: as she lay on her back, I held both feet and moved them over her head to the floor. The next student's feet were far from the floor. I didn't yet know that one person's limits were caused by tight muscles, while another's were due to bone on bone compression. I had never heard of Paul Grilley or the idea of skeletal variation. For now, I was an asana sponge soaking up all the postures and flows that Saul offered.

As the days drew on, Saul would offer more tidbits about the energy aspects of the practice, but he never provided an in-depth, overarching theory. The course was more practical, hands-on learning. He did say that when we are born, we are endowed with a certain amount of energy, which we inherit from our parents, our environment, the planets, etc. He called this our original chi. As we live, we gain energy and lose energy. Regardless of how much original chi we were given—and it varies from person to person—there is a journey towards balance. The healing process is personal. It is not the healer's responsibility to balance the client's chi; all we can do as healers is practice the therapy as safely as possible.

One unusual insight stayed with me: Saul mentioned that body piercings can disrupt the flow of chi. He didn't cite a source but claimed that ear piercings could lead to tinnitus or balance issues, and belly button rings could disturb digestion. "If you must do it," he advised, "get pierced by an acupuncturist."

I remembered something from physics: electricity flowing through a wire generates a magnetic field in a metal ring around the wire. Conversely, moving a magnet surrounding a wire could generate electrical flow in the wire. Could metal piercing the body alter our internal energetic flows? Maybe chi is a kind of bioelectricity. I stored that thought away. It would come back to me years later.

After nine full days of practice, it was time to return home. It had been an intense training, physically and energetically. And yet, I wanted more. Fortunately, Saul announced a level-two course: a deeper dive, scheduled for December 8–13, 2003. I resolved to be ready.

Learning Is Endless

In the meantime, I continued to absorb as much yoga training as my limited time off work would allow. I studied with David Williams, Tim Miller, David Swenson, Shiva Rea, Erich Schiffmann, and Nancy Gilgoff when they came to British Columbia, always with a notebook in hand. In July 2002, a yoga conference titled *Yoga for Living* was held in Olympia, Washington—just a few hours' drive south of Vancouver. The presenters included Beryl Bender Birch, David Life, Judith Lasater, Shiva Rea, Rod Stryker, and Doug Keller. I chose Doug as my primary teacher for the event but also sampled classes from the others. During those months, I also collected and studied dozens of yoga books and videos. I wrote down the sequences these teachers shared and gradually incorporated many of their postures and approaches into my own teaching.

My right knee had healed well, and I returned to my Mysore-style ashtanga practice at City Yoga, guided by Fiona Stang, her husband Julian Decker, and Mike Dennison. But my left medial meniscus remained torn and did not improve. Full lotus still eluded me. Eventually, Dr. Horlick scheduled another surgery for March 2003. This time, I was given a general anesthetic and missed the chance to observe the operation. The procedure was successful, though my recovery was longer than it had been for the right knee. I suspect this was because I didn't have the benefit of nine days of Thai yoga therapy, living and practicing on the floor.

Meanwhile, the bouts of lightheadedness kept returning. I would feel well for weeks, and with that renewed energy, I would ramp up my practice. But inevitably, I pushed too hard. My optimism would outpace my endurance, and I would crash. The cycle repeated itself: long stretches of inactivity, followed by bursts of intense effort, only to collapse again into stillness.

Over time, I learned to sense when a crash was coming—but it was hard to stop. When I felt good, I wanted to move, to live fully, to practice again. But I always overshot my limits. Like Sisyphus condemned to push his boulder uphill, I kept pushing, only to watch it roll back down. Striving, collapsing, recovering. Again and again.

Back to the Lotus—
November to December 2003

"The purpose of sound," said Dave Stringer, "is to lead us to silence. And out of silence, sound arises." Dave had a large presence in the small room where Saul taught the second level of Thai yoga therapy. He also had a large voice that powerfully projected his music.

"The meaning of every kirtan song you will ever sing is either love or god," he continued. "When you hear songs about Radha and Krishna or Sita and Ram, those are about love: love, love, love, love, love! When you hear Devakinanda Gopala, Shiva Shankara, or Saraswati Ma, those are about god: god, god, god, god, god! That's it. Now you can understand every kirtan you'll ever hear."

When we were practicing Thai massage, the room felt spacious. But when the kirtan began, it seemed to shrink. Maybe it was the energy—or maybe it was because Dave brought his band. He sat cross-legged behind his harmonium, flanked by a tabla player, a woman playing rhythm instruments, and if I'm remembering correctly, a guitarist. Saul sat to his left, on keyboard. We students along with some White Lotus staff, formed a semicircle on the floor. A slide projector displayed the lyrics on the back wall.

At the end of each song, the music dissolved into silence. No applause—just stillness. A mini-meditation. Before each song, Dave would share the history of kirtan, which had emerged from the fifteenth-century South Asian bhakti movement: a tradition of ecstatic love poetry. Though directed toward the divine, the object of devotion was often a human form. Bhaktas sang simple mantras in call-and-response, accompanied by drums, cymbals, clapping, and dance. Their message? "Joy." Their instruction? "See the divine in everyone."

After 30 minutes of singing, I noticed I had stopped. I sat still, trying to understand what was happening. Saul caught my eye and silently mouthed, "Bernie, start clapping." I did, and everyone joined in. Halfway through the next chant, I got up and danced at the back of the room. My mind felt as calm and clear as it did after a long pranayama session.

The Cambrian explosion, 540 million years ago, unleashed an unprecedented variety of life. I'd argue that the 1990s and early 2000s saw a similar—if smaller—explosion of yoga forms in the West. Teachers from India were invited, coaxed, and sometimes bribed to share their teachings abroad. While this wasn't new, the soil at the time was especially fertile. Yoga was evolving and branching in countless directions.

Kirtan was one of those branches. It bloomed at conferences, in studios, and at trainings. In Vancouver, I watched it spread quickly. Local yogis held regular sessions. Maalaa Lazar became known for her family-friendly offerings. Wade Morissette, brother of Alanis, recorded an album and toured. Sandra Leigh formed a local band called Give Peace a Chant and enlisted Shakti Mhi's husband, Itamar Erez, to play— though watching Itamar on harmonium was like watching a Formula 1 car coast through a school zone at 30 kilometers per hour.[155]

Meanwhile, international kirtan "rock stars" passed through Vancouver. Jai Uttal played at St. Andrew's-Wesley United Church. Wah! came. Saul brought Jim Beckwith to town. Deva Premal and Miten led a weekend chanting workshop at UBC. Deva's early albums made their way into the Prana Yoga and Zen Centre, where Itamar created a "Prana Song Sheet" to help students sing along.

Something about kirtan made me want to move. Like pranayama, it altered my state—but where pranayama made me still, kirtan made me move. I couldn't yet articulate the link between the two practices. That understanding would come later.

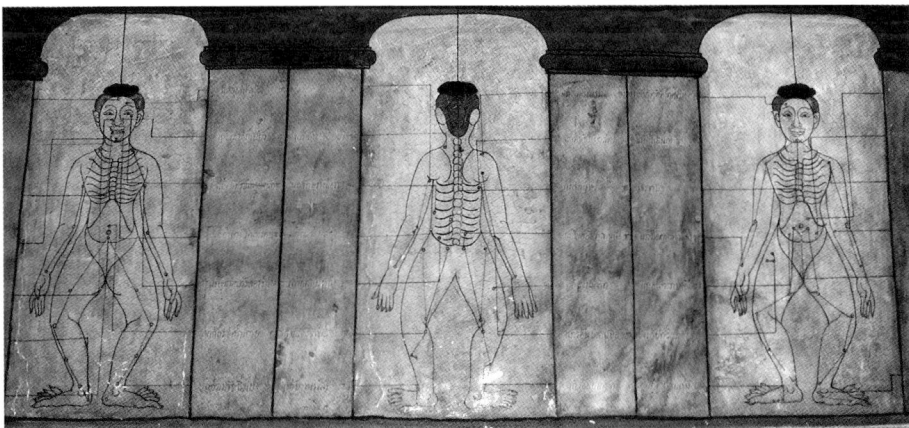

Figure 6: The sen lines of Thai yoga massage, depicted in the Wat Po Temple.[156]

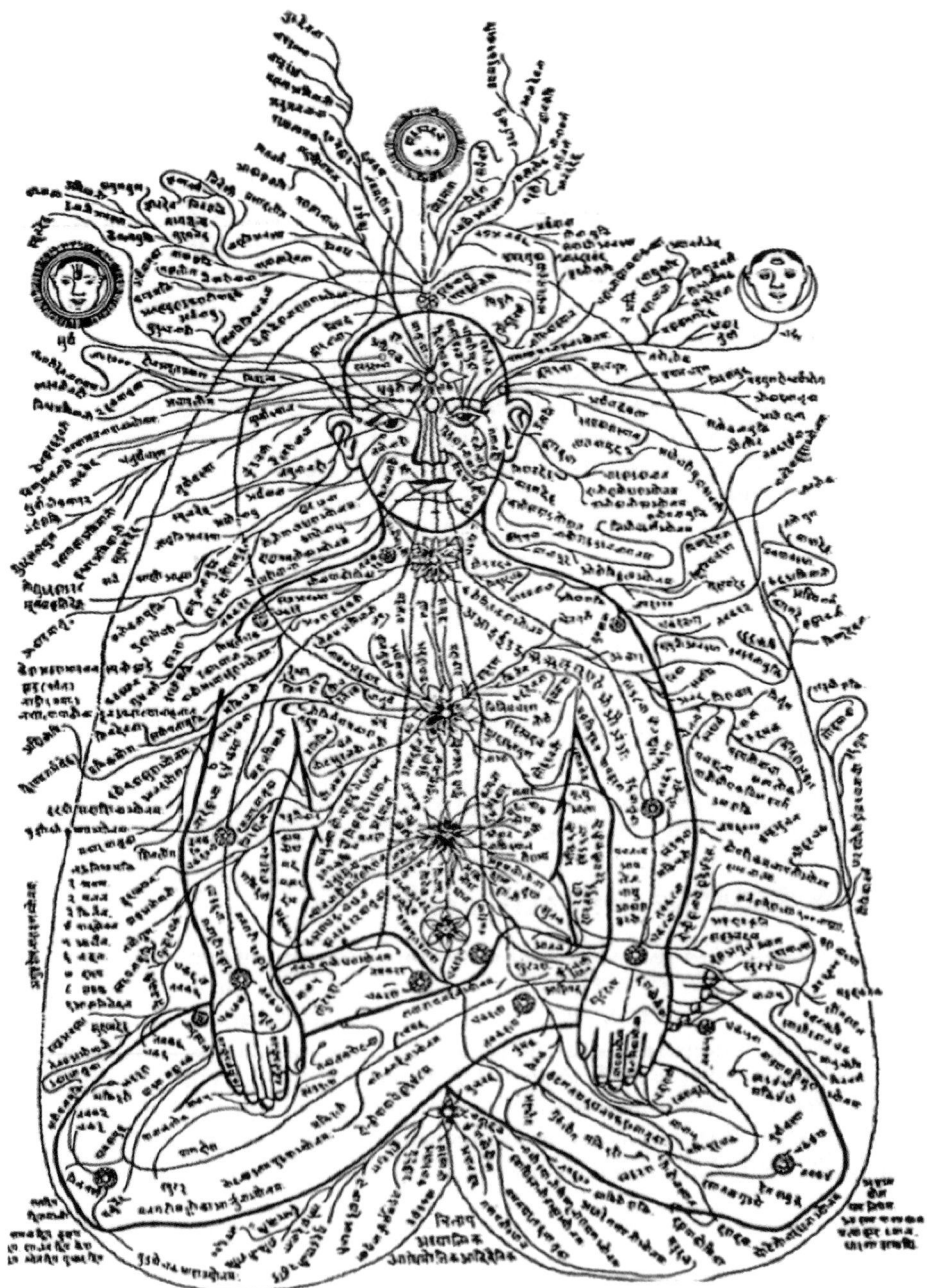

Figure 7: The nadis as depicted by the nineteenth-century Tibetan sage Ratnasara.

Back at White Lotus, the evening flowed—vibrant and musical. We ended at 9 p.m. The crowd was yogic, after all. We still had two full days of the five-day training to go. The Thai yoga practice grew more intricate. We learned new flows with challenging postures.

Saul reminded us that the more depleted a client was, the less pressure we should apply. "A weakened body is like a burned-out house," he said. "It may look fine, but one breeze could blow it down." For such clients, restorative yoga is better. If someone already has hypermobile joints, more opening isn't the goal—use palming and thumbing to stimulate energy instead.

He often returned to the posture of the practitioner. "Guard your energy," he told us. "The energy must move through you—not from you. After each session, do a cleansing. Down dog for five minutes, or some other energetic posture. You can cut the connection with a sharp physical gesture, burn sage, take a shower, or even just run cold water over your wrists." He had other practical advice: "Don't use ujjayi breathing. To your partner, with their eyes closed, you will sound like Darth Vader. Even they shouldn't use ujjayi—it's not a relaxing breath."

Though this training offered a bit more theory about sen lines and meridians, it remained a hands-on learning experience. Thai yoga therapy was clearly a fusion—drawing from Indian and Chinese sources. But my understanding of energy and channels was still in its infancy.

A Taste of Yin

On the second-to-last morning, Saul joked that he was running low on ideas for our morning practice. "How about a yin yoga class?" he asked. I had never heard of yin yoga before, and it seemed no one else in the room had either. Years later, when I told Saul that his yin class had changed my life, he raised his hands and said, "That wasn't really a yin class. I can't take credit for that."

He was partially right. What he taught was more of a yin–yang fusion. But it was the first time any teacher had asked me to hold a pose for minutes at a time. We dangled in uttanasana (standing forward fold) for two minutes, then moved into malasana (squat) for another two—then repeated both. He had us hold a low lunge (dragon pose) for five minutes on each side. More long-held postures followed. I had never been so challenged in any yoga class. Ashtanga was intense. Bikram was tough. But nothing tested me like staying in one pose for five minutes. It was fascinating.

Two days later, the training complete, I prepared to fly home to Vancouver. I stayed overnight in a downtown Santa Barbara hotel and had a free morning before my flight, so I found a copy of the Yellow Pages[157] in my hotel room and discovered a local studio—Santa Barbara Yoga Center—just a few blocks away. They offered a morning kundalini class. I'd never done kundalini before. It was interesting, but not for me: too much fast breathing and quick movement.

After class, I browsed the studio's offerings of books and VHS tapes. One caught my eye: *Yin & Vinyasa Yoga* by Sarah Powers. This was the first time I had heard of her. I remembered Saul's yin yoga class and how deeply it had affected me. I bought the tape.

Over the next three months, Sarah's yin yoga became a regular part of my life. I still practiced ashtanga most mornings—when I felt strong enough—but on the down days, when dizziness kept me home from work, I'd sit on my mat and press play. By early 2004, I had been practicing ashtanga consistently for four years, but one posture still eluded me: *prasarita padottanasana,* the wide-legged forward fold where your head touches the floor. For years, my head had never come close. But after three months of Sarah's yin practice, it touched the mat.

Yin yoga increased my range of motion more than years of ashtanga had. Sarah Powers, clearly, was a star in the yoga sky. I knew I would study further with her. What I would learn through her was more than a new way to do asanas; I would learn much more about prana, which hid within a variety of guises: energy, force, breath, chi, and kundalini.

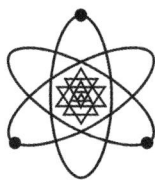

CHAPTER 15:

Kundalini Rising

On a clear November night in 1572, Danish astronomer Tycho Brahe looked sky-ward and saw something that should not have been—a new star blazing in the constellation Cassiopeia. This "nova," brighter than Venus, would soon be visible even in daylight. In Europe, its appearance shattered the ancient belief that the heavens were immutable. Aristotle had taught that the stars beyond the moon were eternal, incorruptible. But Brahe's calculations, using the cutting-edge tools of parallax and trigonometry, proved the nova lay far beyond the moon, demolishing the celestial perfection of Aristotle's cosmos and heralding the dawn of modern science.

In India, where the heavens never had been presumed fixed, such an event did not upend cosmology but still held deep personal significance. For some yogis and tantrikas, the sudden brilliance of a new star could be read as a divine message—an inner awakening mirrored in the sky. For one such woman, long removed from the rituals of temple life, the nova would mark the beginning of her final transformation.

Garima's Arrival

No one was stirring in the ashram just meters away to the south. There was a slight wind stirring the teak branches, but the night was clear. Garima sat and meditated.

Garima was old by anybody's standards, but how old, not even she knew. She had been born here in Guwahati, Assam, far north of where the Ganges enters the ocean. She had lived in the Kamakhya temple, an ancient and revered center of tantric practice—left-hand practice. She took initiation at the age of 14, the day she was married. She had been excited by the prospect of learning the tantric secrets that her older brothers merely hinted at. But her guru told her that she should not seek *moksha*—liberation, at least not in this lifetime. He said to come back in her next life as a man, find him and he would make sure she would reach final freedom in that life.

When her husband died, Garima was given three choices: climb upon the funeral fire and commit *suttee*, joining her husband in the afterlife;[158] remarry quickly; or serve as a consort to unmarried practitioners. On the day she was to be with another man, she chose an unoffered fourth option and fled the temple. She went far to the west, to seek the path of the nath yogis.

Garima eventually made it to Prayag, a place where the Ganges and Yamuna rivers meet. This was where, every 12 years, the Magh Mela would bring together yogis, tantrikas, and people from many religious backgrounds to bathe in the waters, to commune with god, to dance, to sing, to sit, to smoke, to eat, to be with each other.[159] Everywhere there were men. She skirted the masses until she found two yoginis. For years, she lived with them, walked with them, learned from them, and when they passed, she decided to return to Asam. But not to the Kamakhya temple.

Instead, she found a dilapidated hut across from an entrance to the ancient Vasistha ashram in the south of Guwahati. The ashram followed the right-handed path of tantra. The head of the ashram was Paramahansa Purnananda. One morning, while greeting some benefactors at the gate of the ashram, he noticed Garima sitting in lotus pose outside the broken hut. She wore a simple, cotton sari that had faded to a dull grey. Ashes were spread upon her throat, chest, and arms. On her forehead were three horizontal lines.[160]

They did not speak to each other, but Purnananda did bow to her. That evening, he asked his students to find out who she was. By noon of the next day, two chelas, students at the ashram, brought food and water to Garima. They called her "Ma" and stayed to repair the roof of the hut. Every noontime and evening, they would return with food and do other repairs.

Years passed. Chelas came and went. Garima would rise at *brahmamuhurta*, the time of brahma, to do her morning *sadhana*, her hatha yoga practices. Her main *kriyas*, cleanses of the body, and bathing would follow the sadhana. After these practices were complete, she would eat whatever the chelas had brought her. In the mid-afternoon, she would do more pranayama and meditation. The evenings were a time for a light meal and then a final meditation. In this way, the days passed until the day a new star appeared in the northern sky.

The advent of a new star was meaningful, but not in the paradigm-changing way it would be in Europe. The portent was of a more personal, private nature. Garima knew that this new star was important, but exactly why was not immediately clear. It took several days to understand. In 10 days, after the star had passed its peak brightness and started to slowly dim, she could not help but know. A time of change was upon her; Garima's own dimming was beginning.

The next morning, two chelas came to deliver her daily meal. These two young men had been attending her for a few months, but she did not know their names. They knelt before her and placed the bowls on the ground, bowed, and were about to leave when she spoke to them. They froze in surprise. Ma had never spoken to anyone before.

"What are your names?" she asked.

The young men look at each other. The younger one, probably about 16 years of age, spoke. "I am Shankar." The other, perhaps a year older, added, "I am Visvanatha."

"Why are you at the Vasistha ashram?"

"To escape samsara," said Shankar.

"To exhaust our karma," added Visvanatha.

Garima smiled and asked, "What does he have you doing besides bringing food to an old woman?"

"We are participating in a grand task, Ma," said Shankar eagerly. "Paramahansa Purnananda is creating a great composition. It is a shastra that will describe the world as an expression of the divine mother. It is the definitive summary of tantra."[161]

Garima frowned. She had tried that path, and it had led her nowhere. She made an inner resolution and said, "Very good. I will teach you."

This caught the young men by surprise. They had been told by their guru that the presence of Ma was a blessing for the ashram, and by serving her, they were gaining great karma. But they already had a teacher.

Garima read their concern and continued, "Tell your guru what I have said. Come back tomorrow at brahmamuhurta, and we will begin."

Visvanatha and Shankara were still kneeling before Garima, looking at each other in disbelief. Shankara then dared to ask the question they had speculated upon privately. "Who are you, Ma?"

Garima's gaze softened, focused off in the distance and across time. In a quiet voice, she said, "I… was… the consort of Shiva."

That quiet response sent a shiver down Visvanatha's spine, and he dared to ask, "And… who are you now?"

Garima turned to them both, her face fierce with anger, and growled, "Shivoham!"[162]

The force of her words struck them like thunder, and they stumbled backward, shaken. Scrambling to their feet they mumbled apologies about having to get back to their duties, bowed quickly, and hastened away. The next morning, just before dawn, they were back. Their guru had overridden any hesitations they had by saying, "When the goddess calls, you cannot refuse."

A Woman's Life in a Left-Handed World

Shiva's grief was unbearable. In Garima's deep meditation, it came to her as a vision—or was it a memory? Shiva danced across the cosmos with the lifeless body of his beloved Sati draped over his shoulder, his Tandava threatening to unravel creation itself. Vishnu, unable to calm him, hurled his discus. Sati's body was sliced apart, scattering across the world. Where each piece landed, sacred temples rose. The most revered was Kamakhya, where Sati's yoni—her womb and genitals—touched the earth.

Garima saw herself standing inside Kamakhya's sanctum, facing the sacred cleft in the rock. Moist from a hidden spring, this unadorned yoni was the temple's sole image of the goddess.[163] Nearby, red cloth waited to be laid across the stone, destined to absorb the fluid that seeped from within.

The young Garima stood before the goddess. She felt a strange wetness flowing down her legs. Looking past her white sari, she saw a small pool of red. She was having her first menstruation. She was neither afraid nor shocked: she felt fulfilled, as if her destiny was unfolding. When she looked back at the yoni, its fluid too had turned red. The goddess bled, and so did she.[164]

Red and white—menstrual blood and semen—the sacred hues that would bind her life. In the left-handed path of tantra, these were not taboo but fluids of power. On the fourth day of the goddess' menses, pilgrims waiting outside the temple received strips of soaked cloth, believed to contain divine essence. These gifts were cherished, stored as sacred relics in homes.[165]

Garima now saw herself, married, seated for the first time in a ritual chamber heavy with incense, chanting, and anticipation. Around the guru, men and women sat in a circle. Each woman had placed a shawl in a box. At a signal, men drew the shawls and paired off with their owners—not their wives, never that. All the women present were there of their own free will, and yet, as members of the temple since childhood or even birth, was there really a choice?

She sat on her partner's left thigh. They drank wine and bhang, becoming intoxicated. Though vegetarian, they consumed fish and meat—offerings meant to break boundaries. Garima was confused and not sure what to feel.

In that chamber, Garima had no name. She was "Shakti" or "Duti," her partner, the "Sadhaka" or "Shiva." Her sadhaka began chanting mantras while kissing and fondling her. In turn, she began to anoint his penis with sandalwood and saffron. They began the *maithuna*—the ritual union—not for pleasure, but for alchemy. Their fluids mingled to create *yoni-tattva*,[166] the most potent of elixirs, rich in *ojas*: distilled prana.

She saw herself now with her guru and heard his teachings. The sadhaka must retain his semen—his *bindu*—and, if it is released, must draw it back, along with the female fluid. *Vajroli mudra*, the technique for this, demands years of preparation—drawing water through the urethra, inserting rods into the penis to expand the passage, training pelvic muscles for suction. Few ever succeed. Most resort to drinking the mingled fluids instead.

Garima questions her guru, asking what women gain from such practices. He answers with certainty: women are already close to the divine. They practiced *sahajoli mudra*[167] easily, their yonis naturally able to draw in fluids. But their role is to assist men—facilitating their partner's path to *jivanmukti*, liberation while alive. Women cannot awaken kundalini. Not in this life.

Initiation for women, he says, is not for their benefit. A woman becomes *badhya*—bound—sworn to obedience. Should she stray or refuse to obey, misfortune will follow.[168] Garima remembers the sting of those words.

Garima then saw her teachers at the Magh Mela in Prayag. They are offering her food and refuge. They tell her plainly: "You have never met a *jivanmukta*! Those rites in Kamakhya were a diversion. Stay with us. Hatha yoga is the true path. It makes no difference whether you are male or female. You have had your final birth."

The vision ended abruptly, and Garima stirred. The night was still dark, but she knew now what to share with Shankar and Visvanatha: a path beyond ritual and dogma, into the discipline of hatha yoga.

The Alchemy of Effort

The crescent moon was low in the east, preceding the sun, which was still below the horizon. Garima began Visvanatha's and Shankar's instruction with a short, seated meditation. As the sun appeared, she had them do 18 *pranams*. Standing, facing east, they bent forward, placing their hands on the earth. Stepping both feet back, they lowered their bodies to the earth, hands extended overhead. From the earth, they stood up again. The movements were familiar to them; they had been doing these prostrations since childhood.

She told them that the pranams were to honor the sun; they were not asana. Asana was to strengthen the body. But it was more than that, too. She promised to explain later. After the asana practice, it was time for pranayama.

They knew about pranayama, of course, but the practices they had been taught were rudimentary, and they had not progressed very far in their ability to extend the breath. They had not been told that this was the point of the practice. Garima realized she would have to work slowly with them, developing their ability over months. She guided them through a session of alternate nostril breathing while they sat in lotus pose. Much that she'd hoped to teach on this first day she instead skipped, finishing with a short meditation. She told them to go bathe and dismissed them until the afternoon.

When they returned, Garima explained the process they would follow every day. In the morning, they would practice. The afternoons would be dedicated to mastering meditation. In the evenings, they would receive commentary on the practice. Part of the morning would expand to include asanas, mudras, bandhas, and *pratyahara*—closing of the sense doors. These stages would prepare them for the most important limbs, which would follow later in the day: pranayama, *dhyana*—meditation—and *samadhi*, the trance.[169]

Hatha Yoga's Import

On the first evening, Garima sat in lotus, padmasana, on her grass mat in front of the two chelas. A small fire in a shallow pit flickered beside her. Sitting cross-legged on the earth, Shankar seemed agitated. Garima asked him why. He replied with a challenge in his voice, "Why should we bother with your hatha yoga? We are already learning a path which will see us purified and able to join with the divine through devotion and rituals."

Garima looked to Visvanatha to see whether he held a similar view. He responded, in a meeker tone, "Guruji said we must listen to you and do as you request. Personally, I was hoping we could learn the special abilities told in the tales of great yogis. Will you teach us how to achieve siddhis and do magic?"

Garima was not pleased. Clearly, she needed to undo many years of incorrect views. She said, "The purpose of hatha yoga is to achieve liberation, moksha, through perseverance and discipline. The purpose is not to obtain magical powers, although some special abilities may manifest. Those must be avoided and ignored in order to obtain moksha. Set your goal clearly in your heart and mind, and I will guide you through the path to obtain samadhi, from which you will reach moksha."

Strictness in a guru is not unusual, and the students were used to their teachers being very demanding. However, Shankar glared at Ma defiantly. She knew he would not be easy to tame. She allowed him to speak once more.

"Ma… how can a woman teach a man? It is well known that women cannot achieve moksha."

"Do you think Shiva can exist without Shakti?" asked Garima. "Without Shakti, Shiva has no life. Without Shiva, Shakti has no form. How can you hope to achieve your goal without the help of the goddess? The divine union you seek, the liberation I offer, requires you to submit to the goddess!"

Visvanatha was nodding in understanding, but Shankar bit his tongue and said no more. Chelas were conditioned from an early age to put their whole heart into the path they were following. But Garima knew from bitter experience their current path would be fruitless. She stiffened her resolve to help them achieve the ultimate goal.

Awakening the Kundalini

"You may have been taught," Garima began, "that everything you see is illusion. That it is all the play, the *lila*, of the Divine. Whose illusion? Shiva's. And you may have been taught that we are caught in this divine game and must play it out before we are freed, before we reach moksha. You may have heard that Shiva, the formless, has a will to create—*iccha*. That from this will arises knowledge—*jnana*. And from knowledge, the power to act—*kriya*. These, you've been told, are the three powers of Shakti, descending into form until she condenses—like dew on a blade of grass—and hides herself within you as the giver, the surpasser, and the destroyer of life."

She looked around at the boys. They were nodding. Of course they had heard this. Perhaps from Purnananda. Perhaps from a dozen other teachers who quoted sutras and shastras in practiced tones.

"But I am not here to teach you ideas," she said, her voice sharper now. "Not *that* kind of knowing. I am not here to talk about iccha, jnana, and kriya as if they were jewels you could polish and place on a shelf. I am here to train your bodies to hold power. And that power does not come from understanding—it comes from effort."

She stood up, her eyes on Visvanatha. "The Divine hides herself in your body, yes—but not as an idea. She coils herself low in your belly. She is there! You won't free her by thinking. You will free her by sweating. By waking up early. By holding your breath when every instinct tells you to inhale. You will call her not with prayers but with pressure—with bandhas and mudras and the fire of tapas. You want moksha? Then build a body that can hold it."

Garima sat down again and continued. "While in the body, Shakti takes on many names. You may hear her called *Kubjika, Bhujangi, Ishwari, Kundali, Vama, Devi,* even *Prana.*[170] But for our purpose, we will call her *Kundalini.*"

She looked again at Visvanatha. "And do you know why she is called Kundalini?"

He straightened. "She is the serpent—the coiled one."

"Yes," said Garima. "She coils three and a half times at the base of the spine. But why a coil? What does it mean?"

Visvanatha frowned, thinking.

Garima's gaze shifted to Shankar.

He hesitated. "A snake coils when it is asleep… Maybe her name means she sleeps."

Garima's eyes lit with approval. "Yes. Kundalini is not dead, but dormant—coiled like a sleeping serpent. When awakened, she rises, sudden and straight, like a rod of lightning."

She paused, her voice deepening. "This is why so many fear her. To awaken Kundalini is not a game. It is to stir something ancient and dangerous. She is the fire at the root of your being. Once she begins her ascent, there is no turning back."

Garima stood again, lifted her arms, and continued: "Kundalini must rise through the sushumna nadi, the central channel. But for her to rise, it is not enough to sit and chant. You must prepare the path. This is the work of hatha yoga. It is not only postures. It is the work of breath, of effort, and of the sacred fluids within you: bindu, rasa, semen, amrita. Shakti takes these forms. To waste them is to weaken her."

Garima continued, "There are some who speak falsely. There are teachers who say she extends from the feet all the way to the crown of the head.[171] They are wrong. There are gurus who have said that she resides in the head, and from there she is invited to descend to the lower lotus, most often the heart. As she descends, she remains attached to the top of the head and once she arrives at the heart, she can escort the *jivatman,* the individual atman, back to the crown.[172] This teaching will lead you to harm. There are teachers who will say that she lives at the highest center, while other teachers claim she lives in the belly, at the level of the navel.[173] Turn from these teachers.

"There are teachers who will argue and say the Kundalini cannot be asleep! If Shakti sleeps, so must we sleep. If she were not awake, we would fall into a coma. This is false, for prana still pervades the body. In the beginning, Shakti descends, just as prakriti evolves and descends into buddhi, and then into ahamkara, then manas, indriya, tanmatra, and bhuta. The path to moksha is awakening Kundalini so she can reverse her descent, undo her evolution, and rise again toward the most subtle, sukshma, state."

She stood in front of Shankar. "You must learn to unite the opposites. Sun and moon. Left and right. Prana and apana. All of this—every movement, every breath—is directed toward one purpose: the inner marriage of Shakti and Shiva. Without that, no liberation is possible."

She glanced at their faces and saw fatigue.

"That is enough for tonight," she said softly. "Sleep now. Return at dawn. Tomorrow, we begin the real work."

The boys bowed. Visvanatha's gaze lingered on Garima, eyes shining with curiosity. Shankar looked away. Then, they turned and left her.

Rebellion Brews

The days turned to weeks. The chelas grew strong with the practice, which allowed Garima to add more challenging asanas and pranayamas, but the evenings' discourses were often troublesome. Visvanatha was an eager sponge, always thirsting for more. More knowledge, more postures, more abilities. Garima worried that he was becoming proud of his growing abilities. But Shankar… he was a challenge. He accepted nothing without great debate.

After one evening session, Visvanatha remained when Shankar departed, and shared with Garima, "Every night, Shankar tells guruji everything we discuss. Guruji does not seem to mind your wisdom being taught to us, but much of what you say contradicts what he has told us. This bothers Shankar because he respects guruji highly. He presses guruji for comments and ways that he can argue with you. Guruji just shakes his head and tells him to go to bed. But the next day, guruji's own discourse concerns the topics you have presented. I tell you this so that you know it is not just Shankar you are debating."

Visvanatha's confession confirmed what Garima already suspected. She felt that she had three listeners, not two. In person, Garima and Purnananda had never spoken a word to each other, exchanging only looks and nods. Her debates with Shankar were how they interacted. She was not surprised when Shankar challenged her yet again the next evening.

"Ma," said Shankar, "you say the main tool to be used to achieve liberation is the body. You teach us asanas and purifications, and teach that the body is the route to moksha. Guruji teaches the body is sacred and divine, but its main function is as a focal point for our meditation and visualizations. The *padmas*—the lotuses—are the steps to the divine. Each is a seat of a sacred deity. When I meditate upon them, I feel their power guiding me inward, upward. Why do you not teach us to visualize them, to call out the mantras of each chakra?"

Instantly, Garima was taken back in her mind to the hours, days, months she had spent visualizing the devas and devis. She had become so accomplished in the tantrik practice that she could not turn it off. Everywhere she looked, she saw the divine. Her friends complained about her aloofness and avoidance of everyday, mundane chores, of friends and family. All she saw was the goddess. And still, her guru said moksha was unavailable because she was a woman. From bitter personal experience, she knew that this path did not work, at least not for her.

Surprised by this bitter memory, she needed time to compose herself before responding to Shankar. She stalled by testing him. "Tell me what you have learned of these lotuses. You say that Paramahansa Purnananda has composed a great shastra, which you are memorizing.[174] Surely you know everything about them. Explain each lotus!"

The Six Padmas (Chakras)

Shankar had not expected to be put on the spot. He glanced at Visvanatha, who merely shrugged. "Recite," he suggested. So Shankar began to chant the shastra. He was quickly stopped by Garima.

"No," she said. "Tell me in your own words, not his, so I know you understand the words!"

The Muladhara

Shankar's resolve stiffened like a snake that had been struck. In a formal tone, he began, "The main nadi is the sushumna flowing through the spine. Along it are the six lotuses, the padmas, also called chakras, which is why the shastra is called the *Sat-chakra-nirupana*, a description of the six chakras. The first is the root support, the *muladhara*. It is placed below the genitals and above the anus. This lotus has four petals that are red or crimson, but its center—the outer covering known as the pericarp—is yellow and shaped like a square.[175] It is the home in the body of earth, *prithivi*. It has a *bija*, a seed sound, of *lam*.[176] This is the bija of Indra! The goddess living here is Shakti Dakini."

The Svadhisthana

"Above the muladhara is the supreme lingam, the *svadhisthana*, located at the root of the genitals, with six petals of reddish-orange or vermillion. The pericarp of the lotus is white and shining, in the shape of a crescent moon. It is the home of water, the bhuta *apas*. Its bija sound is *vam*. Here is Vishnu in the form of Hari sitting on his bird, Garuda. With him, in divine blue, is the rice-loving Shakti Rakini. Her eyes are as red as blood, her teeth like razors, and in her hands are the battle-axe, spear, drum, and lotus flower."

The Manipura

"Higher, at the root of the navel where it meets the spine, is the lotus of 10 petals, the *manipura*, shining with the color of dark rain clouds. It is the home in our body of fire, *agni*, with its bija of *ram*. The pericarp is a triangle pointing downward. Rudra, the destroyer of the universe, sits beside the dark-blue Shakti Lakini, the benefactor of all. This is the lotus of power, the power to create and destroy."

The Anahata

"Behind the heart is the lotus *anahata*. Like the wish-fulfilling tree, it bestows even more than anyone could ask. Its bija is *yam*; its bhuta is air or *vayu*. Its 12 petals are the color of the bhanduka flower, with its dark reddish hue. Its hexagonal pericarp is formed by the intersection of two triangles of equal size: one facing downward, the other upward. Within this we find Isha, the form of Shiva as the supreme ruler, and sitting on a red lotus is the Shakti Kakini, yellow like ten million flashes of lightning, and excited because she drinks *amrta*, the nectar of the moon as it passes downward towards the sun."

The Visuddha

"In the throat is the lotus *visuddha*, the purity of space, *akasha*. Its bija is *ham*. Its 16 petals are a smokey, purple hue. The pericarp is a circle, white like a full moon or an ocean of nectar. Within, ever beneficent Sada-Shiva sits together with the Shakti Sakini, who is light itself. Sada-Shiva is androgynous—one side is male, white as snow, Shiva, the other side female, golden Shakti."

The Ajna

"Between the eyes is the *ajna*, which means command. This is the abode of mind, *manas*. Manas is beyond all senses. It is commanded by buddhi. The ajna lotus has two petals, white like the moon. Like the moon, it shines through the glory of meditation, dhyana. Inside is the goddess, the Shakti Hakini, with her six heads and six arms. In the circular pericarp, at the center of the lotus, is first a yoni, and within that is Itara, the lingam of Shiva. The bija sound is aum. Guruji says when my focus is here, I should first meditate upon Hakini, then manas, then Itara, and then pranava."

"These," finished Shankar, "are the six padmas."

Garima was impressed. "I saw your mouth open, but I heard your teacher's voice. Still, you did well. Eventually, you will speak with your own voice."

The Nadis

Turning to Visvanatha, Garima asked, "Are you equally learned? What have you been taught of the nadis?"

Shankar sat disgruntled. He was pleased by Garima's praise but annoyed that she had not yet answered his question.

Visvanatha answered, "In the shastra, there is mention of several nadis, also called *siras*. Guruji warned us that many teachers have different names for the same thing, which can lead to confusion. He told us to listen to them politely but rely upon his teachings. The siras and nadis are channels, little rivers within the body. But they are sukshma; they are part of the subtle body, so they are difficult to sense and know. While some pandits say there are 350,000 nadis and others that there are 72,000, we only need to know a few.

"*Sasi* is the moon channel, also known as *chandra nadi* but also as the *ida nadi*. It lies upon the left side of the backbone. *Mihira* is the sun, also known as the *surya nadi* but also as the *pingala nadi*. It lies upon the right side. *Meru* is the grand mountain that lies at the center of the universe, the home of the gods, supporting the whole of creation. In our case, Meru is the *danda*, the rod of the backbone, which supports our body. Within Meru is the sushumna nadi, which houses yet other nadis within.[177]

"The ida and pingala are outside Meru. Now, some pandits teach these are like bows, arching from the scrotum or perineum towards the shoulder. At the level of the heart, the curve of the bow is greatest. At the shoulder, the nadi crosses the middle of the body and ends in the nostril opposite from the side it arose. Both nadis meet with the sushumna nadi at the space between the eyebrows, forming a great braid. The ida nadi is the Yamuna river; the pingala is the Saraswati river; in the sushumna flows the great Ganges river."

Two Paths

"Yes, well said," admitted Garima, smiling at Visvanatha. "But I have not forgotten your question, Shankar! Why do I not teach you visualization upon the padmas? Because these are not mere gates of light or homes of the devis and devas. They are knots—*granthis*. Bound points. They are not stairs you can climb until they are unbound."

Shankar did not understand. "Then why are they described in such detail? With colors, petals, mantras, deities?"

Garima replied, "The mind loves form, and the seeker must begin somewhere. But listen closely: chakras are not to be worshipped. They are to be pierced! The yogi must not decorate the knots; she must unravel them. Visualization can help focus the mind—but it is no substitute for pranic fire. Until the granthis are burned through by the rising force of Kundalini, the lotuses do not bloom. They bind."

Visvanatha was confused and said, "Guruji says visualization purifies the mind and aligns us with the cosmic order."

"Yes. That is the path of tantra," said Garima. "Through mantra, mudra, and mandala, the tantrika attunes to the divine. He brings the gods into his subtle body and moves upward through grace. But the hatha yogi does not beg for grace. She kindles it herself. She does not knock politely at the door of the final padma; she blows it off its hinges."

Shankar's agitation was growing. "Then you are saying we should reject mantra? Reject devotion?"

Garima paused before responding, to allow a breath for Shankar to calm down. "All tools are useful. But not all tools are primary. In hatha yoga, we begin with the body, with the breath. When the prana moves freely through the nadis, the mind becomes still. When the bindu is preserved, the senses withdraw. When apana meets prana, the inner fire awakens. Then—and only then—do the lotuses open. Not by visualization. By experience."

"But what if devotion opens the way?" asked Shankar. "What if mantra melts the knots? Isn't bhakti a fire too?"

"That is the promise. But I have seen many bhaktas fall into despair when their gods did not answer. Their faith was not forged by tapas. The hatha yogi builds from the ground up. We purify the nadis. We awaken the inner serpent. The chakras are not gods to be adored; they are gates to be broken."

A silence settled between them. Finally, Visvanatha softly commented, "They are both paths. The tantrika climbs with mantra and vision. The hatha yogi climbs with breath and fire. Don't both seek the same summit?"

Garima looked at him with affection. "Yes, Visvanatha. Two paths, one mountain. But if you decorate the path and do not walk it, you will never reach the peak. Choose the path you can walk, not the one that flatters your mind. We begin as bodies, not as gods. We are earth and blood and breath. Start there. The rest will come."

The next morning, only Visvanatha appeared for sadhana. Garima was not surprised, but she was disappointed. Visvanatha could only shrug.

The Seventh Level

Garima felt her time growing shorter. Like the star that had shone brightly months ago and then faded completely, she did not have long to finish Visvanatha's training. She worked him harder than ever, especially in pranayama and meditation practices, determined that he would reach samadhi and the *sahasrara*, the ultimate padma. One night, almost a year after the star had appeared, she had a final lesson for Visvanatha.

"You and Shankar once told me what you knew about the six padmas and the sushumna nadi in which they reside. The highest padma mentioned was the ajna, which has two petals. You live in the realm of opposites, of two, not one. Of prakriti and purusha; of sun and moon. In the pit of the belly lives Surya, the sun, with its fierce heat, agni. As the sun bakes the earth, drying out all life, so too does the agni within our belly consume your life's vitality. Within the dome of the skull resides Chandra, the moon. The moon releases the dew each night that revitalizes the earth and renews life. This inner dew, this most important bindu, is called amrta, the nectar of immortality. As long as it drains downward and is consumed by the sun, death is inevitable. You have learned to reverse this flow through inverted asanas such as *viparita karani* and the space-sealing mudra, *kechari*, where the tongue is folded backward to prevent the loss of bindu.

"No doubt, you have heard some pandits teach that there are lotuses above the ajna. This is the domain of ahamkara, buddhi, and prakriti. Above them all is sahasrara—the thousand-petaled lotus. It is not within the body. It is not one of the six chakras. It shines like the full moon. It is cool and moist with nectar, amrta, which constantly flows from it. Inside the circle of the moon is a triangle, and inside that is pure emptiness, the great void, *sunya*. It is as subtle and as hard to see as the end of a hair divided a million times.

"The tantras teach that this is the abode of the divine, the Parama-Shiva; he is brahman and all the atmans. You will hear this place called many names; do not be confused. It may be called purusha-prakriti, parama-purusha, the abode of Hari-Hara, the abode of Devi; but you can know it as the abode of Shiva. Here, the atman is dissolved in brahman; it always was, but you don't realize it until you reach this level. Shiva and Shakti are one; this realization cannot be undone. Liberation is achieved even though the yogi still lives on. Life can continue for as long as the yogi likes, but karma can no longer touch him; he is ever free of the bonds of birth, death, rebirth, re-death, ever free of samsara. Knowing this, you are never-more born again. Here is every form of bliss. This is the tantrik path. I will attest to you that it does not work.

"The hatha yogi, however, through the heat of practice, awakens Kundalini. This occurs when prana is forced from the ida and pingala and clears the path of the sushumna; once she has reached the ajna, the yogi is transformed. You are free from the cycle of death and rebirth—samsara—and all karma is dissolved. You acquire a divine or deathless body—*divya deha*. In this state, the yogi can exercise great powers, siddhis.[178] However, some yogis choose to forgo this state and seek the final dissolution of the body. This is the next part of the journey; the jivatman leaves the body.

"When it is time for dissolution, the yogi, knowing that is it time for prana to leave the body, time to be absorbed into Shiva, like a drop of rain is absorbed into the ocean, will sit in yoga asana and restrain the breath with kumbhaka. The jivatman will move from the heart to the muladhara and awaken Kundalini. The jivatman and Kundalini will be drawn upwards, piercing the lower lotuses and coming to the ajna. All the bhuta, all the levels, all the *tattvas* of Samkhya, gross and subtle, will dissolve, and the jivatman and Kundalini will merge with the bindu.

"Next, in the state of samadhi, the yogi will pierce the final gate, the Brahma-randhra, at the crown of the head, leave the body, and forever dissolve into Shiva. He realizes he is the divine, he becomes Shiva or brahman or whatever you name it. Upon the dissolution of your body, you will become the creator, preserver, and destroyer of the worlds."

Looking fondly at her student, Garima said, "You are ready, Visvanatha. We will mediate together through the night, and you will experience the deepest levels of samadhi. Prepare yourself to sit for a long time."

A Light Goes Out

As the hour of brahmamuhurta approached, Garima looked up to the northern sky where her star had once appeared. When Visvanatha came out of his entranced state, she smiled and said, "You have done well. It is time for me to leave. When I am gone, you may return to your ashram or go into the forest. The choice no longer matters. But wherever you go, whatever you do, remember your practice."

Visvanatha did not understand. He thought Shri Ma meant to wander off into the forest, never to be seen again. He protested and claimed that he was not ready for her to leave. There was still so much more for him to learn from her. He begged her to stay.

Garima shook her head and said, "No, it is time. I will depart."

Alarmed, Visvanatha refused to leave her side. All day he remained with her. He refused to go away, fearing that if he turned his back to her, she would slip away.

She smiled at his fears and finally consented, "Okay, if you wish to stay by my side, sit with me again tonight. We will once more enter samadhi together."

This gave Visvanatha great comfort. As long as he could be with her, Shri Ma would not run away. The moon was still dark as they prepared for deep meditation, sitting upon their grass mats outside Shri Ma's hut. They sat throughout the night in bliss, in samadhi. When Visvanatha stirred in the morning, Ma was still sitting. She sat motionless, not breathing. But she often didn't breathe for hours. Still… something was different. Finally, he sought Paramahansa Purnananda and brought him to her. He looked at her and shook his head.

"She is gone," he said.

"Gone!" replied Visvanatha. "No, she can't be gone. She is just meditating. Can you not bring her back?"

"She is gone," Purnananda repeated, this time with a small smile. He was almost as old as Shri Ma and felt his own time coming to a close. He was pleased that she had been able to leave in the way and at the time of her choosing.

They let Shri Ma sit in meditation for the rest of the day. Everyone from the ashram passed by to bow and pay their respects. Even Shankar came. He and Visvanatha asked permission to bring her to the cremation grounds, but Purnananda said she would not be cremated. Instead, that evening, a great pit was dug in the very spot where she had preferred to meditate. There, she was interred—still sitting upright in her meditation posture.[179] A sacred pipal tree was planted over her body. There would be no further incarnations for Garima. She was free.

Two years later, Shankar and Visvanatha dug another pit a few meters away from Shri Ma. There they interred Purnananda and planted another pipal tree over him. He hadn't completed his grand shastra, the Sri-tattva-cintamani, the Auspicious Gem of Truth, but he did complete the Sat-chakra-nirupana an "Exposition of the Supports of the Inner Body," which Shankar and Visvanatha eventually wrote down and added their own commentaries. The trees grew tall, and their highest branches eventually entwined. But as the years turned and the city around the ashram grew, eventually the trees were cut down. Buildings and roads pushed the forest further and further away. The story of Shri Ma was lost to time, but the words of Paramahansa Purnananda survived, thanks to the teachings of Shankar and Visvanatha.

The Yoga Forest

Imagine a grand tree—ancient, resilient, and still growing. Call this tree "yoga." Its roots run deep in the soil of South Asia, planted so long ago that no one can say exactly when. From its thick trunk, many branches have grown—one of the largest being classical yoga, which took form around 2,000 years ago in a shastra called the *Patanjalayogasastra*, or "Yoga Sutras of Patanjali."[180] Over time, more limbs sprouted—tantra and hatha yoga among them—each giving rise to twigs and offshoots: various schools, styles, and interpretations of yoga.

This image guided my early studies. But a decade later, I had to revise it. There is not one yoga tree, but a yoga forest—sprawling, diverse, and filled with competing voices. Classical yoga didn't evolve from a single pre-classical tradition, and tantra didn't simply grow out of classical yoga. Both have roots in Buddhism, Jainism, tribal rites, and local folk practices. Even hatha yoga, though influenced by tantra, also influenced tantra in return.[181]

Today, many students imagine yoga as a path to peace, light, and spiritual awakening—or at least to toned bodies and calmer minds. This is one sunlit part of the forest. But darker paths also wind through it—paths where ascetics sleep in cremation grounds, where yogis use taboo practices to gain control over others. These aren't modern studio stories. Yet they're part of yoga's long history.[182]

In the story of Garima, we saw one path. Her journey from a left-handed tantric cult to being a solitary hatha yogini reflects the complex and often painful realities of women in tantra. Though fictional, Garima's story is rooted in real places: Kamakhya Temple and the Vasistha Ashram in Guwahati.[183]

The yoga forest is filled with contrasting philosophies.[184] In Patanjali's system, based on Samkhya, yoga is a disunion—separating purusha (soul) from prakriti (nature). Liberation, or *kaivalya*, is achieved when all mental fluctuations cease and the soul stands alone.

Tantric yoga tells a different story. The separation of purusha and prakriti is only an illusion; the divine is everywhere and within. Here, samadhi comes through devotion, visualization, and ritual absorption. To see the divine clearly is to become divine.

Hatha yoga offers another definition. Samadhi is a trance so deep, the yogi becomes insensate—unmoved by heat or cold, sorrow or joy. In some texts, it's described as a merging into sound, or a death-like stillness where even breath stops. The Hathapradipika links samadhi to raja yoga (dharana, dhyana, and samadhi); the Gheranda Samhita identifies six kinds of samadhi, including states of bliss, devotion, and non-dual absorption.[185]

With so many views on yoga and samadhi, it's no surprise that liberation means different things too. Moksha, *mukti*, kaivalya, and nirvana may refer to union with the divine, freedom from rebirth, or even becoming superior to the gods. Some Buddhist schools say there's no self to liberate; others describe a liberated self that transcends the cycles of samsara. There is no consensus on what liberation is, and there is no agreement on what it is that becomes liberated!

Living liberation, becoming a *jivanmukta*, is just as confusing. It became definitive during the formation of *Advaita Vedanta*, especially by Shankara in the eighth century, although its roots were visible earlier. Here, the simple possession of the knowledge that you are brahman and that the world you see is an illusion will liberate you, even while you still live. This is not possible in the teachings of classical yoga. But despite living for a time as a jivanmukta, eventually the body must be dissolved and the self, the atman, will merge with the "interior of heaven."[186]

The Many Views of Prana

So where does prana fit into all this?

We have seen in the ancient teachings that prana can refer to the vitality of life, but also to the air we breathe, to bodily fluids, and to gods and their powers. In Samkhya, prana is just one of the vayus—subtle airs—of the body. In that philosophy, life arises from the proximity of purusha to prakriti, not from prana itself. In both tantra and hatha yogas, prana has been elevated in importance. It has many synonyms: when it is the universal power of the universe, of creation, it is the goddess Shakti; when it is embodied in a person, it is called prana—or Kundalini, when personified—and gives life to the individual. It joins the soul, the atman, to the body. Tantra uses mantra and visualization to awaken her; hatha yoga uses physical effort, breath, and meditation.

In hatha yoga, basic pranayama practices purify the nadis—particularly the ida and pingala. More advanced breath control, including kumbhaka and bandhas, builds heat and power, leading to siddhis or liberation. When the breath is mastered, the yogi may direct the breath to exit the body through the crown, achieving *utkranti*—voluntary exit from the body. This is how Garima chose to die.

The subtle body was thought to contain a network of nadis (channels) and chakras (centers). These allowed the movement of breath, prana, bindu (fluids), and kundalini. The body was still viewed as a microcosmic homologue to the macroscopic universe; what happened in one would affect what happened in the other. The number of chakras varied throughout the yoga forest, with some teachers citing as few as four and others as many as 16.[187] By the time the *Sat-chakra-nirupana* was compiled, most teachers were satisfied with the number six, and from this point forward, six became the standard view, if we assume the sahasrara was excluded from the list.[188] In the nineteenth and twentieth centuries, the chakras would take on an expanded role in both tantra and hatha practices.[189]

Although many yoga traditions require an ascent up the central channel of the body, the sushumna, what exactly ascends is not always agreed upon. Depending on the teaching, what ascends may be the atman, the prana or vayu, the Kundalini energy, or even the bindu (seminal fluid or nectar). Confusion arises here, too, as some teachers claim that amrta must be raised up and prevented from seeping downward, where it will be consumed by the agni in the belly, but in other teachings, the idea is to cause the amrta in the upper body to be released and flood the lower body.[190] The whole conflation of bindu and prana is confusing because bindu, as semen and menses, are real substances, but the kundalini is a psycho-spiritual substance or process. More confusingly, in a text known as the Padmasamhita, compiled around the tenth century, the kundalini is not something that pierces the chakras and rises upward, but rather an obstruction that must be destroyed with heat so that the breath, prana can rise up.[191] The Yoga Yajnavalkya, a classical yoga text compiled sometime between the second and fourteenth centuries CE, also describes kundalini as a blockage preventing prana from entering the sushumna.

Depending on which part of the yoga forest you visit, the goals and practices will vary. Even the words themselves—chakra, samadhi, liberation—can take on entirely different meanings from one tree to the next. If there's a particular path you want to follow through the forest, it's best to find a guide—a guru—who knows the terrain. Garima was such a guide. But notice how her practice of pranayama was fierce, ascetic, and challenging. The modern teacher T.K.V. Desikachar, by contrast, would not have agreed with her approach. In his hands, pranayama became something far gentler, more adaptive, and therapeutic. As we will see, his teaching emerged from a different part of the forest—one where healing, not power, was the goal.

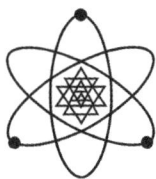

CHAPTER 16:

Hollyhock

In the late 1960s and early '70s, long before Lululemon and City Yoga arrived in Kitsilano—a Vancouver neighborhood named after Chief Xats'alanexw of the Squamish nation—the area pulsed with countercultural energy. The streets were filled with incense and peppermints, psychedelic posters, organic food co-ops, and bookstores brimming with Eastern philosophy, environmental treatises, and political manifestos. On the beaches and in cafes, young idealists gathered to discuss how to fix the world.

In one home, Rex Weyler, Bob Hunter, and Irving and Dorothy Stowe strategized ways to stop US nuclear testing near Amchitka Island, Alaska. Their meetings birthed the "Don't Make a Wave Committee," soon renamed Greenpeace. In 1971, they launched a boat to Amchitka, igniting a global movement.

A decade later, Rex Weyler was at a folk festival in Kitsilano when an elderly Hungarian woman—a singer in a vocal harmony troupe—gave him a cryptic message: he would realize something important when he saw red hollyhocks rising above a hedge. Weeks later, on remote Cortes Island, reachable only by ferry and hours of travel north of Vancouver, Weyler stumbled upon a forgotten garden ringed with red hollyhocks. The land had once hosted the Cold Mountain Institute, British Columbia's answer to Esalen. It had folded six years after its founder's death, and the site had fallen into disrepair.

But Rex remembered the prophecy. He gathered support and, together with others, revived the space as a retreat center dedicated to personal growth, social transformation, and environmental renewal. They named it Hollyhock.

In August 2003, Hollyhock hosted a workshop titled The Symbols of Yoga, led by T.K.V. Desikachar, son of T. Krishnamacharya—the teacher of B.K.S. Iyengar and Pattabhi Jois, and often called the grandfather of modern yoga.

Mythology and symbology had always fascinated me. From childhood through adulthood, I had devoured myths and religious tales. During a difficult period in the '90s, a compassionate friend, Hugh Boyle, introduced me to the writings of Carl Jung, whose teachings on symbols in the unconscious helped me heal. I soon found my way to Joseph Campbell and the archetypal motifs behind mythic stories. So when I heard Desikachar would be teaching at Hollyhock—on myth, symbols, and yoga—I felt called to attend.

I remember our first meeting vividly. Desikachar stood beside his son Kausthub and daughter-in-law Lakshmi, who held their newborn daughter, Shraddha, in her arms. Dressed in white, glasses perched on his nose, Desikachar looked serene and slight of build, his white hair gently tousled. He greeted us in the Raven's Hut, one of two circular buildings on the Hollyhock grounds.

The plan for the week was simple. Kausthub would guide us through morning asana practices, then we would break for breakfast. After eating, we'd gather for Desikachar's sessions, which included mantra, mudra, stories, and reflections on the symbolic language of yoga.

The Breath is the Envelope

Kausthub began our first morning practice with what he called *vinyasa krama*. We started simply: standing tall, we inhaled while lifting the arms overhead, then exhaled as we lowered them. We repeated this basic movement five times, always led by the breath. Desikachar later explained, "The breath is the envelope of the movement. Begin the inhalation, then move. Finish the movement, then finish the breath. Everything is done inside the breath."

From there, we built the sequence step by step. Each stage added a new element: folding forward, halfway lift, lunge, plank, cobra, and finally downward dog—always returning to standing between rounds. Each new movement was introduced gradually, patiently, and then practiced five times before progressing. The full sequence took about fifteen minutes—slow, mindful, almost meditative. It felt deeply yin-like, though I had not yet heard that term.

Later in the week, Kausthub led another variation—one I had first learned from Tim Miller. I wondered whether Tim had studied with Desikachar or arrived at it on his own. Either way, I loved the sequence and had taught it for years in my hatha classes at the Prana Yoga and Zen Centre.

It began in virasana, sitting on the heels. Inhaling, rise to kneeling with arms overhead. Exhaling, return to sitting. In stage two, we added a forward fold into child's pose with arms extended. Then back up to kneeling, then seated again. Stage three brought us onto all fours with the spine dropped low (cow pose) on the inhale. Stage four rounded the spine up (cat pose) on the exhale. Stage five introduced cobra, and finally, stage six ended in downward dog for five breaths before reversing the sequence. Stage seven was a reprise of stage five; stage eight reprised stage four; and so on until we ended sitting on our heels again. Every movement was within the breath. I loved it so much, I set it to Pink Floyd's "Brain Damage/Eclipse." My students affectionately called it the "Pink Floyd Flow," and when timed just right, it lasted exactly five minutes and 21 seconds—just like the track.

During one break, I spoke with Kausthub about the term *viniyoga*, which I'd heard associated with their lineage. But I'd also heard that Desikachar didn't want it used anymore. I asked why.

Kausthub paused before replying. "To my father, branding yoga is a form of murder."[192] Desikachar had once asked his own father, Krishnamacharya, what to call the individualized approach they practiced. Krishnamacharya suggested viniyoga, a word found in the Yoga Sutras, meaning a suitable or appropriate application. But over time, the word had become a brand—a fixed label—which troubled Desikachar. What had once described a flexible, tailored approach to practice was now marketed as a style. So he asked students to stop using the term.

"So what do you call it now?" I asked.

"We don't call it anything," Kausthub said. "But if you must, just call it 'the yoga of yoga.'"

There's No Place Like Aum

One of the main themes of the week was the meaning and importance of Om—spelled more accurately, Desikachar said, as *Aum*. He explained that Aum has four syllables, which one would completely miss if you were to spell it "Om". The syllables are A, U, M, and the silence that follows.

To illustrate, he taught us the *cin mudra*. Holding out our hand, we touched the tip of the forefinger to the thumb. The little finger stood for "A," the ring finger for "U," the middle finger for "M," and the circle formed by thumb and forefinger represented the fourth state—*turiya*—pure awareness, the silence beyond sound, the "master" or "Lord." In India, this mudra is usually done with the right hand, but Desikachar noted that in Tibetan imagery, the Buddha sometimes forms it with the left.

These four states can be symbolically interpreted in many ways. One is body, mind, speech, and consciousness. They can also represent the three gunas. The little finger may be the tamas gune; the ring finger may be the rajas gune; the middle finger may be the sattva gune. These three gunas are always changing. Wrong perception, avidya, arises due to focusing only on these three changeable, impermanent aspects. The first state may represent the creator, or Vishnu. The third state represents the individual atman, or jiva. The second state links the first and third together: it "introduces" the jiva to the creator.

"In order for a mantra to be truly a mantra, it must be placed inside the envelope of Aum," said Desikachar. "Aum begins the chant; Aum ends the chant. If you remove cheese from a pizza, it is no longer pizza. If you remove Aum from a mantra, it is no longer a mantra. When I was young, women were not allowed to use Aum. My own mother was not allowed to chant Aum; instead, she used the mantra Am. But in a departure from orthodoxy, my father, Krishnamacharya, did teach Aum to women and was heavily criticized for this practice. My father pointed out that this restriction was never mentioned in the Vedas and was only a cultural rule, not a spiritual one."

Interestingly, Aum is never mentioned in the Yoga Sutras. The only reference is to *pranava*, a word meaning "that which hums." While many assume this is a synonym for Aum, Desikachar offered a different view. He said the presence—or absence—of Aum signals the nature of a text: if Aum is explicitly mentioned, the text is religious; if not, it may be more secular. He considered the Yoga Sutras to be non-sectarian—which is possibly why the collection is not classified as one of the six orthodox Hindu schools.

Desikachar had a quiet spirituality but not much interest in formal religion. When chanting the Vedas, he insisted on precise pronunciation. When chanting other texts, he allowed more flexibility. "Chanting these texts," he said, "is not prayer, but it can be meditation or therapy."

He also expressed concern about Western yoga students borrowing Hindu practices without understanding their context. He questioned why students in the West, especially ashtangis, observe moon days or skip practice on Saturdays—customs rooted in Hinduism, not yoga. "Why adopt these rituals if you're not Hindu?" he asked. "Would a Jewish person wear a crucifix? Would they tattoo it on their body?" He made a comparison between Aum and the crucifix: "We use the word 'cross' every day," he said, "but that doesn't mean we're referring to Christ. Likewise, many chant Om, but when you wear ॐ, that's a symbol of a Hindu deity."

His plea to us was simple: don't use ॐ carelessly. Write Aum or use the Devanagari script औम् instead—it's a representation of sound, not a sacred icon.

Over our time together, Desikachar told us many stories, and interspersed within them were explanations of their meanings. He explained these stories as metaphors or teachings. We heard several tales about Patanjali, the author of the Yoga Sutras, who was the incarnation of Ananta, the serpent upon which Vishnu sleeps. He told us the story of the churning of the Cosmic Ocean by the devas who sought immortality. This story was a metaphor for the role of the guru in leading the student to libera-tion.[193] We heard stories of King Janaka, who appears in many Buddhist tales as well as in the *Ramayana*. One story involved Janaka waking from a dream and refusing to talk to anyone because he began to doubt what was real. His guru set him straight by pointing out that neither the waking world nor the dream world is real; what is real is the awareness of both. It's the watcher who is real.

Prana and Pranayama

Throughout the week, Desikachar interwove teachings on prana and pranayama into our practices. During these short sessions, I gleaned much of Desikachar's views on prana and pranayama, and this was complemented by my readings in the evenings from his book. I had brought *The Heart of Yoga* with me, which he had first published in 1995.[194] In Desikachar's teachings, pranayama consists of two syllables: prana and ayama. In his view, "ayama" means expansion or extension. He poetically describes prana to be "that which is infinitely everywhere." Prana fills us and keeps us alive and healthy. Desikachar translated prana into the modern Western term "vitality." Thus, prana is the vitality of life.

Citing the Yoga Yajnavalkya, he explained that when more prana is outside the body than inside, illness and fatigue arise. Depleted inner prana leads to listlessness, depression, and disease. The Yoga Sutras says that a disturbed mind causes irregular breathing, which in turn causes more suffering.[195] Pranayama helps collect and circulate prana, keeping it within the body. "A yogi," Desikachar said, "is one whose prana is all within his body."

For Desikachar, pranayama was not about ratios or breath-holding, but about attention. "The whole point," he said, "is to be aware of your breath." You could focus on where you feel the breath—nostrils, chest, or belly—or on the sound of it, such as in ujjayi breathing. But the goal was not to control the breath, only to observe it. Be aware of where in your body you feel the breath, but don't worry about putting the breath there. Be aware of how long you breathe, but don't worry about lengthening or extending it. Be aware of the sound of your breath, but don't worry about creating sounds while you breathe. Over time, observation naturally refines the breath and prepares the mind for meditation.

He suggested reversing the usual pattern of breath awareness. Instead of beginning in the belly and rising upward, we were to feel the inhale start at the collarbones and descend to the abdomen; then, on the exhale, feel awareness rise again. This up-and-down flow mirrored prana and apana—the two currents of energy in the body.

Desikachar said, "Prana flows into us as we inhale, but prana is also the power behind our exhalation. Within the body, it is transformed into various powers that are essential for helping us eliminate what we do not need. When it enters the body, it is called prana, but when it leaves the body, it is called apana. Apana also refers to the lower abdominal area and its functions. Apana can develop as a residual substance after prana has been consumed, and we need to eliminate this refuse. Too much apana prevents prana from developing.

"If you cannot hold your breath, are short of breath, or cannot exhale slowly, you have an excess of apana, and this leads to many physical problems. During inhalation, prana meets apana; during exhalation, apana meets prana. This movement is pranayama. When pranayama assists in regulating the breath, it calms and focuses the mind. Pranayama is breathing consciously. If you can do this, there is no danger in practicing pranayama.

"The most important part of pranayama is the exhalation. If it is done easily, slowly, and quietly, all is well. If not, you are not ready to practice pranayama. It is okay if the inhalation is rough, but an uneven exhalation is a sign of impending or present illness. The reason the exhalation is so important is because it eliminates impurities from the body. When that happens, there is more room for prana to enter. Only once this occurs should the student worry about breath retentions. The purpose of breath retention is to calm and rest the mind."

He emphasized that pranayama should always follow asana practice, but only after sufficient rest. "If the body is not still, the breath cannot be still. And if the breath is not still, the mind will not be still." Postures for pranayama should be effortless. The longer you wish to sit, the easier the posture must be.

"Some students," he said, "will be taught to extend their breath, to breathe with specific ratios of inhalation and exhalation lengths, and other techniques, but these are merely a means to an end, not the end itself. The goal is not to use any technique but simply to observe the breath. When we can do that, we are truly practicing pranayama. When I initially work with a student, I do not mention any techniques. This must be done gradually, because if we gather our energies too quickly, we risk being blown apart."[196]

Seven Bija Sounds

Early on the last morning, I walked into the orchard and stood quietly between the fruit trees, facing east, waiting for the first rays of sun. When they touched me, I began chanting the seven bija sounds Desikachar had taught us. He had not given us spellings—only the sounds themselves. All but the last began with an aspirated "h," and each was chanted as a single syllable.

Facing east, I chanted "h-ram." I turned south and chanted "h-reem." To the west: "h-room." To the north: "h-rhyme." Turning again to the east, I finished the sequence with "h-rome," "h-rum," and finally "raha." I repeated this cycle seven times, then walked back through the orchard to join the group for our final day at Hollyhock.[197]

Recall that Desikachar's definition of prana was the vitality of life. This is a form of the philosophy known as *vitalism*. His teachings offered a felt sense of vitality through breath and movement. But not long ago, in the grand salons of Paris, the concept of vitalism was being dissected with logic, mathematics, and debate.

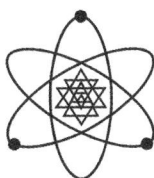

CHAPTER 17:

The Salon

"Oh, there she is!" exclaimed Madame Germaine de Staël in English, looking to the entrance of the salon and the flustered woman who just walked in. She called to the new arrival, "Madame Lavoisier! Over here."

Madame Lavoisier paused, took a calming breath, smiled, and navigated the crowded room to join de Staël and two gentlemen. Madame de Staël's salon was renowned for its influential gatherings. Her critical views on Napoleon had previously led to her exile, but after a year of restraint, she was permitted to return to France. As the regulator, she would see that tonight's conversation flowed toward topics more scientific and worldly, and less political.

The salon, which referred both to the gathering as well as the reception room, was held at de Staël's residence on Rue du Bac, Paris. The elegant mansion was known to the intellectual elite of the early 1800s. About 30 guests lounged on couches and chairs amid Rococo mirrors and paintings by Fragonard and Boucher. Rich fabrics adorned the walls and furniture, while numerous candles cast a warm glow.

Lavoisier greeted de Staël with a curtsey, acknowledged by a nod. She then curtseyed to the two gentlemen—one familiar, the other unknown—who responded with shallow bows.

"I apologize for my tardiness," said Lavoisier, also in English, following de Staël's lead. "My cabriolet broke an axle, and it took some time to secure another."

"Well, life is either boring or suffering," replied de Staël. "No matter. You're here now." She turned to the gentlemen. "You know Monsieur Laplace. May I present our distinguished guest, Count Rumford—General of Bavarian forces, social reformer, inventor, knighted by King George III, and originally from Massachusetts! Quite the résumé, Count!"

Turning to Lavoisier, she continued, "The count is en route to London, with only a brief stay in Paris, yet he graces us tonight. But you, my dear Anne-Marie, probably already know of the count's work in the field of science. His discoveries about the nature of heat would have warmed your late husband's heart. Ah, hearts are strange organs, are they not? They warm more than blood. Some say they warm the soul. But I leave that to the vitalists."

Lavoisier was slightly startled by her friend's informal use of her first name but hid this behind a warm smile. Germaine was clearly in a matchmaking mood—perhaps with reason. The count was tall, handsome, likely in his late forties—about five years her senior. Pierre-Simon Laplace she knew well; he had worked with her late husband and was among Europe's most respected academicians, highly regarded even by Napoleon.

"I knew your husband's work well," said the count. "I was shocked when I heard he'd fallen to Monsieur Guillotine's horrid device. Too many good minds were lost. But, as Madame de Staël has decreed, no politics tonight. She and Monsieur Laplace have told me of your key role in your husband's discoveries. Without your documentation and translations, his work might have vanished like a puff of air. I look forward to hearing more of Antoine's thoughts—and yours." He bowed again, eyes twinkling.

"Well, I've been looking forward to this evening," said de Staël. Turning to the elder gentleman, she said, "Monsieur Laplace, perhaps you can confirm a rumor I've heard."

"At your service, madame," he replied.

"Well," she continued, "Napoleon was reportedly studying your work on planetary orbits and asked why you made no mention of the hand of God. What did you tell him?"

Laplace smiled faintly. "I told him I had no need of that proposition."

Laughter rippled through the group. "Surely you didn't!" Lavoisier said. "Did you really tell Napoleon that God played no role in the heavens? How bold! How did he react?"

"I wasn't quite so bold," Laplace replied, "but he did look puzzled, as if he couldn't fathom what I meant."

Still chuckling, the count asked, "So, Monsieur Laplace—do I take it you're not a supporter of Madame de Staël's vitalism?"

"My vitalism?" said de Staël. "Oh no—I just tossed the word out. I know little about it. Perhaps you can enlighten me."

Lavoisier gave her friend a subtle glance of surprise. Germaine was being mischievous. She had heard her speak on vitalism before—Germaine knew exactly what it was. Clearly, she was baiting the count, steering the conversation to let him lecture. Men did enjoy that.

The Four Elements of Aristotle

"Vitalism?" said the count. "It traces back to the Greeks. Aristotle and Plato believed life depended on pneuma—breath—the source of all movement in the body. Without pneuma, there was no life. Others, like Democritus and Epicurus, held that everything—even the soul, or psyche—was made of atoms. Life, to them, was simply the motion of particles, without any divine purpose. Aristotle also taught that all matter was made of four basic elements: air, water, earth, and fire. But we now know, thanks in part to you, Madame Lavoisier, your husband, and Monsieur Laplace, that this is false. Air—pneuma—is not a single substance but a mix of gases. So how can breath be a vital force beyond its physical makeup?"

"Please explain," said de Staël. "Air is not an element? It seems quite essential. Without it, we don't live long."

Rather than reply, the count graciously turned to Laplace, allowing him a chance to share his experience. Laplace was happy to take up the thread.

"It's a fair assumption," Laplace said, "but our understanding of air has changed. In Sweden, Carl Scheele found that what we call air is actually two gases—one that promotes combustion, one that prevents it. Around the same time, Henry Cavendish in England found similar results. He identified 'fixed air' and 'inflammable air'—what Monsieur Lavoisier renamed carbon dioxide and hydrogen.

"Carbon dioxide was first noticed above beer vats. Joseph Priestley found a way to produce it in quantity—allowing Joseph Schweppes to create the very soda water you're drinking!"

Madame de Staël raised her glass of fruit-laced soda water in salute, while the men sipped red wine.

Laplace continued. "When Priestley placed an animal under a glass filled with carbon dioxide, it quickly died. So too did any flame inserted in the gas. But plants thrived on it." Looking at Lavoisier, he asked, "Do you recall Priestley's visit?"

"Yes," nodded Lavoisier. "It was in 1774."

"Antoine and I studied these two gases for years," said Laplace. "We proved that the one Priestley called 'pure air' sustained life and combustion. Your husband renamed it oxygen in his landmark text.[198] He also renamed other gases Priestley discovered—ammonia, hydrogen chloride, and nitrous oxide. Truly, he helped turn alchemy into modern chemistry."

"And I'd add this," said the count. "Lavoisier disproved the Greek element theory. He showed pneuma was not divine, but just a gas that enabled breath and fire. Democritus was more right than Aristotle."

"So air is not an element—it's a mix of gases," said de Staël. "But surely there's more than chemistry that animates us. If a plant breathes and grows with carbon dioxide, and I with oxygen, is that all that separates us? Does the gas alone make us human?"

Fire Is Not Elemental

"We do not claim that oxygen alone is sufficient for life, but it is necessary," said the Count. "Vitalists, however, claim a special 'something' is sufficient. We disagree. Some point to fire as that essence—but fire is not elemental. Wouldn't you agree, Monsieur Laplace?"

"Indeed. Before Lavoisier's work, a chemist named Georg Stahl proposed that combustion released a substance called *phlogiston*, from the Greek 'to set on fire.' He believed burning caused something to leave the material."

"That sounds reasonable," said de Staël. "Candles give off smoke—something clearly departs in burning."

"You're not alone," said Laplace. "Many believed it. But when we burn a metal, the residue weighs more—so something is gained, not lost. What is gained Is oxygen. For instance, heating mercury forms mercury oxide. No phlogiston is released—oxygen is consumed."

"I understand that air isn't elemental—it's made of gases," said de Staël, glancing at Laplace, then turning to Lavoisier. "But I recall that your husband did include fire as one of the elements in his book."

"That was unfortunate," Lavoisier admitted, turning to the count. "Antoine did list fire as an element, or to be more accurate, he felt the *caloric* to be a physical entity which was elemental in nature. But your studies, Count Rumford, have banished that notion. Perhaps you'll explain?"

"True," said the count. "Caloric was thought to be a fluid carrying heat—more in hotter bodies, less in cooler ones, flowing from hot to cold. But if that were true, heated objects should weigh more. My experiments showed they do not. Think of a bell—its sound continues as long as you strike it. Likewise, motion creates heat. I proved this by boring holes in cannon barrels: friction made them hot. When I stopped drilling, they cooled. Heat isn't caloric—it's motion. And fire is not an element."

"But surely water is?" asked de Staël. "This glass may contain bubbles of carbon dioxide, but the water itself must be pure. No?"

"No, water isn't elemental either," said Lavoisier. "By using electricity, Antoine and I were able to split water into two gases: hydrogen and oxygen, always in a volume ratio of two to one."

"Astounding," said de Staël. "Water comes from air! Can the same be said of earth—does it come from water?"

"No—earth isn't a single element either, but a mix of substances and metals," replied Lavoisier.

The Electricians

"I still don't see why you doubt vitalism," said de Staël. "Are the functions of life purely physical? Surely something non-material is needed for the miracle of life! Oxygen explains breath—but can it explain movement? What if a soul is required for life? How could you disprove that?"

"Not knowing a cause doesn't mean one doesn't exist," said Lavoisier. "Science reveals nature's workings—but answers take time."

"Well said," agreed Laplace. "Invoking soul, spirit or even God to fill gaps in our knowledge is tempting—but it reflects ignorance, not insight. Given time, material answers will emerge."

"I agree, Monsieur Laplace," said the Count. "A few years ago I was in Italy. There, I saw Signore Volta's demonstration of electricity. He learned a trick from Signore Galvani, though he does not give him much credit. Volta attached a severed leg of a frog between two wires of different metals. Once the connections were made, the leg jumped! It seems that electricity can move our muscles. Soul is not required."

"Fascinating," said Lavoisier. "We used Volta's pile to create the electricity that showed water was composed of hydrogen and oxygen."

"Electricity!" said de Staël. "I remember when Monsieur Benjamin Franklin visited us in his role of Envoy to France. He would often attend my salons and talk about it. I believe he called Volta's device a 'battery.' But was he right to think electricity is another fluid—like the discredited caloric?"

"We don't yet know what electricity really is," said the Count. "It may be a fluid, but that's unclear. What fascinated me more than the battery was what Volta ignored. You see, Signor Galvani was the first to tie a frog's leg to wires and cause them to twitch. He discovered that the impulse was coming from *within* the flesh of the frog! Not only can our muscles be activated by electricity, but our body actually creates its own electricity!"

"I knew of Volta's work," said Laplace, "but not of Galvani's success. If he is correct, that's another hole in the vitalist argument."

"What?" said de Staël, incredulously. "You reduce us to twitching frogs. But what of dreams? Of love? Of despair? Show me a voltaic pile that produces those."

"Again," said Laplace, "we don't claim life is only electricity—no more than it is only oxygen. But these experiments show that movement requires electricity, not soul or spirit. So, back to your original question, Count Rumford—yes, I am not in favor of the whole idea of vitalism."

The Count and Madame Lavoisier

Unseen by the men, de Staël gave Lavoisier a sly glance and said, "Gentlemen, you are masters of the measurable. But beware—deny the immeasurable and you flatten the very wonder that makes life worth living. I don't reject your truths, but I doubt they are the whole truth. Was it Rousseau who said, 'Reality may have its limits—imagination does not'? Did not Aristotle say, 'The whole is more than the sum of its parts'? You may name gases and generate electricity, but life resists dissection. Let's revisit this another time. For now, I must borrow Monsieur Laplace. There are a few people that I promised to introduce him to. Count Rumford, may I leave you in Anne-Marie's capable hands?"

Germaine is too much, thought Lavoisier. *How obvious can she be?* Still, the night could be interesting. She let the count escort her to a quiet corner and took a seat on a shadowed divan. A pity he was only passing through.

Back in London, Sir Benjamin Thompson—Count Rumford—found life dull. His commissions and pensions fluctuated with politics, and he lacked the investments to sustain him. He missed the continent's vibrancy and soon returned to Paris. He and Madame Lavoisier moved in together and spent pleasant months traveling through Bavaria and Switzerland. In October 1805, after navigating divorce and death certificates, they finally married—only to discover they were ill-suited. The count wanted quiet retirement and scientific dabbling; Anne-Marie thrived on Parisian society. They parted within four years. She paid him a generous settlement—an annoying but necessary bribe to get him out of her padded and powdered hair.

Man: the Cartesian Machine

The rise of the scientific method during the Renaissance led Europeans to question ancient teachings and find them wanting. The idea of four basic elements was rejected, as was the belief in a vital substance—no pneuma, spiritus, or prana was needed to animate life. While early thinkers like Descartes, Galileo, and Newton accepted the soul's existence, they increasingly dismissed the notion of a magical life-giving vitality.

While the conversation in Madame de Staël's salon, set in 1801, is fictional, all the characters are historical. The mechanistic worldview was gaining ground—a materialist shift that had its roots in Descartes nearly two centuries earlier. Known for "I think, therefore I am," Descartes was a pioneering scientist and philosopher. He unified geometry and algebra, and proposed that matter and mind were entirely separate realms—dualistic but independently real.

Descartes lived in the early seventeenth century—a time of great advances in precision crafting of gears and clocks. These led to the invention of wonderfully animated machines: mobile statues, hydraulic automata that mimicked natural phenomena, and mechanical animals that had no souls yet could move on their own. This caused Descartes to believe animals and humans were similarly mechanical, just more complex.

Descartes was not speaking metaphorically; he thought we *were* machines: machines whose motions are generated by heat—produced, he believed, in the heart.[199] The universe, to him, was a giant mechanism governed by laws and reducible to its parts.

In the philosophy of *mechanism* (also called *mechanistic* or *mechanical philosophy*), the world is naturalistic, atomistic, and deterministic.[200] These features allow the world to be mathematically predictable. Applied to biology, the paradigm assumes that there is a continuity between the non-living and the living and that the whole is determined by its parts. This idea led to the counter-protest, "The whole is more than the sum of its parts."[201]

Descartes proposed a mind–body split in which the soul was not needed for life but was needed for consciousness and reason. He proposed that the pineal gland, buried in the brain, gave the mind control over the body.[202] Further, while animals had life, they did not possess a soul.

Galileo and, later, Newton built upon Descartes's ideas. Where Descartes saw the universe as a combination of matter and motion, Newton added the dimension of space and then developed mathematical equations that predicted how forces, such as attraction and repulsion, govern the universe. Once a force could be characterized and predicted, there was no need to explain exactly what it was or how it came to be. Its existence was deduced from its actions.

Astrology gave way to astronomy. Chemists like Boyle and Lavoisier sought to bring similar precision to their field. Alchemy gave way to chemistry. As physics and chemistry became predictable, many assumed biology would follow—life, too, should yield to mathematics. By 1800, Descartes's idea of the "animal machine" had entered mainstream scientific thought. Lavoisier wrote that life was regulated by respiration, perspiration, and digestion—all describable in physical terms.[203]

Vitalism challenged this reductionism. Vitalists saw life as requiring a "vital force" or soul, beyond mechanics—though undefined and unmeasurable by science. Others saw life not in terms of an added substance, but as an emergent property of complex patterns. In this view, life was not reducible to parts; it arose only from the whole.

Animistic vitalism regained popularity as a reaction against Descartes's machine view of life.[204] Experience tells us that when an animal or person dies, the body—the machine, if it is a machine—remains the same, and yet its heat and life force, whatever that was, has gone. Whatever vital substance endowed the body with life leaves at the moment of death. So, how can life be only a machine?[205] For Stahl, it was clear that what gave life was the soul, which he termed the *anima sensitiva*, similar to Aristotle's psyche.[206] Mechanical explanations are fine for the inanimate world, he felt, but they fail to explain living organisms.

Stahl's views lost favor by the eighteenth century. A new version—*somatic vitalism*—emerged. It posited an internal property, not an external force. Like Newton's gravity, this vital property was known only by its effects.[207] If Newton did not have to describe exactly what a gravitational force was, why did we need to describe exactly what the internal life force was? As one physiologist wrote, this internal life force is "no more strange than the gravity, attraction, and mobility that belong to various bodies."[208] Yet no consensus formed on what this vital force was or how it worked. Was there one force or many? No one knew.

While mechanism took firm and unrelenting hold of the emerging science of biology, the vitalistic views never completely died away. New versions kept surfacing because, despite its great successes, the mechanistic view of life remained unable to unravel all the mysteries of life. A bottom-up, reductionist approach was not and still is not able to explain the properties of an organism as a whole.

Enlightened thinkers in Parisian salons of the seventeenth and eighteenth centuries wrestled with the nature of life, energy, and vitality in the abstract. In the twenty-first century, I was about to discover how these same forces—spirit, prana, and chi—would come to life in my own body, on a yoga mat in Seattle.

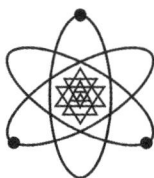

CHAPTER 18:

Seattle

"There are four ways that we can stimulate the movement of chi or prana. The first is through the application of needles, called acupuncture," explained Sarah Powers. "This is the only method we will not use in our yoga practice."

Sarah Powers exuded a calm yet focused energy. With straight, shoulder-length hair and a composed smile reminiscent of the Mona Lisa, she often seemed serene and grounded. Born in California, she had been exposed to a variety of Eastern philosophies while growing up in San Francisco and Los Angeles. In the 1980s, she began doing yoga and dove into ashtanga, Iyengar, and then vinyasa styles of practice. After a decade of mostly asana practice, she still felt restless. Despite reading many books on meditation, she had little inner awareness. Not until she saw a bookstore sign—"Meditation: the only way in and the only way out!"—did she commit to daily practice.

Sarah started attending sessions at a Buddhist monastery and eventually studied mindfulness and meditation in the Zen, Tibetan, and Theravada traditions. As teachers expounded on the methods, philosophies, and benefits of meditation, Sarah would quietly sit at the back of the room, holding yin postures. She discovered, almost by accident, that her meditation was far deeper after practicing yin yoga. As a result of her decades of integrating meditation insights with asanas, Sarah's teaching felt to me like a bridge between the physical and psychological aspects of yoga.[209]

"The other three ways to stimulate chi to flow can be accessed through our yoga practice," continued Sarah from the front of the room. "The three ways are posture, breath, and concentration.

"The posture creates a form of acupressure that works like acupuncture to pull on and pressurize our tissues, coaxing blood and chi to flow through the body to make the tissues we just used more usable in the future.

"The third way to mobilize energy is by deepening and lengthening the breath. This practice creates calmness and clarity and increases the flow of prana harmoniously. The breath is the primary anchor of asana practice. A guiding principle of hatha yoga is the increased distribution of prana throughout the body. We can assist this mobilization of energy through the practice of ujjayi.

"The fourth and final method is by focusing attention. When the mind is distracted, our energy is disorganized and destabilized. When the mind is concentrated, our energy will be even-flowing and stable. *Prana flows where our attention goes.* Like a magnet, a focused and spacious awareness will draw chi to the center of the body. When this happens, we no longer experience the distraction of fragmented energetic and emotional dissonance. We can now move easily into contemplative practices."[210]

I was sitting off to Sarah's left, on the floor of a relatively large conference room in the Seattle Center. It was May of 2004. Over 40 years earlier, the world had come to Seattle to attend the 1962 World's Fair. The grounds were the home of a space-age, mile-long monorail that ferried people from downtown Seattle to the fair, and the soaring, 605-foot Space Needle. There were dozens of other students raptly listening. Sarah's gaze slowly scanned the room, making eye contact with everyone.

Sarah suggested teachers think of their students as fellow yoga enthusiasts. If teachers treat their students as customers, it turns yoga studios into yoga stores and conferences such as this one, the Yoga Festival Northwest, into yoga malls with hundreds of students doing yoga shopping.

While I had attended the first Yoga Festival Northwest in May 2003 to further my knowledge in anatomy, for this year's conference, I specifically wanted to learn more about yin yoga. Picking up more anatomical knowledge would be a bonus. Someone named Paul Grilley was scheduled to present several lectures discussing how bones limit our range of motion. That sounded interesting. I booked two of his sessions, and another session called "Protect Your Knees" by a different teacher.

It was the second day of May, and the second day of sitting close to Sarah. Yesterday, she had taught two long sessions. She began with sun salutations to help her "get to know the bodies in the room." During the yin yoga portion, while the class stayed in the postures for several minutes, Sarah described her philosophical approach to yoga, meditation and the Daoist concepts of medicine and energy. She was extremely articulate. She spoke slowly in a cadence that encouraged full attention. Her voice was like a gentle river carrying us downstream. Around each bend, a new vista opened and a new realization dawned. Her practice blended dharma talks with asanas, gentle pranayama, soft moola bandha, and directed awareness. A constant, reoccurring theme was mindfulness.

Mindfulness of what? So many options! We could choose to be mindful of the body and notice any pain or discomfort or any pleasure and ease. We could choose to be mindful of the mind and the states it takes. Do we detect any clinging or judging? Can we recognize what actually is rather than what we think is? She defined meditation as "bare attention" and "mere recognition."

In the yogic framework of Patanjali, concentration leads to absorption, which leads to samadhi. The Buddha tried the yogic approach and found it lacking. After samadhi ends, suffering still exists. He wanted more. He wanted to end suffering, not wallow in samadhi. Thus, he developed a different approach to meditation, one Buddhists called mindfulness. In the Buddhist framework, concentration leads to mindfulness, which leads, in turn, to insight.

At the end of the asana practices, Sarah guided us through seated meditation. In the first stage of meditation, she asked us to focus on the breath. This was the concentration stage. In the second stage, the mindfulness stage, she directed us to focus on sensations. In the final stage, she asked us to focus on "watching the watcher." She suggested asking questions like, "Who am I?" and "What is this?"

Sarah described the concepts found in Daoist philosophy and in Traditional Chinese Medicine. She explained chi, jing, and connective tissues, including fascia. This was the first time I had heard a yoga teacher mention fascia. Sarah drew a connection between fascia and chi.

It is prana, chi that heals. Coming out of a long-held yin yoga posture gives us the opportunity to sense chi releasing and flowing. It is important to pause after each pose so we can attune to the feeling of chi, to feel the openness, not just physically but also emotionally. Blockages to chi directly affect our health.

These chi blockages occur in the deeper connective tissues; closer to the bones; in the deep fascia, which include our tendons, ligaments, and joints. To be able to affect these areas, we need to relax our muscles. Relaxed muscles allow the pressure from the postures to soak into the deeper layers of the body, reaching the connective tissues that house our meridians.

Sarah talked to us about many forms of chi. There is a yin form of chi, which helps our bones. There are yang forms of chi, organ chi, meridian chi, and others. Each form of chi may exist in different states. There are renegade states of chi, which flow backwards; there is stagnant chi; rebellious chi; deficient chi, which really means there is a lack of chi. One particular form of chi, called *jing*, she described in more detail.

"Jing," she said, "is the essence of chi. It is found in the Kidneys, from which it flows to all the other organs. For this reason, jing is given the 'royal seat.' It helps to strengthen and heal all the other organs and forms of chi. Jing develops the marrow and the bones; it helps to create and strengthen blood, which is produced within the marrow. When jing is weak, the bones of the spine and knees are weak. Kidney jing lubricates the joints. Too much heat can weaken jing, and this can show up as issues in the stomach and heart. When trouble arises in the Kidneys, it can be revealed through the arousal of fear and debilitating doubt. For this reason, Daoist doctors will strengthen the Kidneys first, regardless of which condition or disease a patient has. For all these reasons, it is important to do yin yoga postures targeting the Kidney meridian lines."

Where are the Kidney meridians? Sarah was about to tell us. "The Kidney meridian travels through the sole of each foot, the inside of the legs, and enters the torso near the tailbone. From there, it follows the ligaments of the lower back, connects to the physical kidneys and urinary bladder, and continues to flow upward through the liver, diaphragm, lungs, throat, ending at the root of the tongue.

"The Kidney meridian is yin and is paired with the Urinary Bladder meridian, which is yang. The Urinary Bladder meridian is the longest one in the body. It has 67 unique acupuncture points. The Urinary Bladder meridian begins at the inner corner of the eye, travels over the top of the head, where it meets the body's midline, and then descends along the back, tracing the flow of energy down either side of the spine. Each meridian exists bilaterally, creating symmetry. Where the two Urinary Bladder meridians begin is the location of our sixth chakra. The meridian running down the left side of the spine is equivalent to the ida nadi in the yogic view; the one on the right is equivalent to the pingala nadi. The Urinary Bladder meridians run down the back of the legs and the outside of the feet. At the little toes, they turn around and become the Kidney meridians."

Which postures might apply a physical stress on these meridians, and thus stimulate the flow of chi? Any pose that creates a sensation to the inner legs or lower back. Postures like butterfly or straddle (a seated pose with legs wide apart) will create tensile stress along the inner legs. This stress may stimulate the Kidney meridians and the flow of jing. The point of a long-held caterpillar, a seated forward fold with straight legs, resembling paschimottanasana but without the muscular effort, is not to stretch and lengthen the hamstrings, although that can occur, but to create acupressure along the Urinary Bladder lines.

Just as acupuncture needles are left in place for a long time, up to 30 minutes or more, the stresses produced in the yin yoga postures are maintained for a long time. Sarah gave us three basic rules, principles, or tenets of the yin yoga style of practice:

1. Come into the postures until you sense you have reached an appropriate edge.
2. Once you have arrived at your edge, become still. No muscular effort is required or desired.
3. In the stillness, stay for time. This gives chi time to work into the thicker taffy of the connective tissues.

Time is the magic ingredient. It takes time for the acupressure to activate the flow of chi. This may not be noticeable while you are in the posture, but when you come out, there will be a sense of fragility and a feeling of energy release, indicating the pose has done its work.

The Importance of Alignment

Over the first two days, I spent 12 hours with Sarah. I was torn between staying for all her classes or attending the anatomy presentations. On Saturday morning, I reluctantly skipped Sarah's class. I don't know what I missed, but probably the other meridians and organs of importance. I would have to find other occasions to fill in these pieces. Instead, I went to the session on protecting knees. I was 12 months post-op on my second knee, and it felt fine, but even so, I wanted to learn more.

This teacher's approach to teaching was quite different from Sarah's. Where Sarah would give dharma talks from the front of the room, the new teacher would move about the room, adjusting students and often calling us all over to witness a particular student. This *"come see"* approach was common in the Iyengar community. After giving us a presentation on the anatomical structure of the knee, how it was not a ball-in-socket joint but more of an elaborate hinge joint that relied solely on soft tissues for stability, she had us do standing postures that illustrated the importance of alignment. She warned us that the body will shrink to whatever is our usual range of motion. If you only ever lift your arm to reach a cup in a kitchen cupboard, you will lose a lot of your shoulder's full range of motion. In other words, "Use it or lose it."

Moving the body and loading the joints is essential to joint health. Holding stresses for 90 seconds to two minutes is healthy. Also important is aligning the knee with the hip and the foot. She gave various examples. In warrior postures, we were urged to ensure the knee tracked over the toes and not allow the toes to point outward. She taught us how to engage our muscles to build stability. She taught us to line up the heel of the front foot with the middle of the arch of the back foot. We were trained to make sure the knees did not collapse inward towards each other, a position called genu valgum. We were warned against hyperextending the knees in standing postures, such as triangle poses. We were encouraged to lift our kneecaps to ensure we engaged our quadriceps to avoid any hyperextension.

The teacher repeated what I had learned earlier about using a rolled-up washcloth tucked firmly behind the back of the knees while sitting on the heels in vajrasana. She said this cures nine out of 10 people of the knee pain that occurs when the knees are fully flexed. She also warned us to make sure our feet did not point inwards when we sat on our heels.

I left the class excited to put into practice all her new alignment cues. My excitement lasted for about two hours—the time it took to have lunch and then attend my first Paul Grilley class. My world imploded. All my wonderful alignment cues became as useless as buggy whips after the invention of the automobile. The yoga world was on the verge of abandoning horse-drawn carriages.

Paul Grilley Rocks My World

Paul was a smiling, laughing Buddha of a teacher. He possessed a hairstyle very similar to mine: neither of us had any. He was neither tall nor short, nor as slender as the ashtanga teachers I had studied with. Sarah described him as having a football player's build, but he certainly was not bulky. He sat with ease in lotus pose at the front of the classroom. In one corner of the room was a big black bag filled with a variety of human bones. Behind him was a blank wall upon which he projected computer slides. Most of the time, he was up walking around, telling jokes, laughing with a very unique cackle. Often, he would ask students to come up to the front of the room to demonstrate their uniqueness.

Paul started with some basic principles. There are two reasons we may not be able to do a particular posture: (1) we are stopped by tensile resistance: our tissues, whether muscles or fascia like our ligaments or joint capsules, simply cannot elongate any further. This he called *tension*; (2) our tissues have elongated sufficiently that one part of our body is now coming into contact with another part. This he called *compression*.

Tension can be worked on, and over time, more movement may be available. However, once compression has been reached, we have reached the limit of how far we can go, unless we discover a way to go around that point of compression. Even then, however, we will eventually come to a new stopping point. Once compression is reached and there is no way to go around the restriction, no amount of yoga will "open us up" further. We have opened up as much as we ever will in this lifetime.

The concepts of tension and compression being the limiters of our range of motion was new to me. But Paul was not done. He then introduced the concept of skeletal variation. Every yoga teacher and student I had come across in my seven years of practice had made an unconscious assumption: that under our skin, our bodies were all the same, and our bones looked exactly like the drawings shown in anatomy books.

Paul showed a photograph of two femurs and asked us to notice the differences. One femur had a sharper neck angle. Paul explained how this one difference would affect how much leg abduction was possible. The person whose femur had a large neck angle might easily do the side splits, called *samakonasana*. The other person, with a sharper neck angle, was never going to come close to side splits, no matter how much stretching of their adductors they did, how much ujjayi breathing they did, or how tightly they engaged moola bandha. They just didn't have the bones to do the splits.

I sat spellbound. In the two sessions that I attended with Paul, he showed us the variations in the arms, shoulders, hips, and feet. At one point, he showed us two tibias and explained that every long bone in our bodies has a twist to it. He called it a "torsion." In this case, it was *tibial torsion*. The average person's tibial torsion causes their feet to point outward when the leg is in a neutral position at the hip, even though the knees are pointing straight ahead. In order to bring the feet parallel to each other, he has to internally rotate the femur at the hip socket, which points the knees inward.

Paul asked, "Where should the foot be pointing in mountain pose or warrior pose? Straight ahead? Let's think again."

I could not help remembering the alignment cues I'd learned in the session a few hours earlier: "The foot must point straight ahead, and the knee must be aligned in the same direction." It turned out that these alignment cues I had been collecting were good *for some people*, but not for all people. Indeed, as Paul showed, not for most people! If your intention is to keep the hips and knees in a strong, neutral position where they can most effectively transmit force, the foot will have to be pointing outwards. How much depends upon how much tibial torsion you possess.[211]

"So why," he asked, "are yoga teachers adjusting students and putting their feet into a parallel alignment? In doing this, they are ignoring skeletal variations and inadvertently pulling students out of their own neutral alignment at the hips and knees."

In my mind, I watched all my treasured alignment cues start to evaporate. All the trainings I had taken, learning how to adjust students and place them into aesthetically pleasing alignment, seemed to be wasted money. Why was I trying to align students in the first place? If I adopted Paul's "functional approach," aesthetics would become irrelevant. I needed to teach from a functional viewpoint, which meant having an intention for each pose and then asking the student to pay attention. What was she feeling? It was going to take some time to digest the implications of what Paul was presenting.

In 2003, Paul created a DVD called *Anatomy for Yoga*. Across four hours of video presentations, he described the reality of skeletal variation and its impact on our range of motion. I bought the DVD and devoured it, making copious notes. And I started to share my new understanding with my students. I gave short trainings for the other teachers. But there was still much more to learn, from both Paul and Sarah. Fortunately, they were jointly planning to give a 10-day training in early 2005 at White Sulphur Springs, California.

Of course, I signed up. It was there that I learned about a teacher of both Sarah and Paul, Dr. Hiroshi Motoyama, who was a yoga adept influenced by the teachings of the Theosophical Society. To understand what Dr. Motoyama taught, it is worth investigating the history and views of the Theosophical Society. Its writings and lectures brought the South Asian views of energy, channels, and chakras into the twentieth century.

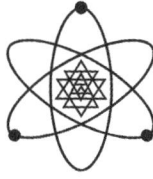

CHAPTER 19:

West Meets East—Theosophy

Flying from Vancouver to India was a long journey. The usual route took me through Hong Kong, with a direct flight onward to Madras. Whether flying east or west, the trip always took about 24 hours, including stopovers—sometimes in London, where I could take the Tube and spend a few hours in Hyde Park, or in Hong Kong, where the layover was shorter but the flight longer. On this trip, I was coming into Madras International Airport. Looking out the window, I could see the river Adyar almost directly below me.

At the airport, I was met by Kshema. Her father, Suresh Nadgir, owned the Malhar Corporation, which represented our interests in India. During the summers, Kshema and her younger sister Padma returned to India from their studies at Bryn Mawr College in Pennsylvania to learn the company's business. Now, both had graduated and were back in India full-time. I was surprised to learn they had taken over. Suresh, now that his daughters were fully grown, educated, and ready to take on the world, had donned the white linens of a forest recluse, leaving behind his children, his wife, and society.

Suresh was following the ancient Indian tradition of *ashrama*, the four stages of life. One begins as a student, becomes a householder, then renounces worldly duties when the children are grown, and finally returns as a teacher or sage.[212] Few today follow all four stages, and though I returned to India six more times, I never saw Suresh again.

In the 1600s, reaching this part of South Asia from London required sailing down Africa's west coast, around the Cape of Good Hope, then up the east coast and across the Indian Ocean. With good weather, the voyage took six months. With bad luck, nine—or worse, it ended at sea. In 1639, the British East India Company acquired from local Nayak rulers a 10-kilometer stretch of land between the Adyar and Cooum rivers. There, they built Fort George. Though small villages already dotted the Tamil countryside, it was British investment that transformed the region into a bustling colonial hub—a city they named Madras.[213] It soon became the administrative, military, and commercial center of British operations on India's eastern coast.

In 1882, the Theosophical Society—founded seven years earlier by Helena Blavatsky and Henry Steel Olcott—abandoned its New York base for what it saw as a more spiritually vibrant climate. Blavatsky, dogged by accusations of fraud in the West, sought a quieter, more sympathetic home in the East. The society purchased 27 acres of land near the mouth of the Adyar River. After Blavatsky's death and Olcott's retirement, a new generation of leaders took over. Annie Besant became president in 1907, joined by Charles Leadbeater—a writer, philosopher, and self-proclaimed clairvoyant.

The Inner Life: A Rooftop Discourse

It was a warm September evening in 1910 as Subramanian Iyengar made his way through the gates of the Theosophical Society's sprawling estate in Adyar. The sun was beginning to set. This was Iyengar's first assignment for *The Hindu*, the nationally renowned newspaper founded by his great uncle decades earlier. He had been chosen for the job because he was a recent graduate from Presidency College, where he specialized in Indian philosophy and religions.

Iyengar had done his research and knew a fair amount about the society. He also knew that tonight's speaker, Charles Leadbeater, had a checkered past. On the one hand, Leadbeater was hailed as a mystic and gifted spiritual teacher; on the other, there were whispers of a hasty departure from London and hushed allegations about inappropriate conduct with young boys under his tutelage.[214] The scandal had forced his resignation, but in 1908, at Annie Besant's invitation, he rejoined the society in India.

The tranquility of the estate stood in stark contrast to the noise and bustle of Madras. Iyengar walked slowly along a winding path, taking in the lush greenery and calm air. At the entrance to the main building, he was greeted by Mr. Narayan Iyer, his host for the evening. Iyer was a kindly looking man in his late 50s, neatly mustached and dressed in a simple white dhoti and kurta. It was he who had invited *The Hindu* to send a reporter to one of their Sunday talks.

As they climbed the stairs to the rooftop, Iyer explained, "We gather every Sunday at sunset for what we call the 'Rooftop Meetings.' It's a chance for members and guests to hear from some of our leading thinkers and to discuss spiritual matters. Tonight, Mr. Leadbeater will speak."

At the top of the stairs, the rooftop opened onto a broad terrace. The Adyar River shimmered in the fading light, and a jasmine-scented breeze moved gently through the crowd. The space was already bustling with people—some seated on wooden benches, others standing in small groups, chatting. The guests were a diverse mix, drawn from many backgrounds.

Iyengar, taking it all in, said, "It's quite a gathering."

Iyer smiled. "Theosophy attracts a wide range of people, all seeking a deeper understanding of life and the mysteries of the universe."

As the last rays of sunlight disappeared below the horizon, a hush fell over the audience. Mr. Iyer led Mr. Iyengar to a spot near the front, where they had a clear view of the makeshift podium. A bell rang softly.

Annie Besant stepped forward to address the gathering. She was getting on in years but still carried an air of commanding presence. Her thick white hair was piled high, and she wore flowing white robes with a long string of wooden beads around her neck.

"Welcome, friends," she began. "The Theosophical Society stands as a beacon of unity and truth in a world too often divided by creed, race, and nationality. Our purpose is to seek the deeper mysteries of life—to explore the wisdom that lies beneath the surface of all religions, philosophies, and sciences. We do not align ourselves with any single creed, for our mission transcends the limitations of dogma. Instead, we strive to synthesize the ancient wisdom of the East with the intellectual vigor of the West, offering a platform for all who are earnestly searching for spiritual enlightenment and the answers to life's most profound questions.

"Our objectives are clear and vital: to form a nucleus of the universal brotherhood of humanity—embracing all people, regardless of race, creed, sex, caste, or color; to encourage the study of the great religions, philosophies, and sciences, both ancient and modern; and to investigate the unexplained laws of nature and the powers latent within every human being. The Theosophical Society calls upon each of you to rise above the divisions that separate us and to engage in the noble pursuit of truth. Through spiritual growth, intellectual development, and ethical living, we can contribute to the evolution of human consciousness and move toward a world of greater harmony and enlightenment.

"Tonight," she continued, "we are honored to welcome one of our most distinguished members, Mr. Charles Leadbeater, who will speak to us on the subject of 'The Inner Life.'" A ripple of anticipation moved through the crowd. "I am certain his words will inspire and enlighten us."

Besant stepped aside, and Charles Leadbeater took the podium. He was tall, perhaps in his late 50s, with a full beard and hair streaked with white. He wore a formal black suit without a tie. A silver cross on a long chain hung across his chest. He looked every bit the intellectual mystic. His voice was gentle yet assured, and he began without preamble.

The Seven Planes of Being

"We all know that we have a body—that much is obvious.[215] What is not obvious, but becomes quickly evident once we begin the spiritual journey, is that the physical body is only the lowest level of our being. It is but the outermost manifestation of our true nature. To one who knows how to look, it becomes clear that we exist on seven planes. The lowest—the gross physical plane—is where our body lives, ages, and dies in accordance with the laws of physics. But in the other planes, different laws apply.

"The seven planes in which we exist are the *physical*, the *etheric*, the *astral*, the *mental*, the *causal*, the *buddhic*, and the *atmic*. Allow me to briefly describe each so we may understand how they relate—and how the inner light flows between them.

"The etheric body is a more subtle form of the physical body, composed of finer matter. It is sometimes called our 'etheric double' and serves as a bridge between our physical form and the higher planes. It is through the etheric body that energy—such as prana—vitalizes and sustains our physical health. Healing occurs through its influence.

"The astral body is our desire body—the seat of emotions, feelings, and psychic energies. It is the source of dreams, instincts, and visions.

"The mental body comes next and has two aspects: the lower and the higher. The lower mental plane is the realm of thought, logic, and reason—the faculties we use to navigate daily life. The higher mental plane is home to intuition, abstract thought, and spiritual intelligence. It is the gateway to insight and realization.

"The causal body exists in the causal plane, which some consider part of the higher mental plane. This is the seat of the soul—the true self. Here we store the experiences and lessons gathered over many lives. The causal body is immortal and continues beyond the cycles of birth and death.

"The buddhic body exists in a plane of unity and spiritual intuition. This is where enlightenment and oneness are realized—where the self dissolves into vast compassion and interconnection.

"Finally, we arrive at the atmic body, the highest and most spiritual of all. Here resides divine will and purpose. It is the soul's destiny to rise beyond physical, emotional, and mental boundaries and unite with the divine."

As Leadbeater spoke, Iyengar jotted down a few observations in a small notebook he had brought. Leaning slightly over his shoulder, Iyer observed the young man write two titles in neat, cursive strokes across the top of a blank page. On the left, he wrote: *Theosophical View*; on the right: *Samkhya*.

Beneath the Theosophical heading, Iyengar listed the planes Leadbeater had described: physical, etheric, astral, mental-lower, mental-higher, causal, buddhic, atmic. Between each, he drew lines with double arrowheads, indicating reciprocal movement or influence. For the higher mental and causal levels, however, he drew a circle around both, perhaps to mark their closeness or overlap.

Under the *Samkhya* heading, he added seven classical categories: bhuta (gross elements), tanmatra (subtle elements), indriya (senses), manas (mind), ahamkara (ego), buddhi/mahat (intelligence), and purusha (consciousness).

Then he began connecting the concepts between columns with lines and arrows—some confident, others tentative. He drew arrows from bhuta to the physical plane;

tanmatra and indriya both linked to the etheric, though the latter was marked with a question mark. Manas received two connections—one to the astral plane and another to the lower mind, each with a hesitant squiggle and more question marks. Ahamkara was tied to the causal plane, buddhi to the buddhic plane—again with a question mark. Finally, he linked purusha to the atmic plane and placed one last question mark beside it. He noted prakriti but seemed unsure where that concept fit in.

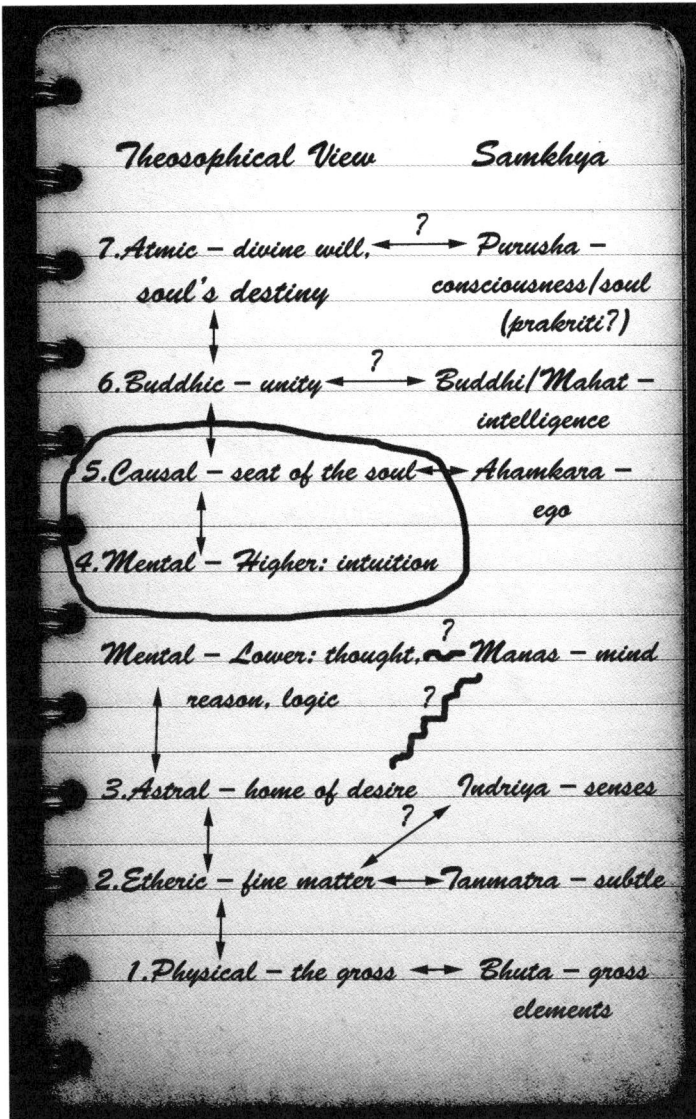

Figure 8: Mr. Iyengar's notes comparing the Seven Planes of Theosophy to Samkhya's Hierarchy.

It was clear to Iyer that his young guest was struggling to reconcile Leadbeater's layered cosmology with the Samkhya system. While the buddhic plane sounded like buddhi, they were clearly not the same. The Samkhya system, Iyer thought, for all its elegance, was primitive compared to the clairvoyantly observed reality that Leadbeater was now revealing.

The Force Centers

Having described the seven planes of existence, Leadbeater paused for a sip of water before continuing. "Within the etheric body are spinning wheels or vortices of energy, which the Mahatmas—those masters of the subtle realms—called chakras. The word chakra means 'wheel' or 'disc' in Sanskrit. I prefer the term, 'force center.' These are not physical objects but, rather, energy hubs through which the life force, known as prana, flows.

"Prana, also called vitality, is a universal life force found throughout nature. It exists everywhere but is especially abundant in sunlight, which radiates it toward us. This vitality fills the atmosphere and is absorbed by all living creatures through the breath."

He glanced around the attentive crowd, then added, "Raw prana enters the body through the spleen—what I call the spleen force center. From there, it is transmuted and distributed throughout the physical body. Prana is refined into distinct currents, each serving different functions to support health and vitality. Clairvoyantly, it appears as a fine, luminous mist—tiny particles of light that permeate the air."

Once again, Mr. Iyer noticed Iyengar jotted down a note: "spleen force center?" Clearly, this term was unfamiliar to him. He began sketching a diagram of the traditional seven chakras along a simple outline of the spine: muladhara, svadhisthana, manipura, anahata, visuddha, ajna, and sahasrara. But he quickly realized that Leadbeater's sequence would not align with this classical model—especially regarding the second and third centers.

Leadbeater resumed: "When prana flows properly, the body remains in health and balance. But if it is blocked or overly intensified, it can cause weakness, agitation, or overstimulation.

"Distinct from prana is another energy, known as the serpent-fire, which the Mahatmas and others have called kundalini. Whereas prana is essential for bodily and subtle health, serpent-fire is spiritual. It lies latent below the first force center and must be awakened with great care. When properly aroused, it vitalizes the chakras and brings about profound spiritual transformation—including psychic abilities such as clairvoyance." His voice grew firm. "But let me caution you: this fire must not be awakened lightly. To tamper with it without guidance is perilous. The breath and the mind must be disciplined under the tutelage of a master."

He then clarified: "Electricity, as we know it, is merely one expression of universal energy. Other forms include heat, light, and motion. Prana is yet another—distinct and not interchangeable with these others. Likewise, serpent-fire may appear similar in the lower planes, but in the higher realms, it is of a different order. It is like liquid fire rushing through the body, spiraling like the coils of a serpent."

He paused, his tone grave. "In the average person, serpent-fire lies dormant at the base of the spine, completely unsuspected. It is far better to leave it sleeping until one has attained sufficient moral development. Only with strong will and purity of thought can one endure its awakening without harm. Uncontrolled, it can cause physical pain, tear tissues, and even destroy the physical body."

Leadbeater paused again, letting the gravity of his words sink in.

Iyengar took the moment to jot another note in his book: "Kundalini = Serpent-fire = Dangerous." Beside it, he added a small checkmark, as though to affirm the warning from his own experience or training.

After taking another sip of water, Leadbeater continued, "The function of each force center is to bring down into physical consciousness whatever quality is inherent in its corresponding astral center."

The Root Center

"The first, the root force center at the base of the spine, radiates in four spokes—like the petals of a flower. These undulate, giving the impression of quadrants with hollow spaces between them, as though marked with the sign of the cross. When fully awakened, this center glows with a fiery orange-red light. It is the seat of the serpent-fire. This force exists on all planes and, once awakened, activates all the other centers. The astral body, initially inert and unconscious, begins to awaken through this force."

The Solar Plexus Center

"The second center, located at the solar plexus in the upper abdomen, has ten undulations or petals. It's associated with emotion and sensitivity to astral influences. Its predominant colors are blended reds and greens. Once activated by the serpent-fire, this center brings the ability to *feel* astral vibrations—though not yet to see or understand them clearly."

The Spleen Center

"The third, the spleen center—lower than the second, on the left side of the abdomen—is the gateway for prana or vitality from the sun. It has six sun-like petals and glows radiantly. This center specializes and distributes vitality throughout the body and enables astral travel, sometimes with partial memory upon return."

The Heart Center

"The fourth, at the center of the chest, is golden in color. Each of its four quadrants is further divided into three parts, creating 12 spokes or petals. When awakened, this center endows the person with empathy—the ability to intuitively understand the joys and sorrows of other astral entities."

The Throat Center

"The fifth, located at the throat, has 16 petals and is mostly blue, with a shimmering, silvery effect—like moonlight on water. Once activated, it enables *clairaudience*, allowing the person to hear voices or music on the astral plane."

The Brow Center

"The sixth, at the brow between the eyebrows, appears divided into two halves: one rose-yellow, the other purplish-blue. Each half contains 48 spokes, for a total of 96 petals. This center awakens *astral sight*—the ability to perceive subtle forms and visions. Early awakening may produce vague shapes or colorful mists; full development brings clear clairvoyance."

Leadbeater paused for emphasis. "The brow center also enables minute physical vision. A fine, flexible tube of etheric matter extends from it, ending in a microscopic eye. This organ can contract or expand, allowing etheric magnification."

The Crown Center

"The seventh, at the crown of the head, is the most resplendent of all—vibrant with indescribable color and vibrating with near-inconceivable speed. Its full awakening completes the development of the astral body. A person whose crown center is awakened can consciously leave and return to the physical body, maintaining awareness through sleep and death.

"For many, the sixth and seventh centers converge upon the pituitary body, a gland in the brain just behind the eyes, which acts as the sole bridge between the physical and higher planes. In others, the sixth remains at the pituitary, but the seventh aligns with the atrophied pineal gland, a small structure near the center of the brain."

Iyengar's Notes and Doubts

As Leadbeater spoke, Iyengar carefully noted the descriptions, comparing them to the teachings he had received. The most jarring difference was the spleen center, which replaced the classical svadhisthana (sacral) chakra. According to tradition, svadhisthana was aligned with the reproductive organs, but Leadbeater had omitted any such reference. He also noted the shift away from spinal alignment. Whereas the yogic chakras were said to rise along the sushumna nadi within the spine, Leadbeater's centers appeared to be positioned according to glands: the spleen, the pituitary, and the pineal. He laid down his pen and simply listened, trying to reconcile the two models in his mind.

Leadbeater continued, "When the serpent-fire has passed through all these centers in a certain order—which varies according to the individual—consciousness becomes continuous up to the entry into the world beyond the end of life. By this, I mean that a person may achieve an unbroken awareness that persists through the transition from physical death, through the astral realm, and into the mental plane—what we call the heaven-world. This represents a high stage of spiritual development, where the soul remains conscious throughout the afterlife process. It is a state of profound peace and spiritual enjoyment before the next incarnation is undertaken."

He paused again, allowing the weight of his words to settle over the rooftop gathering.

"I have heard it suggested," he resumed, "that the different petals of each force-center represent distinct moral qualities, and that the development of those qualities brings the centers into activity. I must respectfully disagree. I have found no evidence to support this theory, nor can I conceive how it would function in reality.

"Beyond sustaining the physical body, these centers serve another function, one that only comes into play when they are awakened. Each etheric center corresponds to an astral counterpart. The etheric vortex lies on the surface of the etheric body, while the astral center is often deep within the astral form. During astral awakening, a man in his physical consciousness remains completely unaware of the changes taking place. To bring these benefits into the physical realm, the awakening must also occur at the etheric level. And this is achieved in exactly the same way: by arousing the serpent-fire—now clothed in etheric matter and sleeping at the base of the spine."

He leaned slightly forward as if to underscore the importance of what came next. "This arousing must be done through determined and sustained effort of the will. When the first center is activated, the force released is so powerful that it vivifies all the others in succession."

Leadbeater drew his remarks to a close. "As I finish my talk tonight, let me summarize the essence of our teaching and our work at the Theosophical Society: *The purpose of human life is spiritual evolution*—achieved through the awakening of higher consciousness, the continuous refinement of our subtle bodies, and the realization of our divine nature. This, ultimately, leads to union with a greater spiritual reality. The tools we use are meditation, breath, and disciplined self-inquiry—but always under strict and knowledgeable guidance. And what I have offered you this evening is not speculation, but the direct result of testable clairvoyant observation."

He bowed his head slightly. "Thank you—and may your evening be filled with peace."

Points of Departure:
Prana, Scripture, and Ethics

When the applause finally abated, Mr. Iyar turned to Mr. Iyengar with eyebrows raised in enquiry. Iyengar smiled and said, "Well, a lot to think about. I confess to some confusion over the descriptions Mr. Leadbeater provided. They do not seem to tally with the classical texts on such matters. For example, the subtle bodies and the chakras are described rather differently."

"While that may be true," admitted Mr. Iyar, "we must remember that Master Leadbeater's descriptions come from personal observation thanks to his years of study, practice, and his unique clairvoyant abilities. I would sooner trust his direct report of these energies and force centers than credit the second-hand words of sages long passed. Where yogis spoke of prana, kundalini, and chakras, in today's world, science has revealed the true nature of energy, vitality, and electricity. According to Master Leadbeater, science is just starting to realize the vast range and forms of energies not yet observable by their advanced instruments. In time, I am certain that all he has stated will be confirmed as accurate. Allow me to introduce you so you can ask your questions."

Mr. Iyar took Mr. Iyengar's hand and walked him over to the small crowd gathered around Leadbeater. They waited politely until the group thinned out, then Mr. Iyar made the introduction.

"Brother Leadbeater, may I introduce you to Mr. Subramanian Iyengar, a reporter for *The Hindu*. He listened quite intently to your talk and has taken copious notes in his journal. He has a few questions for you, if you have the time."

"Certainly!" replied Leadbeater. "I am delighted to meet you, Mr. Iyengar."

Mr. Iyengar resisted an urge to make yet another jotting in his book and instead committed to memory the fact that Mr. Iyar had addressed Mr. Leadbeater as "brother". He had the feeling that he was witnessing the interactions of members of a monastery, or perhaps even a cult. Having made this mental note, he smiled and addressed Mr. Leadbeater.

"I did enjoy your presentation, but I confess to some confusion. I am new to *The Hindu* as a reporter, but I have studied the *darshanas* of Indian philosophy and practiced yoga under the guidance of my guru.[216] Your presentation on prana, kundalini, and the chakras is quite different from what I've learned. For instance, I've been taught that the chakras are aligned along the spine, yet you place them instead in association with glands or nerve plexuses. You've also added a new one—the spleen force center—apparently replacing the svadhisthana, the second chakra, which traditionally corresponds to the genitals."

Leadbeater paused before answering. "You raise a significant concern. The classical yogic texts do describe the chakras as aligned along, or even within, the spine, and I respect that view. However, in my own clairvoyant investigations, I've observed an additional energy center near the spleen, which I call the spleen chakra. It plays a crucial role in the absorption and distribution of prana. While not mentioned in the shastras, my experience suggests it is highly active and integral to our energy system in ways that ancient texts may not have addressed."

"Hmmm," murmured Mr. Iyengar, still unconvinced. "Perhaps we can return to that, but please clarify your view of prana. You claimed that prana comes from the sun. Traditional texts don't identify the sun as the source of prana—prana is the power of life, expressed in multiple forms. Some systems speak of as many as ten *vayus*, though only five are usually emphasized. I didn't hear mention of them in your talk, though I understand time was short."

"Ah, an excellent point," Leadbeater replied. "Prana is indeed a universal life force, but in my observations, the sun acts as a conduit, channeling it toward our planet. Through clairvoyance, I have seen prana absorbed from sunlight—particularly by the etheric body—which then sustains physical vitality. The sun may not create prana, but it facilitates its distribution. This interpretation may differ from the traditional view, but it reflects how prana functions in our solar system."

"And what of the five vayus? Have you observed them?"

"I'm familiar with the classical teachings about the vayus—prana, apana, vyana, udana, and samana—and they are vital for understanding the inner flow of energy. These teachings are beautifully detailed in the Hatha Yoga Pradipika and other texts. But my focus has been to make prana accessible to those without extensive yogic training."

Leadbeater went on, "Vitality—as I call prana—is the life force not only for the physical body, but also for the etheric and astral bodies. Rather than emphasizing internal subdivisions such as the *vayus*, I have chosen to focus on how individuals can work practically with vitality and serpent-fire to stimulate spiritual awakening. The traditional classifications are valuable, but they are not essential to the work I do."

"I see," said Mr. Iyengar slowly. "But in simplifying these teachings to make them accessible, you seem to have abandoned the Vedic framework entirely. There was no mention of the deities, who in tantra are essential to chakra understanding. Nor did you reference the ethical precepts—the *yamas* and *niyamas*—or the authoritative sutras and shastras. I fear that relying solely on personal revelation could lead to self-deception—or what we call *avidya*."

Leadbeater paused, his tone becoming more conciliatory. "I hear your concerns, Mr. Iyengar—and they are valid from the standpoint of a Vedic scholar. It's true that I have not emphasized deities or theological frameworks. But that is not to dismiss them. Rather, I attempt to express the universal principles beneath those frameworks—principles that can speak to seekers of all backgrounds.

"As for the yamas and niyamas, the ethical precepts—they are crucial. But I believe their intent can be conveyed without Sanskrit. Non-violence, truthfulness, purity, and self-discipline are universal values. In my view, working with the force centers and higher planes naturally awakens these ethical faculties. The path inward demands a pure heart and a steady mind."

"And the scriptures? The Vedas, the Upanishads, the Yoga Sutras?"

"They contain profound wisdom," Leadbeater acknowledged. "But my work is not meant to replace them—it is meant to inspire people to explore both the outer teachings and their inner experience. My observations come from deep spiritual inquiry. They are not a substitute for tradition, but a complement—an invitation to look again at what has always been present."

He paused briefly. "And your concern about avidya is well taken. That is why I emphasize discipline and guidance in awakening the serpent-fire. The spiritual path must always be approached with humility and care—no matter what tradition one follows."

Mr. Iyer, recognizing that the hour was growing late, interjected to forestall further questions. "I am sure you must have many other questions, Mr. Iyengar, and perhaps we will have the chance to see you in future rooftop sessions. But I know Brother Leadbeater has had a long day, and there are still others here he must meet. So perhaps we can bid him a good evening and return to your carriage?"

"Yes, yes, of course," said Mr. Iyengar. He too felt the urge to leave—not out of rudeness, but from a deep desire to sit down and transcribe the many thoughts swirling in his mind. He had a deadline to meet and would need the quiet hours of the night to shape his notes into tomorrow's article. "Thank you both for your kind invitation and stimulating conversations. I do hope to return again in the future."

As soon as Mr. Iyengar took his leave, Mr. Leadbeater was approached by Madame Besant and taken to meet another guest. Mr. Iyer walked Iyengar back to the main gate in silence—for which Iyengar was grateful. The stillness gave him space to organize his reflections, to weigh Leadbeater's revelations against the teachings of his own tradition. They said their farewells quietly at the gate.

Headline News

Early on Tuesday morning, Mr. Iyer brought the newspaper directly to Brother Leadbeater's quarters. In the bottom half of the front page, a column appeared with the following:

The Theosophical Society: Bridging East and West or Straying from Tradition?

By Subramanian Iyengar

In a thought-provoking rooftop talk this past Sunday at the Theosophical Society's headquarters in Adyar, Charles Leadbeater offered his unique interpretation of ancient yogic concepts of chakras, prana, and kundalini—raising both curiosity and concern. While Leadbeater's ideas have captivated many with their accessibility and universal appeal, his omission of traditional Vedic elements—such as the gods and goddesses, the yamas and niyamas of ethical conduct, and the reliance on scriptures—leaves one wondering whether his teachings drift too far from the roots upon which they are based.

Continued on page 34

A New Chakra Epoch

In 1858, the British Raj officially took control of what was then called India, encompassing today's India, Pakistan, and Bangladesh. Nearby colonies like Ceylon (now Sri Lanka) and Burma (now Myanmar) were also under British rule. With this colonial presence came Western scholars eager to learn the languages, philosophies, and spiritual traditions of South Asia. This exchange of ideas wasn't one-way. Teachers from India—most famously Swami Vivekananda, Swami Rama Tirtha, Swami Abhedananda, and Paramahansa Yogananda—also traveled westward, introducing Indian spirituality to new audiences.

Vivekananda, in particular, championed Vedanta and raja yoga, while also adapting his message to resonate with Western listeners. The flow of ideas became a two-way current. Western seekers—some with spiritual intent, others with imperial motivations—also began shaping how Indian concepts would be interpreted abroad.

Among the most influential groups seeking to merge Eastern and Western traditions was the Theosophical Society. Claiming to synthesize the world's spiritual wisdom, Theosophy presented itself as a path to universal truth. However, it was plagued by scandal from the outset. Blavatsky claimed to be in contact with mysterious beings known as the Mahatmas, who allegedly guided her teachings. Critics, including French metaphysician René Guénon, considered these claims fraudulent and dangerous.[217]

Guénon viewed Theosophy as a corruption of authentic traditions—an incoherent mix of Hinduism, Buddhism, and Western occultism divorced from sacred lineages. He believed that Annie Besant and Charles Leadbeater, who took over the society's leadership in the early twentieth century, led it even further astray. Leadbeater's teachings on chakras and kundalini, according to Guénon, lacked grounding in any classical source and were little more than imaginative fiction dressed up in spiritual garb.

For centuries, yogic and spiritual teachings in India had been passed down through lineage (*parampara*) or documented in authoritative scriptures. In contrast, Theosophical teachings relied on clairvoyant revelations and personal visions. This lack of standardization raised red flags, particularly because Leadbeater's teachings were shared broadly, without the protective framework of a guru–disciple relationship.

In traditional yogic systems, awakening kundalini energy is considered a serious undertaking that must be done under the supervision of a realized teacher. Leadbeater, by contrast, offered his teachings to the general public through books and lectures. To many critics, this democratization of secret knowledge was irresponsible at best, dangerous at worst.

Yet, as later scholars point out, Guénon's views—while rigorous—may have been overly dismissive. Theosophy did play a meaningful role in introducing Hindu and Buddhist ideas to Western audiences. Even if it distorted the source material, it helped spark a broader interest in Eastern spirituality during the esoteric revival of the late nineteenth and early twentieth centuries.

Regardless of whether Theosophy is viewed as a legitimate movement or a misguided one, its influence is undeniable. Leadbeater's writings were instrumental in bringing the terms prana, kundalini, and chakra into Western vocabularies—though often in ways that diverged significantly from classical interpretations. Alongside him, Sir John Woodroffe (1865–1936), writing as Arthur Avalon, helped usher in "a new epoch in the development of the chakra system."[218]

Woodroffe lived a dual life as a British judge in Calcutta and a scholar of tantra. Unlike Leadbeater, Woodroffe based his work on Sanskrit texts such as the Shat-Chakra-Nirupana. His 1919 book *The Serpent Power* offered a more faithful, albeit academically filtered, interpretation of the traditional chakra and kundalini teachings. While Woodroffe and Leadbeater approached the subject from different angles—one as a translator of scripture, the other as a self-proclaimed clairvoyant—both were instrumental in shaping how chakras would be understood in the West.

From Mysticism to Modern Wellness

Kurt Leland's *Rainbow Body: A History of the Western Chakra System from Blavatsky to Brennan* traces how the chakra model evolved throughout the twentieth century. From the beginning, there was no consensus on how many chakras existed or what their roles were. Leadbeater's *The Hidden Side of Things* (1913) and *The Chakras* (1927) introduced a seven-center system based on his own clairvoyant experiences, complete with vivid, colored illustrations and psychological associations.

Woodroffe's *The Serpent Power*, released between Leadbeater's two books, remained rooted in classical tantric texts. Yet even his interpretations were shaped by his colonial context and scholarly method. These two streams—Theosophical vision and academic translation—would converge over the decades into the modern Western chakra model.

By the mid-to-late twentieth century, authors like Anodea Judith helped establish the version most yoga students now know: seven energy centers aligned with the spine, each assigned a color from the rainbow and linked to human needs such as safety, creativity, love, and spiritual awakening. Neither Leadbeater nor classical texts described this color-coded system. Leland wryly notes that any system with seven parts today—from endocrine glands to musical notes—can be mapped onto the chakras.

Leadbeater's emphasis on chakras as emotional and psychological centers found fertile ground in the West, particularly among those interested in holistic health. The idea that blocked or unbalanced chakras could lead to physical or emotional issues became widespread, particularly in New Age and alternative healing communities. Depth psychologist Carl Jung added to this framework by interpreting chakras as symbols of psychological archetypes and stages of personal development.

What once had been a metaphysical framework for awakening divine consciousness gradually became a tool for therapeutic self-inquiry and personal growth. This shift—from transcendent liberation to psychological integration—marks a major turning point in the chakra model's evolution.

As with the chakras, the concepts of prana and kundalini were simplified and reinterpreted in the West. Traditionally, prana is understood as an air that moves through nadis (energy channels), governed by five main vayus (currents) and directed by breath and posture. In Leadbeater's version, prana becomes a form of vitality absorbed from the sun through the spleen chakra and distributed throughout the body—much easier to grasp for a Western audience unfamiliar with hatha yoga's intricacies.

Similarly, kundalini in classical texts is portrayed as a latent, potentially perilous force that must be awakened with care. Leadbeater reframed it as a spiritual energy that could be accessed through inner development and clairvoyant practice. This framing helped move kundalini into the realm of personal empowerment and psychic development, eventually making it a cornerstone of the New Age movement.

By mid-century, both concepts had largely detached from their roots. Prana became synonymous with "life energy" and kundalini with personal awakening—often stripped of the rigorous preparation and moral frameworks emphasized in classical yoga. With a desire to map current science to yoga philosophies, yoga teachers began to graft modern medical theories onto the branches of traditional yoga. This trend manifested in the teachings of Dr. Motoyama and influenced his melding of the Eastern views of prana, nadis, chi, and meridians with the new Western views of Energy Medicine.

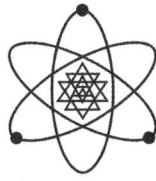

CHAPTER 20:

Energy Medicine

Sarah Powers stood before us in the main room. It was the morning of January 4, 2005—the first full day of the ten-day Yin & Yang yoga teacher training intensive at the White Sulphur Springs retreat center in Napa Valley, California.

Around me, students sat on cushions—some with notepads, others with only the white binder Sarah had just handed out. Also present were her husband, Ty, and Paul and Suzee Grilley. After going over course logistics and readings, Sarah outlined the three main objectives of her yin yoga teaching:

- to explain the concepts of yin, chi, and meridians;
- to teach how to move chi through breathwork and pranayama;
- to introduce us to Buddhist psychology.

What struck me most was how seamlessly Sarah blended Daoist, Buddhist, and yogic traditions into a single, integrated teaching. For example, she explained that *pratyahara*, the fifth limb of Patanjali's eightfold path—typically understood as closing off the senses—can take on different flavors. In its fully yin form, it means complete withdrawal from sensory input. But in a yin–yang version, the senses remain open, yet there is no inner reaction to what arises.

"This," she said, "is the realm of psychotherapy."

Yoga alone, she cautioned, doesn't integrate the whole personality. Asana can't resolve early trauma or ingrained emotional patterns. Her words rekindled my desire to know my own mind more deeply—and to recommit to meditation. But I was equally fascinated by her insights into the Daoist view of energy.

"No one English word or phrase can adequately capture Qi's meaning," claims Ted Kaptchuk, author of *The Web That Has No Weaver*,[219] which Sarah recommended.

Unlike prana, which is more often linked to breath and vitality, qi or chi is the underlying nature of everything—animate and inanimate, including thoughts and emotions. Poetically, Kaptchuk calls it "the pulsation of the whole cosmos."

Chi is not a substance. It's not energy or matter. It's the ground of being and becoming. It doesn't "cause" change—it is the transformation itself. Chi doesn't arrive or depart; it shifts form. Chi is relational. One form of chi can resonate with another to activate potential. The chi in a seed resonates with the chi in the soil, the sun, the rain—and the plant grows. In this way, chi is both yin and yang.

Chi has several sources. We are given a measure of chi before we are even born. This is termed prenatal chi. Consider this like your genes and DNA; you had no say in what you inherited, but these gifts will have a big role to play in your life, growth, health, and death. The second source is the chi we obtain after birth, called postnatal chi. We receive this through our food, called grain chi (*gu-qi*), and from the air we breathe (*kong-qi*). While prenatal chi is fixed—like a trust fund account you can only withdraw from—grain chi and air chi function like a checking account. To prolong life, it makes sense to draw primarily from this postnatal chi and preserve the original reserve as long as possible.

Daoist theory describes five vital substances or "textures":
- *chi* (life force)
- *jing* (vitality)[220]
- *shen* (spirit)
- *Blood* (broader than the Western concept)
- *fluids* (everything from saliva to semen to bile)

Blood, in this model, moves not just through arteries but also through meridians. The term shen is especially nuanced. It encompasses multiple aspects of spirit or soul, including:
- *zhi*: willpower or innate drive, akin to fate—an unconscious movement toward one's path.
- *yi*: intention or reflective thought, close to the yogic viveka (discernment).
- *po*: the somatic, instinctual soul tied to the body and extinguished at death—like Aristotle's animal soul.
- *hun*: the ethereal soul that survives death, beyond the purview of medicine and into the domain of priests.
- *shen proper*: the relational spirit housed in the heart, guiding our social and spatial connections.

Shen, Jing, and Chi

To Sarah, there is a hierarchy between shen, jing, and chi: shen is the essence of jing, and jing is the essence of chi. "Jing," she said, "is birth energy—it brings us into being. It's associated with the water element and housed in the Kidneys."[221]

According to Ted Kaptchuk, jing is the texture specific to life. Much like prana in traditional Indian thought, jing is the vitality that governs the entire arc of existence.

In women, jing unfolds in seven seven-year cycles. At age seven, adult teeth replace baby teeth. By 14, the "dew of heaven" arrives—the onset of menstruation. At 21, maturity peaks. At 28, the body is at its strongest. But from there, decline begins: at 35, the face darkens and hair begins to thin. At 42, whitening begins. At 49, the "waters of heaven" dry up—menopause arrives.

Men experience eight eight-year cycles, with similar patterns of growth, peak, and eventual decline. By 64, according to the ancient model, hair and teeth are gone, and life nears its end.

Sarah went on to repeat much of what she had discussed at the festival in Seattle. Jing governs growth, development, and decay. If it is weak, decline comes early; if abundant, vitality is extended. Both chi and jing involve movement. Jing governs long-term processes, while chi animates shorter-term functions. Jing, as the "root of life," is the source of prenatal chi. From it, chi arises—hence Sarah's claim that jing is the essence of chi.

Where Are the Meridians?

Sarah showed us the general routing of the meridians and which postures might stimulate the flow of chi through them. Fortunately, we weren't training to be acupuncturists—we didn't need to memorize all the acupuncture points. Instead, we learned the general paths of the major meridians and how they related to sensation during long-held postures. If a pose created stress across or along the line of a meridian, it might be enhancing chi flow through that channel.

Using illustrations from Kaptchuk's *The Web That Has No Weaver*, Sarah introduced the twelve main meridians. The six lower-body meridians include the yin channels—the Spleen, Liver, and Kidney—running along the inner legs; and the yang channels—the Stomach, Gallbladder, and Urinary Bladder—running along the front, sides, and back of the legs and torso. The six upper-body meridians include the Heart, Lung, Large Intestine, and Small Intestine, along with two channels that don't correspond directly to Western organs: the Pericardium and Triple Burner. These flow through the arms and hands.

"It's impossible to work with something you're not aware of," Sarah said. "And it's hard to become aware of something if you're resisting it. What's required is curiosity and interest." These, she emphasized, are foundational tools of mindfulness.

"If we want to stimulate chi flow, we must learn mindfulness. While there are physical and psychological benefits to our yoga practices, from an energetic perspective, the benefits include generating communication signals, which are constantly being sent to all tissues. These signals help to heal and maintain the meridian system. Our practice also removes the dams, which are energy blockages in the energy's riverbeds. In turn, this enhances the flow of chi, increases vitality, and harmonizes energetic activities."

The image of rivers is apt. While meridian charts resemble maps, meridians are more like watersheds: each major channel is fed by countless tiny tributaries. Every cell in the body needs chi, and just as arteries branch into arterioles and capillaries, meridians subdivide to reach even the smallest cells.

Paul reminded us not to mistake acupuncture charts for the whole system. The lines shown are only the surface meridians—those accessible by needle. Beneath them lie deeper and broader energy channels. These "reservoirs of chi," as Paul called them, send energy to the surface and back again. With training, one can learn to feel chi moving through muscles, bones, and even internal organs.[222]

Still, I wondered, *Are meridians real? Do they physically exist?* To explore that question, I would need to study one of Sarah and Paul's key teachers: Dr. Hiroshi Motoyama.

A Modern Shaman

In the late 1970s, Paul Grilley had come across *Autobiography of a Yogi* by Paramahansa Yogananda—the same book that would later inspire Saul David Raye's pilgrimage to India. In it, Yogananda recounts tales of Indian adepts with extraordinary powers, some of which Patanjali describes in the Yoga Sutras as siddhis or *vibhutis*: levitation, healing, bilocation, telepathy, materialization of objects, and control over bodily functions beyond ordinary limits.[223] He sent off a request for information to the organization Yogananda had founded, the Self-Realization Fellowship (SRF), and they duly replied.

Paul also visited a bookstore in his small Montana town, hoping to learn more about yoga. Of the three books available on the topic, one seemed way too complicated. He chose the simplest offering. From these sources, Paul began his yoga practice. A few months later, a friend showed him a book by Bikram Choudhury that featured a photograph of Yogananda and his brother, Bishnu Charan Ghosh—whom Bikram claimed as his teacher.[224] Yogananda had reappeared in Paul's life.

In the 1980s, making a living through yoga was unthinkable, so Paul pursued anatomy studies, thinking he might become a chiropractor or physical therapist. After moving to Los Angeles and enrolling at UCLA, he began studying with Bikram and opened his own yoga studio, sometimes practicing for up to six hours a day. Eventually, a falling out with Bikram led him to David Williams, who was sharing the ashtanga sequences he had learned from Pattabhi Jois. With David's guidance, Paul worked through Jois's third series and rediscovered the book he'd once dismissed as too complex—*Light on Yoga* by B.K.S. Iyengar. He set himself the goal of mastering every pose in it.

Later, as his understanding of anatomy deepened, Paul realized the limits imposed by skeletal compression and individual bone variation. No one, he concluded, can do every yoga pose. In his push to go deeper, he had injured himself. Clearly, yoga was about more than asanas. Yogananda himself had barely mentioned postures. His emphasis was on breathwork and subtle energy control, using simple movements to direct prana for meditation—not to achieve physical feats. Eventually, Paul stopped pursuing ashtanga and other practices aimed at unbridled flexibility. Instead, he crafted and popularized the style today known as yin yoga.

Yogananda passed away in 1952; Paul never had the chance to meet him. But one day, he discovered *Theories of the Chakras: Bridge to Higher Consciousness*, by Japanese mystic and scientist Dr. Hiroshi Motoyama, published in English in 1981 by the Theosophical Society. In it, Paul found events similar to those described by Yogananda. Awakening of the heart chakra (anahata) allowed Motoyama to perform psychic healing, during which, he claimed, his "astral body entered another person to effect curative changes."[225] He also described levitation through activation of the muladhara chakra.

In this book, Motoyama explained each chakra and the abilities and risks that arise with their activation. He said he had developed powers such as clairvoyance, telepathy, and the ability to perceive and interact with subtle energy fields. He also described experiences involving kundalini and the ability to see chakras and nadis. All these abilities echo the power of the primal shaman: to leave the body, to fight malignant forces and restore health for a stricken person, to journey to the spirit realm and return with boons for those existing in the physical dimension.

But Motoyama was not only a mystic. He held doctoral degrees in philosophy and clinical psychology and served as head priest of Tamamitsu Shrine in Tokyo—a position he had inherited from his adoptive mother, Motoyama Kinue, a renowned spirit medium, yogic adept, and founder of the Tamamitsu Church in 1937.[226] His early training combined rigorous yogic disciplines with traditional Shinto practices, including cold water immersion, fasting, and sleep deprivation.

Among his influences were Swami Satyananda Saraswati (who wrote the introduction to *Theories of the Chakras*), Charles Leadbeater, and Sir John Woodroffe. Motoyama's writings paralleled those of Leadbeater and Woodroffe in many respects, though he clearly distinguished his own experiences and interpretations.

He also offered a compelling historical theory: Chinese meridian theory, he wrote, arose during the Warring States period (ca. 500–400 BCE). Earlier Chinese records mention neither meridians nor chi. During this period, knowledge flowed from South Asia and the Middle East into China through Khotan and Kashmir. Motoyama believed this influx introduced the yogic ideas of prana and nadis to Chinese medicine, which evolved into the concepts of chi (or *ki*, as he spelled and pronounced it) and meridians.[227] To him, these weren't merely similar—they were the same.

Motoyama argued that chakras were directly linked to organs, and thus to the meridians. Just as the Upanishads taught that the human being is a microcosm of the cosmos, Chinese cosmology posited that the same laws govern both macro and micro. While he acknowledged that maps of nadis and meridians might evolve, he believed they pointed to the same subtle energy system—and he cautioned against conflating these channels with the nervous system. For instance, the spinal cord does not extend to the crown of the head, whereas the sushumna nadi does.[228]

Although Paul never met Yogananda, he traveled to Japan in 1989 to study with Motoyama. Later, Sarah also trained with him in acupuncture and meridian theory. "It was like learning to be my own acupuncturist," she said, "but without the needles."[229]

Theosophical Influence

Motoyama taught that humans possess three bodies, each with an associated mind, inhabiting distinct dimensions of existence—just as Charles Leadbeater had proposed. These dimensions are:
- the physical body and its sensory mind
- the astral body, which perceives emotion and desire
- the causal body, the seat of intelligence and wisdom

Each dimension is sustained by a form of prana. Though we may conceptually separate these bodies and minds, they form an organic whole, interconnected through the chakras and a subtle network of nadis, which regulate energy flow.

Paul Grilley summarized this in his book *A Yogi's Guide to Chakra Meditation*: "The causal dimension is the 'Realm of Ideas'. Our thoughts and beliefs reside here. Not just facts, but beliefs in what is right, proper, good. These are the ideas that create our personality. Here are our opinions and beliefs about life. This is the dimension which unconsciously governs our behavior. This is the most powerful dimension, as shown by the fact that people will die for their beliefs despite the harm they may cause their physical body.

"The astral dimension is the home of our feelings in the guise of emotions. This is the home of our personal wants, called the 'Realm of Form and Desire.' Here we plan and work towards fulfilling our hopes and dreams. This is the dimension of 'I,' 'me,' and 'mine.'

"The physical dimension is the world we sense and experience through our physical body and its senses. To a materialist, this is the 'real' world."[230]

Within the physical body, Motoyama recognized familiar anatomical structures—veins, arteries, nerves—as well as meridians, which he asserted were physical but distinct from nerves. Each dimension has corresponding channels and centers. As he wrote: "a chakra works as a center of interchange between the physical and the astral, and between the astral and the causal dimensions. Through the chakras, subtle prana in the astral body can be transformed... into energy for the physical dimension.... Thus the chakra is seen to be an intermediary for energy transfer and conversion between two neighboring dimensions of being."[231] In other words, chakras are the bridges between the dimensions.

For Motoyama, the purpose of spiritual practice is the evolution of consciousness—both individual and collective. To achieve this, we must understand and develop the subtle body, including the chakras and nadis, to facilitate the flow of prana. By purifying the energy channels, awakening the chakras, and mastering the flow of energy, practitioners can deepen spiritual consciousness and overcome ego-driven limitations. He recommended a synthesis of meditation, yoga, and devotional practice to harmonize body, mind, and spirit.

Asana, he taught, plays three vital roles: increasing and balancing prana; strengthening the sushumna nadi; and sharpening concentration on the chakras. Only when prana flows freely through the sushumna can kundalini rise, awakening the chakras fully. Some modern yoga teachers, notably Paul Grilley, have expanded on traditional views of prana by integrating concepts from subtle energy research, particularly those developed by Dr. Hiroshi Motoyama.[232]

Sarah's teachings also reflected Motoyama's understanding. She would often structure a class to deliberately target and affect specific organs and their associated meridians. Motoyama said that asanas increased chi flow and brought balance to the various conditions of energy. Sarah employed these ideas to explain how postures could stimulate chi flow through the meridians to nourish the organs. She offered flows that targeted the Kidneys, Liver, Gall Bladder, Stomach, and others.

Much of what Motoyama taught and wrote, and indeed what Paul Grilley would also discuss and share, was chakra meditation. The goal was always to awaken a chakra, but this was not without its risks. Motoyama gave many examples of how he overused his stomach and heart chakras. The manipura is the main chakra for *receiving* chi, while the anahata is the main chakra for *emitting* chi. If your manipura is out of balance, it may be due to an imbalance between your upper energy, *prana*, and your lower energy, *apana*. This may cause stomach and intestinal problems and emotional issues.[233] If your anahata chakra awakens, you will become capable of spiritual healing. Overusing this chakra may lead to heart disease, heart attack, and an early death.

To avoid such imbalances, Motoyama offered several strategies: use asana to regulate chi via the meridians; enter samadhi while maintaining devotion to the divine; and practice *shoshuten*.

Sarah explained, "Shoshuten is Japanese and means 'circulation of light.' It gathers scattered energy into a corridor of light, amplifies it into an 'energy egg,' and sends it out to drench the meridians and nourish the organs."[234] Shoshuten is also known as the *microcosmic orbit*.[235] In Daoist inner alchemy, mastery of this orbit leads to the formation of the "Golden Flower"—a radiant, immortal body born of yin–yang integration.[236]

Measuring Chi

My notebooks from those 10 days with Paul and Sarah are filled with observations. I wrote phrases like Paul's: "Yoga's basic premise is to move all the major joints through their full range of motion, safely, each day to promote energy flow." Again and again, our discussions returned to the energetics of yoga.

One statement stood out: *chi flows through connective tissue*. If that's true, then chi is not merely symbolic—it's physical. And if chi is physical, it should be measurable. It should be trainable. "Our connective tissue," Paul said, "should be called our meridian tissue!"

The reason meridians were not observed in anatomical dissections is because fascia is routinely removed and discarded—considered inert packaging material, irrelevant to the study of muscles, organs, or nerves. Motoyama believed the watery layers within fascia conduct energy. Since movement stimulates these layers, practices like yoga, massage, and t'ai chi can influence the flow of chi. But Motoyama wasn't content with speculation—he wanted evidence.

To test his ideas, Motoyama invented two devices. The first, thankfully abbreviated to AMI, was a computerized electrical meter.[237] It mapped low-resistance electrical pathways through the body—distinct from nerves or blood vessels. Motoyama believed these were the meridians and nadis of Eastern medicine. The AMI used 28 electrodes placed on the fingers and toes—specifically, on traditional acupuncture points. A low-voltage current (around 3 volts) was passed through these points, and the electrical resistance was measured.[238] Strikingly, if electrodes were even slightly misaligned, the current wouldn't flow. But when correctly positioned, electricity flowed with ease.

Motoyama claimed these low-resistance paths correlated with organ function. A blockage indicated an imbalance; free flow meant health.[239] While not the first or last to explore bioelectric diagnostics,[240] his work was pioneering.

Motoyama's second invention was more ambitious: the Chakra Instrument. It measured electromagnetic activity and light emissions, using a copper disk and a photo-electric cell in an electrically isolated dark room. He tested 100 subjects—grouped as having "active," "inactive," or "partially active" chakras—and claimed he could measure light and electrical changes when subjects meditated on specific chakras.[241] Motoyama said his research "points to the possibility that... energy working in the chakras can extinguish or create energy in the physical dimension."[242]

In Motoyama's model, one he shared with Charles Leadbeater, chakras correspond to organs and nerve plexuses. For example, the anahata (heart) links to the circulatory system; the manipura (solar plexus) relates to digestion; the svadhisthana (sacral) aligns with reproductive function.[243] Unlike Leadbeater, who thought traditional chakras were symbolic and the real energy centers were the glands, Motoyama believed the classical chakra model was real—albeit operating across subtle dimensions.[244]

I admit to some skepticism about Motoyama's chakra detection. He grouped subjects into categories of chakra activity based on intuition, not hard criteria. His publications didn't share raw data or define signal-to-noise ratios. And while it's plausible that focused attention can affect electrical activity or even trigger light emissions (called biophotons), this doesn't necessarily mean a chakra is "active." It could simply reflect increased blood flow or nervous system stimulation.

That said, Motoyama's instruments intrigued me—especially the AMI. It offered empirical evidence that low-resistance pathways exist in the body, and these loosely match traditional meridian maps. This doesn't prove that chi is electricity, or that nadis are real in the way nerves are, but it's suggestive. There is more happening under the skin than classical anatomy has accounted for.

When pressed for more information, Paul pointed me to articles and books to study and people to contact. He turned me on to the early research of Robert O. Becker, who studied the effects of electromagnetic fields on the development and repair of tissues;[245] he suggested I read Gerry Pollack's work on cells, gels, and the engines of life;[246] he strongly suggested I read James Oschman's summary works on energy medicine and the scientific views of what was happening when Eastern practitioners worked with energy.[247] He also told me about research carried out in the laboratory of Helene Langevin and her experiments showing, from a Western perspective, how acupuncture might work.

Fascia Fascinations

Acupuncture meridians traditionally are believed to constitute channels connecting the surface of the body to internal organs. We hypothesize that the network of acupuncture points and meridians can be viewed as a representation of the network formed by interstitial connective tissue.[248]

In their 2002 paper (in which the above quotation appears), Helene Langevin and Jason Yandow proposed that acupuncture meridians correspond to the interfaces between muscle groups. Picture your upper arm: the biceps and triceps are wrapped in fascia called the *epimysium*, which separates them from one another. Above that is the *deep fascia*, and just beneath the skin lies the *superficial fascia*. A thin film of water lubricates these layers, allowing tissues to glide past one another. Langevin and Yandow found that many acupuncture points lie in *cleavage planes*—not in muscles, but between them.[249] When they mapped the traditional meridian lines, 80% of the time, the lines tracked along fascial boundaries.

Motoyama had shown that acupuncture points were entry sites to low electrical resistance pathways. Langevin and Yandow demonstrated that these same points followed the folds of fascia throughout the body. By following their hypothesis, we can predict:

- The Stomach meridian parallels the lateral edge of the *rectus femoris*.
- The Spleen meridian follows its medial edge.
- The Kidney meridian tracks the medial border of the *rectus abdominis*,
- The Bladder meridians flank the lateral edge of the *erector spinae*,
- The Gallbladder meridian follows the *iliotibial band*,

And so on. The ancient maps make modern anatomical sense.

Fascia is everywhere. It envelops and invests all other tissues—organs, bones, muscles, nerves, and vessels. It interconnects everything. Due to this organizational continuum, the outside of our body is intimately connected to the inside.

During embryonic development, a layer within the developing embryo called the *mesodermal* layer becomes our muscles, bones, ligaments, tendons, and fascia, forming an interconnected and continuous network.[250] This network organizes our superficial structures, like skin, and connects them with the deepest structures, such as our organs. Not only does it serve as a physical support to the invested tissues, but it may form a physically interconnected communication system intimately involved in biomechanical signaling as well as bioelectric transmissions.[251] With this image in mind, it is easy to visualize that distant, superficial points on the fingers and toes are connected to organs far away.

Everything is part of one whole. All of our cells (save for a few migratory ones, like immune and blood cells) are embedded within this living scaffold. If energy flows through the body, it likely follows the paths laid by fascia.

Today, we have the tools to more precisely define prana and chi. We can ask, *What is chi? Is it electricity? Or something more?*

Mechanotransduction

In 1892, the German anatomist and surgeon Julius Wolff discovered that bones subjected to mechanical load would strengthen along the lines of stress. This became known as Wolff's Law: bone adapts to the stresses placed upon it. With regular loading, bone becomes denser; without stress, it weakens. A similar principle, Davis's Law, describes how soft tissues—like ligaments, tendons, and fascia—respond by lengthening or strengthening when appropriately stressed.

Both laws reflect a broader biological process called *mechanotransduction*: the transformation of mechanical forces into biochemical signals. In simple terms, physical stress triggers cellular responses. These forces may include tissue deformation, shearing, hydrostatic pressure, or tensile loading. Depending on the strength and duration of these stresses, mechanotransduction can trigger processes like embryonic development, tissue repair, wound healing, or nerve regeneration. But it can also have harmful effects—such as fibrosis, tumor growth, or treatment resistance.[252]

Most cells are physically connected to the fascia and to one another. When we stretch, twist, or compress tissues, the forces ripple through this network, deforming cell shapes, altering their inner support structure (cytoskeleton), and even impacting gene expression via changes to the nuclear membrane. This mechanical cascade—starting from fascia and reaching the cell's interior—can influence nearly every biological system.

Acupuncture and mechanotransduction intersect in fascinating ways. One of Dr. Helene Langevin's core hypotheses is that acupuncture works not via mystical energy flow, but through mechanical signaling in connective tissue. When a needle is inserted and rotated, the practitioner often feels the tissue "grasp" the needle—an effect called *de qi*, essential in traditional acupuncture. Langevin showed that this grasp reflects fascial fibers winding around the needle, producing mechanical stress.

Within the fascia are fibroblasts, cells that produce proteins like collagen and elastin, enzymes like collagenase and protease, and hydrating substances like hyaluronic acid. When fibroblasts are physically deformed for 20 minutes or more, they shift their shape and begin to secrete chemical messengers. These signals propagate through the tissue, potentially affecting cells several centimeters away.

In Langevin's words: "We propose that acupuncture needle manipulation produces cellular changes that propagate along connective tissue planes. These changes may occur no matter where the needle is placed but may be enhanced when the needle is placed at acupuncture points."[253] This reinterprets acupuncture as a fascia-based therapy, grounded not in invisible energy lines but in biomechanical and biochemical signaling—a view that bridges traditional and modern paradigms.

Acupressure Is Acupuncture Without Needles

Dr. Helene Langevin observed that the effects produced by acupuncture needles can also be achieved by simply holding a stretched position for about 30 minutes—the typical time needles remain in place during treatment.[254] Her research showed that when fibroblasts are loaded for this duration, they reorganize their cytoskeletons, reduce tissue stress, and secrete signaling molecules—some of which are known to reduce pain. She proposed this as a key mechanism underlying the benefits of many physical therapies, from massage to stretching, in reducing scar tissue, inflammation, and pain.

Her team explored this further. In one experiment, inflammation was deliberately induced in the lower backs of subjects. A control group received no further intervention, while a test group was given full-body stretches—held for 10 minutes, twice a day. After 12 days, the stretched group showed markedly less inflammation, reduced pain, and improved mobility.[255] The subjects in this experiment were not humans; they were rats, who apparently enjoyed the whole body stretches.

In another experiment, breast cancer cells were injected into the backs of mice. After four weeks, those who received a daily 10-minute stretch had tumors half the size of the control group. Their immune responses were also significantly stronger.

The researchers concluded that daily stretching helped reduce fibrosis, inflammation, and immune dysfunction—factors known to support cancer growth.[256]

Most prior cancer–exercise studies had relied on aerobic exercise, which can be too intense for patients. However, gentle movement practices like yoga, t'ai chi, and qi gong are generally well tolerated. Langevin's team suggested that these forms of exercise provide sufficient physical stress to stimulate fascia and the embedded fibroblasts—eliciting therapeutic effects.

While most yoga postures aren't held for 10 minutes, especially in more active styles, yin yoga—which emphasizes longer holds and passive stress—may approach this cumulative effect. Through repeated postures targeting a specific area, yin yoga can create sufficient *time under stress* to generate benefits similar to acupuncture. In this sense, yin yoga may function as a form of acupressure, stimulating fascia and chi flow without the use of needles.

This supports an emerging view that physical practices, even gentle ones, generate intercellular signals through mechanical stress, fluid dynamics, and tissue stiffness. Whether these signals correspond to chi or prana is still debatable. A century ago, such ideas would have seemed implausible. But the movements and postures prescribed by yoga and Daoist practice do, undeniably, have measurable physiological effects.

That said, questions remain. I find it hard to imagine how a needle placed near the fingernail of the little finger exerts a direct *tensile* effect on the heart. While a fascial continuum between these points may exist, no Western research has yet shown such long-distance mechanical linkages. Even if plausible, can physical stress truly travel such distances through connective tissue alone? I suspect not. If these channels are real, then perhaps they also transmit something else. If not merely mechanical stress, maybe electrical energy? Or maybe something subtler?

The Body Electric

Since the time of Signori Galvani and Volta in eighteenth-century Italy, we have known that the body is both a conductor and a producer of electricity. There are two main types of electricity: the movement of ions and the movement of electrons. Atoms are normally electrically neutral, but when an atom loses an electron, it becomes positively charged; when it gains one, it becomes negatively charged. Such charged atoms are called *ions*. Our bodies are full of ions—we could not live without them.

In physics, like repels like: negative charges repel negative charges, and positives repel positives. Opposites, however, attract. This is why most atoms remain neutral—any imbalance in charge compels movement to restore equilibrium. When electrons move, they generate an *electrical* current. When ions move, they produce an *ionic* current. While both are forms of electricity, the distinction is important when looking at the body's cellular activity.

Every cell has a membrane potential—a voltage across its surface. Inside the cell is a surplus of negatively charged ions, such as chloride, phosphate, and certain proteins. Outside are positively charged ions like calcium, sodium, and magnesium. This separation creates a kind of electrical tension, or potential energy, similar to a ball held above the ground. In cells, this voltage typically ranges between −40 to −90 millivolts.[257]

Though it may sound abstract, ionic currents are vital to life. Without them, neurons could not communicate. These currents regulate gene expression, protein synthesis, cell growth, motility, and even programmed cell death. Every cell functions like a tiny battery, with energy stored in its membrane potential powering many biological processes.

Because of this, cells are exquisitely sensitive to both electric and magnetic fields. In the 1960s and '70s, Dr. Robert O. Becker conducted experiments on limb regeneration in animals. Salamanders, for instance, can regrow a severed leg. Flatworms like planaria can regenerate an entire body from just a slice. Becker showed that by altering the body's electrical fields, he could influence this regeneration—causing salamanders to grow an arm where a leg should be, or planaria to grow multiple heads instead of a tail.

This line of research continues today. Dr. Michael Levin, a biologist at Tufts University, studies what he calls *bioelectrical communication*—a key mechanism in embryonic development and regeneration. How does an embryo know where to grow a head or a heart, feet or hands? Genes alone don't explain it. Levin's research suggests that cells respond to electric fields that envelop the embryo, helping to guide complex pattern formation.[258]

Levin has shown that cells are linked by electrical connections, forming "nanowire networks" that transmit information across long distances. He found that *all* cells—not just neurons—can process information in ways similar to neural networks. These discoveries, he says, may have "transformative implications for advances in regenerative medicine, bioengineering and synthetic biology."[259]

All this depends on ionic currents. Our heartbeat arises from ionic flow. So does nerve conduction, muscle contraction, and even perception. Most of the body's electrical activity is due to ions—but we also generate another form: electron flow. This is the same type of electricity that powers homes and smartphones—and it's also at work in our bones and sensory systems.

Piezoelectricity and Streaming Potentials

Many kids have them—those shoes that light up with every step. And yet, no parent ever needs to buy batteries. So where does the electricity come from? The answer: *piezoelectricity*. The word literally means "electricity from pressure." It shows up in many modern technologies: sonar, ultrasound, quartz watches, even the spark you get when lighting a gas stove. Whenever certain crystals—like quartz or even some metals—are compressed or bent, they generate an electric charge.

Amazingly, our own bodies are also piezoelectric.[260] The collagen fibers in our bones, tendons, skin, and fascia are structured like soft crystals. When these tissues are bent, stretched, or compressed, they generate small electrical currents—brief pulses of moving electrons. These are not ionic currents, like those that fire neurons or regulate the heartbeat. These are electrical currents created by the mechanical deformation of crystalline proteins.

The most famous example of biological piezoelectricity occurs in bone. When bone is mechanically stressed—during yoga, walking, or resistance training—it generates piezoelectric currents that stimulate osteoblasts, the cells responsible for building new bone. This phenomenon is a key mechanism behind Wolff's Law, mentioned above. The stress-induced current is a signal, telling bone cells: "Strengthen this area."[261] The greater the load placed on a bone, the more robust it becomes—provided that stress is safe and not excessive.

Piezoelectric effects are not limited to bones. When cartilage is compressed, or when ligaments and tendons are stretched, the collagen structures in these tissues also generate piezoelectric charges. These may play a role in tissue maintenance, repair, and even regeneration.[262] Some researchers believe this is why practices like yoga, massage, and t'ai chi—which regularly deform connective tissues—can have therapeutic effects.

Even blood vessels and soft tissues exhibit piezoelectric-like responses. Endothelial cells lining our arteries respond to pressure waves in blood flow, triggering electrical signals that regulate vessel stiffness and blood pressure.[263] Mechanosensitive ion channels like *Piezo1* play a central role in vascular development, showing just how intimately our biology is tied to mechanical forces.[264] It's now widely accepted that most biological tissues exhibit some form of piezoelectricity, whether fleeting or sustained.[265]

However, piezoelectricity isn't the only way mechanical stress generates electricity in the body. When stress is sustained over time—such as in a long-held yoga posture or through acupuncture—ions inside the tissues are physically displaced. This creates strain-generated electrical potentials (SGEPs), also called *streaming potentials*. Unlike the quick bursts of electrons from piezoelectricity, SGEPs are longer-lasting ionic currents that persist for as long as the stress remains.

SGEPs arise when stress causes a fluid flow or deformation in a tissue that separates positively and negatively charged particles. This separation creates an ongoing electrical potential—a kind of battery—that informs nearby cells. Cells respond by altering their behavior: they may deposit more collagen, remodel connective tissue, or initiate repair processes. These longer-lived signals are particularly important in processes like cartilage regeneration, ligament healing, and fascial remodeling.[266]

There is debate in the literature about whether the brief, electron-based piezoelectric currents or the longer, ionic SGEPs are more biologically important. The likely answer is both are important. Piezoelectric signals may serve as quick "wake-up calls," while SGEPs may provide the sustained instructions that drive cellular adaptation.

Interestingly, many of the functions that traditional Chinese medicine or yoga philosophy ascribe to prana or chi—like tissue healing, organ nourishment, or energetic realignment—correspond to what scientists now observe when tissues are subjected to physical stresses. If we broaden our definitions of chi and prana to include these bioelectrical effects, their healing roles seem less mystical and more physiological.

As yoga practitioners, bodyworkers, or energy healers, we may be tapping into these bioelectrical systems—knowingly or not—every time we stretch, hold, press, twist, or breathe. Whether we call it chi, prana, or streaming potential, the body listens—and responds—to pressure.

The Healing Response

When a house catches fire, help doesn't come from the federal government in a remote capital—it comes from neighbors and the local fire department. Similarly, when tissue is damaged—whether by a tear, a crush, or a cut—the healing response isn't directed by the brain or central nervous system. It's local.

Just as each cell maintains a voltage across its membrane, tissues maintain an electric field—typically around 45 millivolts. When injury occurs, damaged cells lose ions, and the local voltage drops to zero. This voltage disparity between injured and surrounding healthy cells generates a flow of electricity called the *injury current*.[267]

This current peaks around 40 minutes after the injury—interestingly, about the same length of time acupuncture needles are commonly left in place—and gradually diminishes. Within six hours, the electrical field returns to normal. The strength of this current is correlated with the speed and success of healing. Applying external electrical fields or enhancing ionic transport through pharmaceuticals has been shown to accelerate repair. In contrast, tissues with reduced electrical capacity—such as in diabetic ulcers or bedsores—tend to heal poorly.[268]

Bioelectricity also operates at the cellular level. From plant cells capturing sunlight to muscle contraction in animals, bioelectricity is essential.[269] Our DNA and cytoskeleton are electrically conductive.

Genes matter, but they are not in charge. As cell biologist Richard Strohman put it: "The genes are important but not on top—just on tap."[270] Genes provide the *how*, not the *what*—like recipes, which still need a baker. In our bodies, the baker is the cell, making decisions based on signals it receives—chemical, physical, or electrical. Electrical signals travel through the extracellular matrix—the water-rich scaffolding of fascia—and along fascial fibers that connect cells. These signals enter the cell and can influence gene expression within the nucleus.[271]

Prana: the Energy of Communication

Imagine you are preparing a birthday dinner for a close friend. For the occasion, you've bought the largest turkey you could find and placed it in the oven—only to realize you're unsure of the temperature setting. You call your mother, who advises you: 325°F (163°C) for five hours.

That five-hour roast consumes a lot of energy—but the phone call that made it possible used almost none. And yet, without your phone's energy of communication, the oven would never have been turned on. We can feel and measure the heat from the oven, but to detect the tiny power of the phone call, we'd need sensitive scientific instruments.

The same is true within the body. The energy needed for transportation and transformation (like digestion, movement, or healing) is large and obvious. But the energy required for communication is subtle. And without it, cells don't act—or they act randomly and chaotically.[272]

We've already seen how dependent the body is on electricity and magnetic fields, but these are only part of the picture. Cells also communicate through hormones, neurotransmitters, cytokines, chemokines, growth factors, and exosomes. These messages might stay local—affecting nearby cells—or travel far away, as hormones do. Sometimes, they only affect the cell that produced them. In other cases, adjacent cells interact directly via surface receptors. Even electrical fields can guide movement—a phenomenon known as *electrotaxis*. Cells such as *exosomes* are also known to release tiny bubbles or bags called *vesicles* that carry instructions in the form of RNA, proteins, and lipids; these are like mail packets passed between neighbors.

According to James Oschman, our cells may also communicate using light—biophotons, which are faint flashes that may pass information between cells. DNA may emit and modulate these pulses of light.[273] More recent studies continue to explore the possibility that light is a medium of intercellular communication. Neurons may communicate via photons in ways faster than electrical synapses allow.[274]

If we think of prana or chi as the energy of coordination and communication, then its scope far exceeds ionic currents or chemical messengers.[275]

The Hands of a Healer

In the early 1800s, the link between electricity and magnetism was firmly established. Scientists like Ampère, Faraday, and Lenz showed that a changing magnetic field could induce an electric current—and that a moving electric current could generate a magnetic field. By 1865, James Clerk Maxwell completed the picture with a set of equations describing electromagnetic waves. Electricity and magnetism were revealed to be two sides of the same coin: when an electron moves, it produces a magnetic field; when a magnetic field moves, electrons flow.

In the 1960s, the development of an exquisitely sensitive device called the super-conducting quantum interference device—or SQUID—made it possible to detect extraordinarily tiny magnetic fields.[276] James Zimmerman refined the SQUID, which became a key tool in medical imaging. By the end of the decade, David Cohen used this technology to measure the magnetic field of the human heart, producing the first magnetocardiogram.[277]

To give a sense of scale, the Earth's magnetic field is between 0.25 and 0.65 Gauss. The human heart's magnetic field, as measured by Cohen, is a million times weaker—around 0.0000003 Gauss.[278] The brain's field is a thousand times weaker. Despite their faintness, these fields are biologically significant.

With this technology in hand, another researcher—John Zimmerman (no relation to James)—measured biomagnetic fields emanating from the hands of energy workers practicing therapeutic touch. What he found was both fascinating and controversial. To understand why, we must take a brief detour into the field of *pulsed electromagnetic field therapy*—PEMF.

Fields That Heal

The voltage potential across a cell membrane—created by differences in ion concentration—is essential for cell function. As mentioned earlier, Dr. Robert O. Becker spent decades documenting how weak electric and magnetic fields influence living tissues. His research showed that the body naturally generates low-level electromagnetic fields that regulate growth, healing, and regeneration.[279] These natural fields are vital for bone repair, nerve healing, and wound closure.

In the 1970s, Dr. Andrew Bassett pioneered the clinical use of PEMF, especially in treating non-union fractures—broken bones that refuse to heal. His work demonstrated that low-frequency magnetic fields induce subtle electrical currents in bone tissue that stimulate repair and cell regeneration.[280] In 1979, the US Food and Drug Administration (FDA) approved PEMF therapy for bone healing.

Subsequent research showed that certain frequencies are more effective than others. One study found that 15 hertz (Hz, 15 pulses per second) was ideal for promoting osteogenesis—bone growth.[281] Other sources suggest 7–8 Hz may be optimal, though field strength, treatment duration, and target tissue type also matter.[282] Frequencies from 1 to 30 Hz are now utilized in treating everything from acne to tinnitus.[283] Some experiments subjected an injured area to PEMF for 20 minutes daily for weeks, while other experiments prolonged the daily exposure for up to 8 hours.

John Zimmerman's experiments with therapeutic touch practitioners took a surprising turn. He found that their hands emitted measurable biomagnetic fields, often hundreds to thousands of times stronger than the heart's magnetic field. More strikingly, these fields were not constant—they were pulsating within the same frequency range used in PEMF therapy: 0.3 to 30 Hz, with a peak clustering around 7–8 Hz.

A Japanese research team led by Dr. Tsuyoshi Seto confirmed these findings using a less sensitive but still effective magnetometer system.[284] Seto's team recorded extraordinarily large biomagnetic fields emitted from the hands of practitioners of Qigong and other energy modalities. The frequencies mirrored those observed by Zimmerman.[285]

We know that devices generating these low-frequency electromagnetic fields have been shown to promote healing. And it appears that energy workers may emit fields in the same therapeutic range. Does this prove that Reiki, Qigong, and similar energy modalities work? Not quite—correlation is not causation. While the data are suggestive, rigorous clinical trials are still needed to determine how, when, and whether these fields directly promote healing. But these discoveries offer an extraordinary possibility: that the hands of a healer may act as living PEMF generators.

West Explains the East

Paul's and Sarah's introduction to the world of energy—and their pointers to researchers like Motoyama, Becker, and Zimmerman—opened my eyes to a possibility I hadn't considered: that we may not need new scientific theories to explain prana and chi. Perhaps we just need to look at Eastern experiences with an open mind, and ask whether the sciences we already have can help make sense of them.

As I began exploring Western explanations for Eastern energy-based therapies, I was struck by how equivocal the field was. Many studies made bold claims about proving the reality of chi or prana, but their methods were often flawed, their samples small, or their conclusions premature. Even the work of John Zimmerman and Dr. Tsuyoshi Seto—often cited in energy medicine circles—was far from definitive.

Seto's experiments, for instance, involved 37 volunteers. But only three of them produced pulsed electromagnetic fields strong enough to register on his magnetometer. All three were seasoned practitioners who claimed to have cultivated the ability to generate and direct chi. In 2012, a team attempted to replicate Seto's 1992 findings and came up empty-handed.[286] Why the discrepancy?

The researchers weren't sure, but they speculated that the shielded room they used may have been the issue. The room was designed to block ambient electromagnetic fields—including the Earth's magnetic field. That's important, because Seto had a theory: the practitioners in his study weren't producing strong electromagnetic fields on their own but were instead tapping into the Earth's magnetic field, acting like a kind of step-down transformer. They allowed the earth's larger field to flow into their bodies and out through their hands.

This idea fits surprisingly well with long-standing beliefs among many healing practitioners—that energy isn't generated from within but channeled from the world around us. The practitioner is a conduit, not the source. I remember Saul David Raye, during my first Thai yoga therapy training, saying, "We are conduits of grace."

Seto's theory also aligns intriguingly with what we know about the rhythms of the earth's magnetic field. In 1952, physicist Winfried Otto Schumann proposed that lightning strikes could generate electromagnetic waves that bounce between the earth and the ionosphere, forming standing waves. The fundamental frequency of this resonance turned out to be 7.83 Hz—confirmed two years later by Herbert König using magnetometers.[287] These standing waves, now known as Schumann Resonances, pulse through the atmosphere at frequencies within the range of those recorded by Seto's subjects: 7–10 Hz.

If Seto's theory is correct, and his subjects were resonating with the earth's own magnetic heartbeat, then placing them in a shielded room may have unintentionally silenced the very field they were trying to access.

Despite the tantalizing nature of such studies, no scientific consensus has emerged. As a 2021 review of non-contact energy healing methods concluded, "While there is some evidence of measurable effects, the field remains highly heterogeneous, and more rigorous, standardized methods are needed."[288] Still, even the most cautious researchers allow for the possibility that something real—though not yet fully understood—may be at play.

Proof Is Elusive

While the therapeutic use of PEMF has been demonstrated in numerous studies, controversy remains around its overall effectiveness. Even the FDA-approved application of PEMF for treating non-union bone fractures has not gained universal acceptance.[289] Similarly, while many studies have explored whether humans can generate measurable biofields,[290] the results have been inconsistent. The most ambitious claim—that practitioners can both generate and direct biofields in ways that stimulate healing—remains unproven by mainstream medical standards.[291] Though anecdotal reports of success abound, rigorous, double-blinded, randomized controlled trials remain sparse.

One of the greatest challenges in proving energy medicine's efficacy lies in study design. In a standard randomized, double-blinded, controlled trial—the gold standard of modern medicine—neither the recipient nor the provider of the treatment is supposed to know whether the intervention is real or a placebo. But how can a touch therapist be blinded? They know when they are actively providing a treatment. While some researchers have developed clever workarounds, the inherent limitations in blinding energy healing studies lead review organizations to default to conservative conclusions. Often, they determine that while such treatments may show promise, the evidence is not yet sufficient to warrant changes to standard medical practice.[292]

This caution is reasonable. Medical professionals have a duty to ensure that any intervention is, above all, safe—and ideally, more effective than placebo. None of this, however, matters to someone who has undergone an energy treatment and experienced positive change. A powerful personal experience can eclipse abstract debates about statistical significance. For the individual, the transformation is real.

It has been over 20 years since Paul and Sarah first sparked in me the idea that prana might be tangible—measurable, even—and that it might play a role in healing. Since then, I've followed the research and debates with what I hope has been an open mind. I remain skeptical of many claims made by energy healers, and I acknowledge the scientific shortcomings in much of the supporting literature. Yet, I've also witnessed a growing understanding in Western science of the many ways the body uses subtle energies to heal, grow, and regulate itself. We now know that cells communicate not only through chemical messengers and neural impulses but also through physical forces, electrical fields, magnetic shifts—and perhaps, light.

It's also clear that earlier generations—stretching back thousands of years—could not have understood these energies in modern scientific terms. Prana, as imagined 2,000 years ago, was not electricity. It was not a "life force" in the energetic sense we speak of today. These concepts didn't exist. But the idea of an inner breath, an animating vitality that departs at death, was both intuitive and powerful in the context of ancient understanding. Today, most yoga teachers define prana more broadly—as the energy of life itself. And in that sense, they're not wrong: life requires energy in countless forms.

I hedge my bets. I'll say that a yoga pose *may* stimulate chi along a particular meridian. I can't say it *does*, as there's no definitive proof. But I believe the hypothesis has merit: that applying physical stress—whether through stretch or compression—triggers cellular cascades involving mechanical, chemical, and electromagnetic signals that may travel through the body to affect distant tissues. I find Dr. Motoyama's idea persuasive—that prana or chi may flow through the water-filled spaces in our body as bioelectricity.

Of course, none of this depends on the student or teacher understanding the science. The mechanisms may be mysterious, but the effect can still be real. The more important question is: *How do you feel?* After the practice, an hour later, the next day? If you feel better, something has happened. And if a skeptic says it was just a placebo—well, does that diminish the benefit?

Scientists do care whether an intervention works, and they have good reason. There's an old maxim in medicine: "The dose makes the poison."[293] Any treatment—no matter how natural or subtle—can become harmful in excess. That's why it's essential to determine whether an intervention is truly effective or merely a placebo. Patients and students deserve full transparency, especially when they are placing their trust in a teacher or therapist. Placebos can be powerful, but they don't always work. If someone forgoes a more effective treatment because they've been told—with certainty—that an unproven therapy works just as well, but haven't been told it might be a placebo, that's not just misleading—it can be dangerous.

The reality is, no treatment or technique works for everyone. Human variation is simply too vast. Even something as commonplace as aspirin can be harmful to some. This is why I now choose to say that a yoga posture or a massage technique *may* be helpful, rather than insisting it *will* be. That small shift in language acknowledges the limits of our knowledge and respects the individuality of each person. Most well-run yoga teacher trainings emphasize this truth by teaching the contraindications for each posture. No pose is universally safe. I wish someone had told me that years ago, when I was earnestly practicing "1,008 rounds of kapalabhati to reach enlightenment." I wasn't told that overdoing it could lead to physical or psychological distress.

Prana Today

When ancient sages used words like prana, pneuma, spiritus, or chi, their language was direct, experiential, and, they believed, descriptive of reality itself. Today's language of science is analytical, precise, and replicable. Yet both traditions have been pointing towards the same mystery: the subtle vitality or force that animates life, guides healing, and promotes wholeness. Today, we can measure many such forces—bioelectric currents, biomagnetism, piezoelectric charges, streaming potentials, and even cellular light emissions. We now know that cells speak to each other in a vast, multidimensional language of touch, pressure, ions, chemicals, and light. The energies of life, or life energy, is not a superstition. It is a scientific reality—just not yet fully mapped. As our tools and understanding evolve, so too must our respect for the wisdom of the past. Prana may no longer need to be explained through symbolic language, but it still moves us in ways that science is only beginning to grasp.

In healing, as in life, balance matters. Even the gentlest energies—prana, chi, touch, breath—can overwhelm when pushed too far. The art lies not just in accessing energy, but in listening for when enough is enough. In my own healing journey, I learned the hard way to listen to my body.

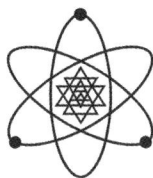

CHAPTER 21:

The Life of Breath

A few years after my 10-day training with Sarah and Paul, I found myself sitting in a dim hotel ballroom, listening to Professor Luciano Bernardi. What he said helped me finally understand what may have happened to my health years earlier. The professor stood at the front of the room, casually dressed, with white hair that stopped short of his ears and was thinning in front. He looked to be about my age, maybe early to mid 50s. I learned that he was a medical doctor from Italy who had conducted many studies on the effects of breath on the heart and our cardiovascular system.

His first comments took me back to my youth, when my mother would insist that all my brothers and sisters had to come to mass each Sunday. My mother loved her rosary, which Bernardi explained came to Europe in the hands of Crusaders returning from the Middle East in the twelfth and thirteenth centuries.[294] They returned with beads on strings, bought or stolen from Sufis and everyday Muslims. Some strings had 33, 66, or as many as 99 beads. The beads were used as aids in the recitation of the names of Allah. Bernardi believed the Islamic prayer beads were derived from the japa mala beads common in South Asia, which often would have 108 beads looped into a circle. These were similarly used to keep track of how many times a mantra was chanted. Once in Europe, the Eastern prayer beads evolved into the modern rosary, from the Latin "rosarium," which means a rose garden. A rosary contains 59 beads, divided into five decades or groups of 10.

The reason Bernardi mentioned any of this was because chanting, whether the Ave Maria on a rosary or an Eastern mantra while in lotus pose, slowed our rate of breathing. Often, these chants evolved to hit a frequency of about six breaths per minute. This rate of breath, which yogis obtain through a four-second inhalation, one-second pause, four-second exhalation, with another one-second pause, mimics something called the Mayer effect, during which our blood pressure rises and falls as we breathe. Inhalation causes blood pressure to rise; exhalation causes it to fall.[295] What may feel like spiritual practice—chanting, pranayama, breath control—is also a biological intervention. A rhythm of regulation. Yogic breathing changes our blood, organs, and brain.

The presentation I was raptly listening to was part of the Symposium on Yoga Therapy and Research, also known as SYTAR, organized by the International Association of Yoga Therapies. It was the weekend of March 5–8, 2009. The lineup of instructors was impressive: Dean Ornish, Timothy McCall, Loren Fishman, Ellen Saltonstall, Leslie Kaminoff, Doug Keller. I had read many of their books and respected their work. Still, it was Bernardi's talk that struck the deepest chord.

The Physiology of Breathing

Imagine flying by helicopter to the top of Mount Everest. You hop out for a picnic at 29,000 feet—and within minutes, you pass out and die. Why?

Bernardi walked us through the physiological cascade: *chemoreceptors*, specialized cells, detect oxygen and carbon dioxide in the blood.[296] If oxygen drops (*hypoxemia*), we instinctively breathe faster and deeper. But, if this rapid breathing expels CO_2 too quickly, a state of *hypocapnia* is created. With too little CO_2 our blood becomes too alkaline (*alkalosis*), and our brain, heart, and muscles begin to malfunction. Paradoxically, breathing faster to get more oxygen actually starves the body of CO_2— especially the brain—throwing off our blood chemistry.[297]

He said something that made me sit up straighter: "CO_2 is more important than O_2!" If we are in both a low-oxygen and a low-CO_2 environment, a condition we find at the top of Mount Everest, what does the body do? According to Bernardi, at first, we will breathe deeper and more quickly due to chemoreceptors' response to the lack of oxygen.[298] But this will cause a dangerous lowering of our CO_2. When that happens, other chemoreceptors will activate to slow down the breathing rate in order to rebuild CO_2 levels. Of course, with slower breathing, we take in less oxygen, which soon leads to our demise.

If we over-breathe and deplete our CO_2 levels, bad things happen.[299] Blood calcium levels drop, which causes our muscles and nerves to become hypersensitive and overly reactive. Our electrolyte balance is disrupted, which can cause the heart to develop arrhythmias and beat slower. Blood pressure drops. We twitch, spasm, and tingle. In severe cases, tetany sets in and the muscles become rigid, paralyzed. Increased pH levels can lead to lightheadedness, brain fog, and fainting. We may feel nauseous. If this continues over a long period of time, we can damage our nerves, heart, and muscles.

Training the Breath Safely

Bernardi conducted experiments with climbers where he taught one group a simple 10-second, three-part yogic breathing technique, which they would do for an hour every day. A control group received no instructions. The result: people who learned to slow their breath down to six breaths a minute lowered their *chemoreflex response*.[300] After two weeks of training, slower breathers had greater blood levels of both oxygen and CO_2; their ventilation reserves and efficiency were significantly greater—and all this despite their resting respiration rates being about one-half of the untrained climbers'.[301]

A 10-second breath has a multitude of benefits: improved exercise tolerance; higher blood oxygen saturation; improved heart rate variability (HRV); and improved *baroreflex*.[302] Baroreflex is the body's ability to adjust blood pressure. A properly functioning baroceptor reflex will detect when blood pressure has dropped or increased and will send the appropriate signals through the autonomic nervous system to speed up or slow down the heart, contract or dilate blood vessels, and increase or decrease blood flow through the heart.

I have always had low blood pressure: I feel a little faint whenever I come up too fast from a forward fold. Tim Miller once called this effect "seeing the yoga faeries." Come up too fast and Tinkerbell flutters about your head while you see stars and feel dizzy. I learned that one way to avoid the yoga faeries is to keep my arms overhead for a few breaths after I come up. I visualize that this allows the blood in the arms to fall to my head and diminishes the faeries. If I lower my arms too quickly, the blood will flow from my head to the arms, which exacerbates the problem.

Bernardi had another suggestion: while we inhale, we are creating a negative pressure within our lungs relative to the outside air pressure. This negative internal pressure results in our blood pressure increasing. This is the Mayer effect mentioned earlier. If you know you are going to feel faint when standing up too fast, try lengthening the inhalation so your respiratory system prolongs the negative pressure state, thus increasing your blood pressure.

Heart rate variability refers to the fact that our heart does not beat with metronomic regularity. As we inhale, the heart rate increases; as we exhale, it decreases. These changes are due to signals from the vagus nerve. If our HRV is high, it indicates that our vagal tone, a measure of how well the vagus nerve is functioning, is also high. When we are young, HRV is naturally high, but it drops with age and with poor cardiovascular conditioning. If you have a low HRV, if your vagal tone is poor, slow breathing will improve it. The vagus nerve is responsible for more than just beating your heart and controlling your breath; almost all of our internal organs are stimulated by the vagus nerve.[303] Slowing your breath rate improves HRV, which means it improves vagal tone, which in turn helps our organs function more optimally.

Slowing the breath rate increases the oxygen saturation of our red blood cells. That alone may not be significant, as the O_2 saturation level is usually 95–100%,[304] so there is little more to be gained.[305] I recalled that some yoga teachers claimed that pranayama practices will "supercharge the body and fill you with oxygen." This is not an accurate statement. Pranayama may increase your O_2 saturation by a few percent, but once you get to 100%, the red blood cells are full and cannot carry more oxygen.

But that is only a non-factor when we are resting. When we are exercising, the demand for oxygen grows, and the heart has to pump faster to maintain this level of saturation. If the blood becomes saturated more quickly and fully due to the increased availability of oxygen from slower breathing, then the heart does not have to work as hard. This is what Bernardi observed: slower breathing improved exercise tolerance.

Counterintuitively, slowing the breath actually allows more air to enter the lungs! And the air goes more deeply into the lungs, where there are more blood vessels. This makes gas exchange easier and more efficient. Alternatively, a yogi may choose to not breathe as deeply and instead reduce the effort of breathing. They may be content to take in the same amount of usable air as an untrained person, but since they are breathing slower, they won't have to work as hard. Slower breathing saves energy.

According to Bernardi, we can either 1) slow down and still use the same amount of effort in each breath, which will give us 21% more gas exchange,[306] or 2) reduce the effort, not breathe as deeply, and keep the same level of gas exchange.

Also important is the way we breathe: Bernardi recommends breathing through the nose. The nose and sinuses are narrower passages than the mouth. Nasal breathing automatically causes us to slow down the rate of breathing. This is what ujjayi breath accomplishes. By constricting the throat, which reduces how fast we can inhale, we are forced to slow down our breath rate. Bernardi's lesson is—slow your breath to 10-second cycles and breathe through the nose. You do not have to breathe more deeply; just ensure it remains unhurried.[307]

A 2013 study of yoga-naive volunteers compared a 10-second breath cycle—with and without ujjayi—to a standard four-second breath.[308] The researchers confirmed Bernardi's findings that baroreflex improves with slower breathing. Additionally, this study looked at two different ratios: 1) inhalations of three seconds with exhalations of seven seconds (about a 1:2 ratio) and 2) both inhalation and exhalation of five seconds (a 1:1 ratio). They found the 1:1 ratio improved baroreflex and lowered blood pressure more than the 1:2 ratio. However, the researchers determined that the difference between the 1:1 and 1:2 ratios was not really significant. They also examined employing ujjayi breath and concluded that ujjayi breathing had minimal impact on outcomes. They suggested that practitioners choose the ratio that feels most comfortable.[309] That was a key finding: do what feels most comfortable! Ujjayi? Yes, if you like.

I sat spellbound during Professor Bernardi's presentation.[310] I'd never heard any of this before. In my mind, connections were being formed and questions asked. How often had I unknowingly hyperventilated during my pranayama practices? Did this affect my brain? Was chanting for an hour or more during a kirtan also doing this?[311]

Normally, after bhastrika or kapalabhati pranayama, I did kumbhakas, holding my breath. But was I holding the kumbhakas long enough? Could the states of mind I experienced be the result of blood chemistry? Was I altering my electrolyte balances? Did my pranayama practices contribute to my health crashes? For the first time, I understood the causal relationship between breathwork and health. While listening to Bernardi, the warning I cited earlier against unsupervised pranayama practice came to mind: "Just as lions, elephants, and tigers are controlled by and by, so the breath is controlled by slow degrees, otherwise it kills the practitioner himself."[312]

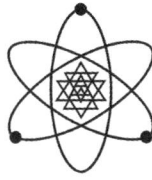

C H A P T E R   2 2 :

The Road to Recovery

After returning from White Sulphur Springs in early January of 2005, I was housebound for the better part of a week. Something in me had changed. My body, once strong and flexible from years of asana and athleticism, had become fragile. I had no choice but to change my practice. While I still loved ashtanga yoga, it no longer loved me. Even walking two blocks left me gasping, dizzy, spent.

After resting for a few weeks, my energy returned slightly, and I began to ramp up my activities again—too soon, as it turned out. Within a month, I crashed. And so began the cycle: rest, partial recovery, return to activity, crash. Again and again.

Simple things would set me off—sweet foods, exercise, social gatherings, even time in front of a screen. I couldn't work more than an hour at a time. My body had become hypersensitive to stimuli I'd once considered harmless. I was a stranger in my own skin.

Out of concern, my company arranged for me to visit the Mayo Clinic in Phoenix, Arizona. I spent several days undergoing tests and consultations. The results? Normal. They taught me some cognitive behavioral therapy techniques and sent me home with little more than a shrug.

My own doctors in Vancouver had been just as mystified. A specialist in internal medicine dismissed my symptoms as psychosomatic and advised me to "get more exercise." I turned to other paths. I consulted with Dr. Shiva Varma and his partner, Dr. Susan Barr, my Ayurvedic physicians. Susan prescribed a sugar-free diet, added more animal protein, and began a *Candida* cleanse. No change. I tried parasite cleanses. Heavy metal detoxes. Chelation therapy. I had the mercury removed from my dental fillings. I tried intravenous vitamin drips, acupuncture, PEMF, massage, supplements, cognitive therapy—you name it.

I even underwent diagnostic testing with a different version of Dr. Motoyama's AMI device, called the Prognos.[313] Based on the findings, my naturopath prescribed various supplements and lifestyle changes. I was trying so many things at once that if anything did help, it was impossible to know which did the trick. Looking back, I think the strongest medicine I took—the one that truly worked—was time. And an unexpected companion: surrender.

In those early months, a typical day would find me sitting on my sofa, looking out at the Vancouver skyline and the mountains beyond. I remember thinking: *This might be what aging is like.* Not dramatic or tragic, but quiet and still. I made a vow: "When I can no longer do what I love, I will learn to love what I can do."

That vow—to love what I could do—changed me. On days I couldn't walk, I could still sit. I could still listen. I could still breathe. I began to cultivate the second of Patanjali's niyamas: *samtosha*, contentment. And slowly, through stillness and simplicity, contentment grew.

I learned to find awe in the ordinary—sound, silence, the brush of air against my skin. My yoga practice changed. I no longer aimed to pass my edge. In fact, I stopped thinking in terms of edges at all. I became more yin-like. I began to embrace the middle path. Like Goldilocks, I found power in not too much, not too little.

Healing came quietly and slowly. Time, it turned out, was not a thief, but a teacher. Hippocrates, Osler, Voltaire—all echoed the same truth: the art of medicine lies in supporting nature's healing, not in replacing it. Sometimes, what the body needs is not to be fixed, but simply to be heard. And held.

The Teacher Appears

As I regained some strength, I returned to work and resumed my studies. I attended silent retreats with Sarah and Ty Powers—gentler now, more yin than yang. Then I encountered the teachings of a Vietnamese Zen master, Thich Nhat Hanh. His students called him Thay, or "teacher." Thay didn't teach rigorous Zen. His path was simpler—mindfulness in every moment. To Thay, meditation meant mindfulness. Not escape. Not effort. Just presence.

Where Patanjali's meditation points inward—toward seclusion and transcendence—Thay's mindfulness opens outward. To breathe, to walk, to eat, to wash the dishes—all could be sacred, all were yoga, if done with awareness. Meditation was not about changing states, but about being fully present with what is.

In 2006, a friend (Diana Batts) and I visited Thay's Plum Village in France for a retreat called Scientists in the Field of Consciousness. Bells rang randomly throughout the day, calling everyone to pause for three mindful breaths. One afternoon, I was just about to eat an ice cream cone when the bell sounded. I watched, smiling, as the ice cream began to melt, and then, with presence, resumed eating. It was one of the best cones I've ever had.

The following year, we joined Thay in Vietnam for a three-week pilgrimage of reconciliation. It was April. The heat soared above 30°C (86°F). My body, which had struggled since India with high temperatures, braced for another collapse. But this time, I came prepared. Dan Friedman had suggested I try electrolytes—just a few drops in my water bottle. While this was before I had heard Professor Bernardi's lecture on breath, blood, and electrolytes, I had long suspected that some unseen imbalance in my chemistry was contributing to my crashes. But I hadn't found a reliable way to restore balance. I tried Dan's idea. Something shifted. With the added support of electrolytes, I felt steadier, clearer, and less vulnerable to the heat. I still avoided the sun, wore a hat, and listened carefully to my body's signals. But I didn't collapse. I traveled, practiced, walked, and meditated in the heat.

It wasn't just the electrolytes, of course. It was my whole approach: awareness, pacing, presence, and care.

The Long Transition

While I was slowly regaining my health, I was also slowly reshaping my life. My ongoing challenges had taught me I could not stay in the business environment forever. I gave Dan a one-year notice of resignation. By the time the year was over, he suggested that I did not need to fully leave MDA; instead, I could consult one day per week and help train my successor. Teaching yoga full-time wasn't going to pay many bills, so I agreed to Dan's suggestion, hoping a part-time consulting role might bridge the transition. Strangely, that "one day a week" gig never quite materialized. After six months, I realized I was still working four days a week. "This is not leaving," I told Dan. "This is called staying!" He just grinned.

It wasn't until 2014 that I finally stopped working at MDA, but the hours per week did diminish gradually. During those years, MDA paid the bills while I taught yoga, studied philosophy, mythology, anatomy, and physiology, and deepened my teaching practice. The slow change in my career mirrored the slow healing of my body. Both called for patience. Both required letting go.

Vancouver's yoga scene was also changing. In 2005, City Yoga expanded to a second location, near UBC. Diana and I both taught yin yoga there, but by early 2006, the economics no longer worked, and both studios closed. Gloria Latham's Semperviva Yoga Studios took over the main location and folded it into its growing network. Along with the mats and props came Diana and me—we became Semperviva yoga teachers. I taught power vinyasa, yin, and hatha and led meditations across several of their locations. My favorite was the Sea Centre on Granville Island, with its views of False Creek, seagulls, and bobbing boats.

In 2006, Shakti Mhi opened the Prana Urban Monastery in the heart of Vancouver, but unfortunately, it only lasted one year. Though I was no longer teaching weekly classes at Prana, I continued to offer yin yoga workshops and teacher trainings through her. Eventually, she started training teachers abroad, especially in Thailand and Israel. In 2010, she sold the Prana studio. It was renamed Exhale and offered Pilates, Zumba, and burlesque. Shakti opened a new location where she taught only yoga teachers. Times were changing.

Shakti decided to return to Israel in 2013. She sent out her final email from Vancouver in March, reminiscing about her arrival and sharing her departure. Her last words to me were: "I'm sure we will meet sometime in the future—if not on earth, then for sure in the heaven of yoga, eating sushi together like in the old times." Our paths had diverged, as they sometimes do for friends. But she was my first teacher. The first to introduce me to prana. The one who opened a doorway I've been walking through ever since.

What Healed Me?

So, what healed me? Was it yoga? Ayurveda? Electrolytes? PEMF? Acupuncture?

Perhaps. But if I had to name the medicines that made the deepest difference, I would say: slowness, stillness, surrender, and time. I had to stop fixing, stop striving, stop grasping—and instead, start listening. It wasn't about doing more. It was about doing less—and *being* more. I had been called into a different rhythm, one that honored chi, prana, and life itself, not as something to control, but as something to trust.

Each crash felt like a failure—a failure of the body. But within that failure was a chance to listen, to learn, and to rebalance the soul. My crisis had stripped away the layers of ambition and identity I had long wrapped around my practice. In their place came something quieter, but truer. A deeper yoga. A softer breath.

My experience of healing wasn't linear, scientific, or tidy. It wasn't provable. But it was palpable. It was real. My energy returned. My vitality returned. Not all at once, and not forever—but enough.

That is what life offers us: not perfection, but possibility.

And still I sit, every day. One day, that will be all I can do. Sit. Watch the sky, birds, children. Practice contentment. To sit and breathe, with awareness and care, is not a retreat from life—it is a return to it.

Perhaps this is what the ancients intuited when they spoke of *prana*. Not a force to command, but a breath to receive.

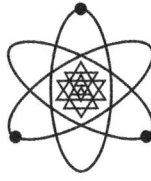

E P I L O G U E :

What is prana?

"Why prana?" was the question I asked Shakti long ago. Her answer was typical of yogis in our time: "Prana is life—it is the energy that gives life." But as we've seen, that's not the answer a yogi living in a forest in South Asia would have offered 3,000 years ago. The meaning of prana has changed—understood differently in different times and places.

To primal cultures, the source of life was breath. If you were breathing, you were alive. The air around us gave us life. Call it the wind, if you like.

To agricultural societies, water was the key to survival. Without it, nothing grows. Water is life, and it appears in many forms. Anything liquid could be seen as a counterpart or homologue of water: semen, blood, menses, rain, rivers, dew. The word "lifeblood" reflects this view—life is in the blood; the blood is life. Water was the sustaining element.

Life, like rain, came from the gods. The dew from heaven—or the moon—was life returning to the earth. Prana, too, was a gift from the gods, and sometimes even a god itself. Prana was the source of all movement and action. Since breathing is a movement, prana was also breath. The breath of the creator god. Indra called himself prana. Prana as water was the semen of Shiva.

As civilizations developed, so too did religion and philosophy. The concept of life began to separate from the concept of soul. The soul—atman, psyche—was who we were. The spirit—prana, pneuma—was what linked that immaterial soul to the material body. Both were needed to be truly alive, but it was spirit, prana, that animated the body. When it failed, the soul had to leave.

Prana became more than just air in the lungs. It was the subtle substance that filled the sky and stirred the heavens. A grand realization arose in ancient agrarian cultures: as in heaven, so on earth. The microcosm was linked to the macrocosm. The air that fills the sky also fills the body. The life-giving waters that fall from heaven also course through our veins.

The gods and heavens influenced events on earth—but the reverse was true as well. What we did in our small, embodied world could affect the gods above. That was the whole point of sacrifice. It was barter: we fed the gods so they would heed our prayers.

With the rise of science, our concepts evolved again. The gods were no longer "out there." We've been out there—and didn't find them. Nor were they "down below." We looked and saw nothing. The gods moved as we grew. They moved inward, to a hidden place few dare to explore.

Prana, as a spiritual energy, moves us toward awe and transcendence. It can shatter our worldview—and reassemble it into something new. Like any form of technology, prana can be used for good or ill. It can lead to insight or delusion, enlightenment or psychosis.

Through the process called science, we have learned that life, in all its forms, depends on energy gradients. Whether it's the simplest virus or a vast aspen forest, without energy, there is no life. If someday we create artificial life made of silicon, it too will need energy. This energy takes many forms—chemical, mechanical, electrical, magnetic, optical, and more. If prana is a life force, it manifests through all of these forms of energy.

This book began with the question, "What is prana?" To answer that it is "life energy" invites the deeper question: "What is life?" Science has not yet answered that definitively. And until it does, we cannot fully define prana either. The understanding of life is still evolving, and so is our understanding of what sustains it.

Until that day comes, change will remain the only constant. And our view of life—and prana—will continue to grow.

Endnotes

Endnotes for Departure, Chapter 1 and Chapter 2

1   I have used simplified English spellings of Sanskrit terms (e.g., *pranayama* rather than prāṇāyāma) for the ease of general readers. Diacritical marks have been omitted unless needed for clarity, consistency, or distinction between similar terms.

2   Throughout this book, "spirit" refers to prana, pneuma, or vitality—the animating force of life—while "soul" refers to atman, psyche, or the witnessing self. These meanings often overlap in other texts but are kept distinct here for clarity.

3   Hebrews 4:12.

4   According to this Biblical image, it is the breath that confers life and soul. Later Christian thinkers debated when the soul enters the body, and over time many came to believe ensoulment happens earlier—perhaps even at conception.

5   According to the Online Etymology Dictionary, *etmen is the source also of Old English æðm, Dutch adem, Old High German atum which all refer to "breathe," See https://www.etymonline.com/word/atman accessed May 6, 2024.

6   The Chinese character for chi 氣 originally depicted steam or vapor rising from rice, combining elements for *air* (气) and *rice* (米).

7   In this book, organ names related to Traditional Chinese Medicine (TCM) such as "Liver," "Heart," and "Urinary Bladder" are capitalized when referring to their meridian or energetic functions, as distinct from their anatomical counterparts. This convention helps distinguish between the broader systemic roles described in Chinese medical theory and the physical organs understood in Western medicine.

Endnotes for Chapter 3

8   For an interesting but controversial view of pre-history, see David Graeber and David Wengrow, *The Dawn of Everything: A New History of Humanity* (Picador, 2023).

9   Mircea Eliade, *Shamanism: Archaic Techniques of Ecstasy*, trans. Willard R. Trask (Princeton University Press, 1964).

10   Manvir Singh, "The Cultural Evolution of Shamanism," *Behavioral and Brain Sciences* 41 (2017): e66, http://doi.org/10.1017/S0140525X17001893. Manvir Singh is an assistant professor of anthropology at the University of California, Davis, where he directs the Integrative Anthropology Lab.

11   James W. Moore, "What Is the Sense of Agency and Why Does it Matter?" *Frontiers in Psychology* 7 (2016): 1272, http://doi.org/10.3389/fpsyg.2016.01272.

12   A seminal 1944 study by Fritz Heider and Marianne Simmel demonstrated our tendency to assign agency and emotion to inanimate shapes. Subjects viewed a 90-second animation of a triangle, circle, and square interacting. Rather than describing geometric motion, most saw a story with characters exhibiting desires, plans, and feelings. See Fritze Heider and Marianne Simmel, "An

Experimental Study of Apparent Behavior," *American Journal of Psychology* 57, no. 2 (1944): 243–59, https://doi.org/10.2307/1416950.

13 Robert M. Sapolsky, *Why Zebras Don't Get Ulcers: The Acclaimed Guide to Stress, Stress-Related Diseases, and Coping*, 3rd ed. (Henry Holt, 2004).

14 Shamans operate where chance, ritual, and belief intersect. Success enhances their reputation; failure is typically attributed to angry spirits, disobedient participants, or opposing forces. In this way, shamans' influence is preserved, and they remain vital mediators between the known and the unseen.

15 Singh, "The Cultural Evolution of Shamanism." However, Rouget does note that there are differences between ecstasy and trance. He describes ecstasy as involving immobility, silence, solitude, no crisis, sensory deprivation, recollection, and hallucinations, while trance is characterized by movement, noise, being in company, crisis, sensory overstimulation, amnesia, and no hallucinations. See Gilbert Rouget, *Music and Trance: A Theory of the Relations Between Music and Possession* (University of Chicago Press, 1985).

16 Even in ancient Egypt with its grand tombs called pyramids and its many complicated philosophies of the afterlife, it was thought that the body must somehow survive and be revived after death.

17 In the oldest books of the Old Testament, it is clear that the ancient Hebrews held this belief. Sheol was the term used for the grave or tomb. This was not a hell or any place of continued existence. It was the place of the dead. See Bart D. Ehrman, *Heaven and Hell: A History of the Afterlife* (Simon & Schuster, 2020).

Endnotes for Chapters 4&5

18 "Mythology is not a lie. Mythology is poetry, it is metaphorical. It has been well said that mythology is the penultimate truth—penultimate because the ultimate cannot be put into words. It is beyond words. Myths are metaphors pointing to spiritual truths. They are not facts; they are metaphors." Joseph Campbell with Bill Moyers, *The Power of Myth*, ed. Betty Sue Flowers (Doubleday, 1988), 5.

19 Seal of Gudea, led by Ningishzida, in William Hayes Ward, *The Seal Cylinders of Western Asia* (Carnegie Institute, 1910), https://archive.org/details/sealcylindersofwoowarduoft/page/24/mode/2up. The image is in the public domain and available at https://en.wikipedia.org/wiki/Gudea#/media/File:Seal_of_Gudea,_led_by_Ningishzida.jpg.

20 On the left: Libation vase of Gudea. Originally published by Ernest Coquin de Sarzec in *Découvertes en Chaldée* (Ernest Leroux, 1886). Image is in the public domain, https://en.wikipedia.org/wiki/Gudea#/media/File:Girsu_Gudea_libation_vase.jpg. On the right: "Fig. 29. Scheme of decoration from a libation-vase of Gudea, made of dark green steatite and originally inlaid with shell. *Déc.*, pl. 44, Fig. 2; cf. Cat., p. 281," in Leonard King, *A History of Sumer and Akkad* (Chatto & Windus, 1910), https://www.gutenberg.org/files/49345/49345-h/49345-h.htm.

21 At any one time in Sumer, there were between 300 and 1,000 gods. "The gods who formed the assembly of the gods were legion." Thorkild Jacobsen, *The Treasures of Darkness: A History of Mesopotamian Religion* (Yale University Press, 1976), 95.

22 It is from the Sumerian astronomers that the world's fixation on the magic number seven arises. In South Asia, we find the number used over and over again: the seven chakras, the seven ancient rishis, seven pranas or vayus, the seven steps of the Buddha, and of course, the seven days of our week. See Thomas McEvilley, *The Shape of Ancient Thought: Comparative Studies in Greek and Indian Philosophies* (Simon and Schuster, 2002), 89.

23 Ur was the birthplace of the Biblical Abraham, the father of all the Jewish and Islamic peoples. It was located about 300 kilometers southwest from present-day Baghdad.

24 Sumer featured multiple snake deities, including Basmu, often linked to fertility and rebirth. Like Ningiszida, Basmu was depicted with horns and a serpentine form. See Joshua J. Mark, "The Mesopotamian Pantheon," in *World History Encyclopedia* (February 25, 2011), https://www.worldhistory.org/article/221/the-mesopotamian-pantheon. The Biblical demonization of the serpent contrasts with its earlier life-giving role in Sumer. See Campbell, *The Power of Myth*.

25 The seal is now in the British Museum. The image is from George Smith, *The Chaldean Account of Genesis* (Scribner, Armstrong & Co., 1876), 91, available at https://en.wikipedia.org/wiki/Adam_and_Eve_cylinder_seal#/media/File:Adam_Eve_cylinder_Smith.jpg.

26 McEvilley, *The Shape of Ancient Thought*, 266.

27 Diane Wolkstein and Samuel Noah Kramer, *Inanna, Queen of Heaven and Earth. Her Stories and Hymns from Sumer* (Harper and Row, 1983).

28 Elements of this story, which was perhaps first told around 3,000 BCE or even earlier, echo down through the ages. Traces of these tales appear centuries later in the Bible. These are ancient stories that predate our written records.

The Sumerian creation story: Before anything was, there was water. Her name was Nammu. Nammu brought forth two children, her son An—the sky—and her daughter Ki, the earth. An and Ki were joined together, forming Anki, the whole universe. From this union came their son, Enlil, the god of air. Air got between An and Ki and forced their separation. Enlil lifted An high and called him the sky (which people today refer to as heaven), but he kept Ki low and called her the earth. In between the earth and the sky lived Enlil, in the dark. To relieve his loneliness and give light to existence, he and his wife, Ninlil, created Nanna, the Moon. Nanna, with his wife Ningal, created their son, Utu, the Sun. Just as Enlil was more powerful than his parents, Utu outshone Nanna; thus, the daytime was brighter than the night.

Enlil joined with Ki, and thus was begotten Enki, the god of water, vegetation, and wisdom, and the lord of the universe. Enki gathered together part of Nammu, the primordial sea, and squeezed her into two great rivers, the Tigris and Euphrates. He caused the creation of cattle and fish, marshes teeming with life, and enriched the soil so it would be fertile.

Now, many of the gods, who physically looked very much like the humans that would follow, settled on the dry land and began to work it. They mined the earth for metals and toiled in the soil to bring forth food. They dug canals to channel the life-giving waters. They worked hard and long and complained constantly. So Enki and his half-sister Ninhursag decided to create a new race who would serve the gods. But life can only come from life—so to summon the new, old life first had to be given. The god Geshtu-e, he who was blessed with supreme intelligence, was chosen.

Ninhursag took clay from the earth and mixed it with the blood of Geshtu-e. All the gods spat upon the mixture as well. Ninhursag formed the clay and pinched off 14 pieces, which she put into the womb goddess, Nintu. After nine months had passed, Nintu gave birth to seven men and seven women. These new beings were born to serve the gods, and they and their descendants became slaves to the gods.

29 From Genesis 1:2: "And the earth was without form, and void; and darkness was upon the face of the deep. And the Spirit of God moved upon the face of the waters" (Authorized King James Version). The Hebrew word for "the deep" is Tehom (תְּהוֹם *tǝhôm*), which also describes a primeval ocean. In Babylon, the primeval ocean was called Tiamat. In Sumer, it was Nammu.

30 Genesis 1:20: "And God said, Let the waters bring forth abundantly the moving creatures that hath life, and fowl that may fly about the earth" (Authorized King James Version).

31   The Adda Seal is housed in the British Museum. A detailed description of it can be found here: https://www.britishmuseum.org/collection/object/W_1891-0509-2553.

32   Leviticus 17:11 reflects a later echo of Sumerian views: "the life of the flesh is in the blood."

Endnotes for Chapter 6

33   See Swami Niranjanananda Saraswati, *Prana and Pranayama* (Yoga Publications Trust, 2009), 113.

34   *Hatha Yoga Pradipika*, trans. Pancham Sinh (Oriental Books Reprint Corp., 1980), 2–15.

35   B.K.S. Iyengar, in page 113 of his book *Light on Pranayama*, gives a slightly different interpretation. He states that time refers to the length of the inhalation and exhalation; number, or condition as he translates the term, can refer to both duration and cycles of inhalation, retention, exhalation, and retention; see B.K.S. Iyengar, *Light on Pranayama* (The Crossroads Publishing Company, 1985).

36   Niranjanananda Saraswati, *Prana and Pranayama*, 155.

37   Unfortunately, Swami Niranjanananda does not cite any source or reference for this study of the 102-year-old yogi; see *Prana and Pranayama*, 137.

38   Swami Niranjanananda distinguishes between *anuloma viloma* as a beginner's form of alternate nostril breathing (without breath retention) and *nadi shodhana* as a more advanced practice that includes specific kumbhaka ratios. In contrast, B.K.S. Iyengar uses the terms interchangeably, applying retention and ratios under both names. See Niranjanananda Saraswati, *Prana and Pranayama*, 240–1, and Iyengar, *Light on Pranayama*, 179–82.

39   Niranjanananda Saraswati, *Prana and Pranayama*, 141.

40   Niranjanananda Saraswati, *Prana and Pranayama*, 140.

41   While Shakti shared with us five pranayama during our month with her, other Sivananda teachers cite nine practices. They are categorized by their effects:

Energizing: *bhastrika, kapalabhati*

Calming: *bhramari, ujjayi*

Heating: *surya bheda, murcha*

Cooling: *chandra bheda, shitali*, also called *shitkari*

Balancing: *nadi shodhana*

42   Niranjanananda Saraswati, *Prana and Pranayama*, 273.

43   Beginners often overdo *kapalabhati*, leading to shoulder lifting, pelvic rocking, or facial tension. We were taught to pace them slowly, encouraging soft shoulders, still hips, and relaxed faces. Verbal cues or light touch (e.g., on the shoulders) helped build awareness. Only the belly should move—with active exhales and passive inhales. Ten breaths per round was the norm for beginners. After each round, we rested by bowing forward and emptying the lungs. At the end, we sat tall, held a gentle breath, and waited for the natural impulse to inhale.

44   The form of kundalini yoga referenced here was developed by Yogi Bhajan—a controversial figure who was at various times a customs officer, spiritual teacher, and entrepreneur. After moving from India to Toronto in 1968, he relocated to Los Angeles in 1969, where he founded the 3HO (Healthy, Happy, Holy Organization) and began widely promoting his own brand of kundalini yoga in the West. His teachings emphasized bhastrika (which he called "breath of fire") as a central practice.

45   Niranjanananda Saraswati, *Prana and Pranayama*, 273.

46 *Hatha Yoga Pradipika* 2:66.

47 Iyengar wrote, "[Kapalabhati and bhastrika] should not be performed by ... women, since the vigorous blasts may cause prolapse of the abdominal organs and of the uterus while the breasts may sag." See *Light on Pranayama*, 179.

48 A final form of pranayama that Shakti taught us was a way to stay cool in the August heat. It is called *shitali* (or *sheetali*, as she spells it.) Not everyone has the genes to do this: curl your tongue into a tube and breathe in through it. You will instantly feel the coolness. If you can't curl your tongue, stick your tongue out a little way and breathe in with lips almost closed. This version is called *shitkari*. Breathe out through the nose. If the day is too warm for either kapalabhati or bhastrika, do shitali or shitkari.

49 Mula bandha is also spelled moola bandha. The Gheranda Samhita lists 25 mudras. Ashvini mudra (also spelled ashwini mudra) is the repeated contraction of the anal sphincter and is claimed to awaken the kundalini serpent, while curing diseases of the rectum and invigorating the whole body.

50 The six classical cleansing practices (*shat kriyas*) of hatha yoga are:

– *Neti*: nasal cleansing using water (*jala neti*) or thread (*sutra neti*) to clear the sinuses;

– *Dhauti*: digestive tract cleansing, such as stomach washing (*vamana dhauti*) or cloth swallowing (*vastra dhauti*);

– *Nauli*: abdominal massage using isolated rectus abdominis contractions to stimulate digestion and detoxify internal organs;

– *Basti*: yogic enema using water or air to cleanse the colon;

– *Kapalabhati*: rapid breathing technique to cleanse the lungs and energize the mind;

– *Trataka*: steady gazing at a fixed point (like a candle flame) to sharpen concentration and purify the eyes.

51 Iyengar, *Light on Pranayama*, 89.

52 David Swenson, *Ashtanga Yoga: The Practice Manual* (Ashtanga Yoga Productions, 1999), 9.

53 Niranjanananda Saraswati, *Prana and Pranayama*, 325.

54 Paul Grilley, *A Yogi's Guide to Chakra Meditation* (Cardinal Publishers Group, 2019), 52.

55 Shakti recommends waiting two to four hours after eating before doing uddiyana bandha, to allow the stomach to empty.

56 Iyengar, *Light on Pranayama*, 91.

57 Niranjanananda Saraswati, *Prana and Pranayama*, 330.

58 Maha mudra or maha bandha should only be attempted once each individual bandha has been mastered. Begin with applying the chin lock, then lift the belly in and up, and finally suck up the anal flower. To release a bandha, breathe a little further in the direction that you entered: for example, if you are doing a kumbhaka on empty lungs, breathe out a little more, straighten the body, and then breathe in. If you are doing a hold with lungs full, straighten the neck, head, and spine, sip in a little more air, then release the breath.

Endnotes for Chapter 8

59 In Sanskrit, the phrase "You are that" is "Tat tvam asi." It is found in the *Chandogya Upanishad*, chapter 6, verse 12.3. See *The Principal Upanishads*, translated and edited by Swami Nikhilananda (Dover Publications, 2013).

60 A Kshatriya is one of the four varnas, which were part of a social hierarchy outlined in ancient texts like the Rigveda and later reinforced in texts such as the Manusmriti. Over time, a rigid caste system evolved from this framework. It consists of: *Brahmins* – the priestly and scholarly class, responsible for religious rituals, teaching, and preserving sacred knowledge; *Kshatriyas* – the warrior and ruling class, responsible for governance, military defense, and upholding justice; *Vaishyas* – the merchant and agricultural class, responsible for trade, commerce, and farming; and *Shudras* – the laboring class, responsible for service-oriented and manual work, often supporting the other varnas.

Outside of this were the outcasts, the untouchables, known as the Dalits. They were often assigned the most menial and ritually "impure" tasks, such as handling dead bodies, cleaning latrines, or dealing with animal hides. Their position in society was deeply marginalized, as they were considered *avarna* (without varna) and were subjected to severe social discrimination.

61 While Sat, brahman, and purusha are sometimes used interchangeably in Indian philosophy, they reflect different conceptions of reality. Sat (truth or being) is often used in the Upanishads to denote pure existence. Brahman, particularly in Vedantic systems, is the singular, impersonal ground of all being—beyond name and form. Purusha, in contrast, is the term favored by Samkhya and yoga systems to describe an individual, witnessing consciousness. While Vedanta sees the self (atman) as identical with brahman (tat tvam asi), Samkhya posits many purushas—each distinct and uninvolved with prakriti, the material world.

62 The association between Kapila's village and the historical city of Kapilavastu—said to be the birthplace of Siddhartha Gautama (the Buddha)—comes from later Buddhist tradition. While this link is widely accepted in popular accounts, modern scholarship remains divided. Several archaeological sites in present-day Nepal and India have been proposed as the true location of Kapilavastu, but no definitive identification has been made. See John Strong, *The Buddha: A Short Biography* (Oneworld, 2001) and Michael Witzel, "Early Sanskritization: Origins and Development of the Kuru State," *Electronic Journal of Vedic Studies* 1, no. 4 (1995): 1–26.

63 Rig Veda X.90.

64 Atharva Veda XI.4.1–26.

65 William Davies, "The Teachings of the Upanishads," *The Atlantic* (August 1893): 178–90.

66 Karl Jaspers, *The Origin and Goal of History*, trans. Michael Bullock (Routledge Classics, 2021; first published 1953 by Routledge).

67 In traditional accounts, Yajnavalkya is considered a real historical figure. Some sources suggest that Uddalaka Aruni was his teacher, though primary texts do not explicitly confirm this. Yajnavalkya became a renowned philosopher and is known for surpassing many scholars in debates, particularly in King Janaka's court.

68 From the Satapatha Brahmana, X.3.3.5–8: "What is the fire which is this universe? In truth, prana is this fire." Also see the Chandogya Upanishad, IV.10.4, which says, "Life [prana] is Brahman, Joy is Brahman, Ether is Brahman."

69 *Kaushitaki Brahmana Upanishad*, trans. E.B. Cowell (Calcutta: Baptist Mission Press, 1861), accessed March 27, 2023 at http://www.pushtisahitya.org/sanskrit/Generic/Upanishads/Kaushitaki_Brahmana_Upanishad.pdf

70 *Kaushitaki Brahmana Upanishad*, III.3.

71 McEvilley, *The Shape of Ancient Thought*, 544.

72 Arthur Avalon (Sir John Woodroffe), *The Serpent Power: The Secrets of Tantric and Shaktic Yoga* (Dover Publications, 1974), 65.

73 McEvilley, *The Shape of Ancient Thought*, 544.

Endnotes for Chapter 9

74   Later ashtanga teachers offered six separate series, but according to both David Swenson and David Williams, originally there had been only four. It seems the last two of the original sequences were too long and thus were broken into two each.

75   David Williams is the author of *My Search for Yoga* (self-published) and *The Complete Ashtanga Yoga Syllabus Poster* (self-published).

76   David Swenson, *Ashtanga Yoga: The Practice Manual* (Ashtanga Yoga Productions, 1999), 9–10.

77   Georg Feuerstein, *The Shambhala Encyclopedia of Yoga* (Shambhala Publications, 1997), 94.

       Richard Freeman advises that the eyes should not be focused on the tip of the nose or between the eyebrows, because this creates tension. Rather, the direction of the gaze is to, and through, these points; Richard Freeman, *Ashtanga Yoga: The Primary Series Video Handbook* (Delphi Productions, 1993), 13.

78   Swenson, *Ashtanga Yoga*, 12.

79   David Swenson, *Ashtanga Yoga Teacher Training Course*, Costa Rica, February 1–11, 2001.

80   Freeman, *Ashtanga Yoga*, 12.

81   *Shambhala Encyclopedia*, 313.

82   *Hatha Yoga Pradipika*, 2.51–53.

83   Scott Lamps and Ida Jo, "Modern Misunderstanding of Ujjayi," Ghosh Yoga [Blog post], July 14, 2021, https://www.ghoshyoga.org/blogs/modern-misunderstanding-of-ujjayi.

84   Sri K. Pattabhi Jois, *Yoga Mala* (Eddie Stern/Patanjali Yoga Shala, 1999), 30, 39. Jois does recommend that pregnant women who are past four months should stop doing asana, but they can do ujjayi until their seventh month of pregnancy.

85   B.K.S. Iyengar, *Light on Yoga* (Schocken Books, 1979), 441–3.

86   According to David Williams, yoga requires constant engaging of the three bandhas. This makes the asana practice a moving meditation. One must intensely concentrate to maintain the constant mula bandha as strongly as possible. As soon as the mind is gone, the mula bandha is gone. In his view, yoga is not something one does. It a state one is left in from proper inward-looking practice.

87   Tim Miller told me this in July of 2004.

88   *Shambhala Encyclopedia*, 140. Different teachers have different names for the same thing. T.K.V. Desikachar called this the cin mudra.

89   Be aware of pain! Or, as David Williams told me, "If it hurts, you are doing it wrong. Hurting yourself more will not make you hurt less. The idea of ignoring pain and calling it an 'opening' is the most idiotic, nonsensical thing I have heard in my life." You can learn more about David Williams's journey and evolution in his memoir *My Search for Yoga* (David Williams, 2019). It chronicles his early fascination with yoga at age 20, through his travels to India and his studies with Pattabhi Jois, focusing on the years 1970 to 1977. The book is available for purchase directly from his website: ashtangayogi.com.

90   "...the 'ha', the moon's coolness." This is not a typo. Mark, echoing Desikachar's statements in his book, said that "hatha" is made of two syllables, "ha" and "tha," which mean moon and sun! Most yoga teachers reverse these and think "ha" is sun and "tha" is moon. However, Sivananda, Satyananda, and Desikachar claim the opposite. I long ago gave up being surprised by different teachers' varying definitions of yoga terms.

91   Black and white Sri Yantra by N. Manytchkine https://upload.wikimedia.org/wikipedia/commons/a/a2/Sri_Yantra_256bw.gif.

Endnotes for Chapter 10

92   According to Plato, Socrates was officially charged with impiety and corrupting the youth—specifically, introducing new gods and not honoring the city's gods. His criticism of democracy and traditional values was seen by many as a dangerous influence. The trial and execution of Socrates are documented in Plato's *Apology*, *Phaedo*, and *Crito*.

93   See Luciano Canfora, "The Fate of Aristotle's Library," trans. James Kierstead, in *Antigone* (n.d.), https://antigonejournal.com/2022/06/aristotle-library-alexandria.

94   Carlo Rovelli, *Anaximander and the Birth of Science* (Riverhead Books, 2023).

95   Stephanie Lynn Budin, "Phallic Fertility in the Ancient Near East and Egypt," in *Reproduction: Antiquity to the Present Day*, edited by Nick Hopwood, Rebecca Flemming, and Lauren Kassell (Cambridge University Press, 2018), 25–38; image appears on page 37.

96   See Plato's *Timaeus*.

97   Plato, *Timaeus*.

98   Aristotle, *On the Soul*.

99   McEvilley, *The Shape of Ancient Thought*, 210.

100   Aristotle's views on delayed ensoulment seem to have changed over time. His two main texts disagree on the exact timing. "On the Generation of Animals" (*De Generatione Animalium*) cites the soul arriving in a male fetus at the 40th day and the soul in a female fetus on the 90th day. In "On the Soul" (*De Anima*), written about 15 years later, Aristotle says ensoulment occurs 40 days after conception, regardless of sex, but here he seems to be referring only to the nutritive or vital soul, not the rational soul. The 40 days after conception date for ensoulment became the baseline belief for many early Christian theologians up to the time of Thomas Aquinas. Notably, Aquinas cites an 80-day point for female ensoulment instead of Aristotle's 90th day.

101   Noel Si-Yang Bay and Boon-Huat Bay, "Greek Anatomist Herophilus: The Father of Anatomy," *Anatomy and Cell Biology* 43, no. 4 (2010): 280–3. https://doi.org/10.5115/acb.2010.43.4.280.

102   Robert Herrlinger and Edith Feiner, "Why Did Vesalius Not Discover the Fallopian Tubes?" *Medical History* 8, no. 4 (1964): 335–41, https://doi.org/10.1017/s002572730002980x.

Endnotes for Chapter 11

103   *Hatha Yoga Pradipika*, verses 46 and 49.

104   The idea that one can "open the hips" is strange. The intention is not to literally pull the head of the femur out of the hip socket. Rather, it is meant more poetically or figuratively. "Opening the hips" means to increase the range of motion between the femur and pelvis. More specifically, it refers to increasing external rotation and abduction. It was my lack of external rotation which required me to twist the tibia around the femur to get my feet on the opposite thighs in lotus pose. Thus, I worked on increasing the external rotation of the femur in the hip sockets, which many yoga teachers refer to as "opening the hips."

105   *Yoga Mind and Body* was released in VHS format by Warner Home Video on October 19, 1994.

106   Joel Kramer, "Yoga as Self-Transformation," *Yoga Journal* (May/June 1980), 1–10, https://joeldiana.com/downloads/writings/YogaAsSelfTransformation.pdf.

107   The five lines were along the legs (two), along the arms (two more), and along the core from perineum to head.

108   Two decades later, Erich clarified for me what caused his knee problems. He said, "I was trying to do mulabandhasana [an advanced posture requiring sitting on the feet in a butterfly (baddha-konasana) with the toes pointing backwards], one foot at a time, turning the foot over to get the inner ankle to the floor. My knee made a loud pop! I was stuck and couldn't straighten my leg. But somehow, I used my hands to fling my leg straight and it popped back in. I've never wanted to do that pose since that happened! I did finally have my knees X-rayed, and there was a significant ACL tear."

109   Erich reported to me in 2025 that he has not had any knee problems for over 20 years.

Endnotes for Chapter 12

110   See F. R. Freemon, "Galen's Ideas on Neurological Function," *Journal of the History of Neuroscience* 3, no. 4 (1994): 263–71. https://doi.org/10.1080/09647049409525619.

111   See Charaka Samhita SA5.5 for the metaphorical use of gods as mental states—Indra (ego), Soma (joy), Rudra (agitation).

112   Kaustav Chakraborty and Rajarshi Guha Thakurata, "Indian Concepts on Sexuality," *Indian Journal of Psychiatry* 55, suppl. 2 (2013): S250–5, https://doi.org/10.4103/0019-5545.105546.

113   Chakraborty and Thakurata, "Indian Concepts on Sexuality."

114   There are 10 vayus in total, but only the five major ones are discussed. The five minor vayus not discussed are *naga, kurma, krikala, devadatta,* and *dhananjaya*: Naga vayu – Governs belching, hiccups, and burping. It helps release excess air from the stomach and is linked to digestion and speech. Kurma vayu – Controls blinking and eye movements. It protects the eyes, maintains moisture, and supports vision. Krikala vayu – Responsible for sneezing and clearing nasal passages. It aids in expelling irritants from the respiratory system. Devadatta vayu – Manages yawning and sleep regulation. It plays a role in relaxation and replenishing energy levels. Dhananjaya vayu – Governs post-mortem bodily functions and is said to linger in the body after death. It also influences heart function and sustains muscle tone.

115   "The word yang originally meant sunshine, or what pertains to sunshine and light; that of yin meant the absence of sunshine, … shadow or darkness. In later development, the yang and yin came to be regarded as two cosmic principles or forces, respectively representing masculinity, activity, heat, brightness, dryness, hardness, … for the yang, and femininity, passivity, cold, darkness, wetness, softness, … for the yin. Through the interaction of these two primary principles, all phenomena of the universe are produced." Y.L. Fung, *A Short History of Chinese Philosophy* (Free Press, 1948), 155.

116   Traditional Chinese cosmology describes the evolution from Dao to qi to yin/yang to the five elements (water, wood, fire, earth, metal). Each element interacts through a generation and control cycle. Water generates wood, which feeds fire, creating earth, which yields metal, which then feeds water. Control: metal cuts wood, wood parts earth, earth dams water, water quenches fire, fire melts metal.

117   The Chinese term *zhēn* refers to acupuncture, while *jiǔ* refers to moxibustion—the application of heat using dried mugwort (*Artemisia*), known as moxa. Together, they form a primary intervention in Traditional Chinese Medicine.

118   The concept of "five shen" is not universally accepted in early Daoist medical texts. The *Huangdi Neijing* ("Yellow Emperor's Inner Canon") primarily mentions shen, hun, and po. Later interpretations added zhi and yi to represent will and intellect.

119 The concept of reincarnation in Buddhist philosophy is complex and often contested. While the Buddha generally accepted the cosmology of his time—which included *samsara* (the cycle of birth, death, and rebirth) and *karma*—he introduced the doctrine of no-self (*anatta* in Pali, *anatman* in Sanskrit), which asserts that there is no permanent, unchanging self to be reborn. What persists, rather than a fixed soul, is the momentum of one's actions—often compared to one candle lighting another. Over time, however, the idea of reincarnation became more firmly established in Buddhist traditions. In the Mahayana school, which was developing around the same time as our story in Taxila, we encounter the ideal of the *bodhisattva*—a being who vows to return again and again, reincarnating across lifetimes, until all sentient beings are liberated from suffering.

120 See David Gordon White, *The Alchemical Body: Siddha Traditions in Medieval India* (Chicago University Press, 1996), 15–29, for his view on the three aspects of human and divine, plus the mediating structure in between.

121 This requires a seven-stage process of gradual refinement of ingested food. The seven fires of digestion are called the *dhatvagnis*. They turn the food into the seven tissues of the body, called the *dhatus*. As Dhanvantari explained, the dhatus are chyle (the digested essence of food), blood, flesh, fat, bone, marrow, and finally the most refined and pure, semen. In women, the seventh is menstrual blood and breast milk.

122 White, *The Alchemical Body*, 25.

123 White, *The Alchemical Body*, 46.

124 White, *The Alchemical Body*, 184–7.

125 While the Vasubandhu in this vignette is fictional, there was a well-known Buddhist philosopher in Gandhara around this time called Vasubandhu who wrote extensively on Buddhist philosophy, logic, and metaphysics. However, this historical Vasubandhu was not a physician. There was also a famous historical Greek physician named Menecrates, but he lived hundreds of years earlier and far to the west.

126 David Wootton, *The Invention of Science: A New History of the Scientific Revolution* (Harper Collins, 2015), 62.

127 From the King James Version of the Bible.

128 Wootton, *The Invention of Science*, 70 and 560.

129 In the 1600s, Jean Baptiste van Helmont wrote, "If a soiled shirt is placed in the opening of a vessel containing grains of wheat, the reaction of the leaven in the shirt with fumes from the wheat will, after approximately 21 days, transform the wheat into mice." See Louis Pasteur, "On Spontaneous Generation," an address delivered by Louis Pasteur at the "Sorbonne Scientific Soirée" of April 7, 1864, available at *Pasteur Brewing*, https://www.pasteurbrewing.com/on-spontaneous-generation/; translation by Alex Levine.

130 This idea of spontaneous generation is described in Aristotle's book *History of Animals*. While this seems fantastical to us today, we must remember that scientists still do not know how life first arose out of nonliving matter. How did the first cells arise? How did the first strands of DNA come to be? These questions remain delightful mysteries. See Stephen Mann, "Systems of Creation: The Emergence of Life from Nonliving Matter," *Accounts of Chemical Research* 45, no. 12 (2012): 2131–41, https://doi.org/10.1021/ar200281t.

131 See Kurt Leland, *Rainbow Body: A History of the Western Chakra System* (Ibis Press, 2016).

132 Shigehisa Kuriyama, *The Expressiveness of the Body and the Divergence of Greek and Chinese Medicine* (Zone Books, 1999), 105–40.

133 *Chandogya Upanishad* 8.6.6.

134 *Brihadaranyaka Upanishad* 4.2.3. Note in most translations of this verse, the word nadi is rendered as "vein" or "artery," but that applies to an ancient word a modern concept that probably was not available at that time.

135 Domenico Ribatti, "William Harvey and the Discovery of the Circulation of the Blood," *Journal of Angiogenesis Research* 1 (2009), 3, http://doi.org/10.1186/2040-2384-1-3.

136 Francisco López-Muñoz, Jesús Boya, and Cecilio Alamo, "Neuron Theory, the Cornerstone of Neuroscience, on the Centenary of the Nobel Prize Award to Santiago Ramón y Cajal," *Brain Research Bulletin* 70, no. 4–6 (2006): 391–405, https://doi.org/10.1016/j.brainresbull.2006.07.010.

137 Ancient Ayurveda considered the nadis to be physically real. The Charaka Samhita (c. 300 BCE–200 CE), an authoritative Ayurvedic medical text, states that the human body has hundreds of nadis, some of which carry blood (*rakta*) and others that are responsible for conveying life energy (*prana*). The Sushruta Samhita (c. 600 BCE) provides one of the earliest descriptions of surgery and mentions sira (veins) and dhamani (arteries). It distinguishes between siras, which carry blood and are linked to kapha (phlegm), and dhamanis, which pulsate and are linked to pitta (bile). The description of dhamani suggests an early awareness of arterial pulsation, though it was not understood in the circulatory sense we know today.

Endnotes for Chapter 13

138 According to the Oxford English Dictionary, transubstantiation is "the conversion of the substance of the Eucharistic elements into the body and blood of Christ at consecration, only the appearances of bread and wine still remaining."

Wikipedia has a good summation of the history of transubstantiation and the current position of the Catholic Church that the bread and wine are, in fact, transformed by the priest into the body and blood of Christ. See also Nathan Busenitz, "Did the Early Church Teach Transubstantiation?" [blog post] The Master's Seminary, April 21, 2016, https://blog.tms.edu/did-the-early-church-teach-transubstantiation.

According to a Pew poll in 2019, only a third of US Catholics believe that transubstantiation really occurs; see https://www.pewresearch.org/short-reads/2019/08/05/transubstantiation-eucharist-u-s-catholics.

139 "And as they were eating, Jesus took bread, and blessed it, and brake it, and gave it to the disciples, and said, Take, eat; this is my body. And he took the cup, and gave thanks, and gave it to them, saying, Drink ye all of it; For this is my blood of the new testament, which is shed for many for the remission of sin." Matthew 26:26–28, King James Version.

140 *Ananta* is usually translated as endless but can also be rendered as infinite or unending. *Shesha*, also spelled Śeṣa, can mean remains or residue.

141 The source of the creation myth is based loosely on the Vishnu Purana, which was compiled and written in layers with many unknown contributors. Its date of creation is unknown and perhaps unknowable, as it accreted layers over hundreds of years. It may be based on stories dating as far back as 1000 BCE. Some historians do not believe it reached its completed state until the ninth century CE.

142 If you're wondering how in the world to pronounce chthonic, pronounce the first two letters as a "kuh" and then say "thonic." Thus you have "kuh-thonic."

143 White, *The Alchemical Body*, 216.

144 A naga is a mythological serpent being found in Indian, Buddhist, and Southeast Asian traditions, often depicted as a powerful cobra or part-human, part-serpent entity. In early South Asian

cosmology, nagas are associated with water, rain, fertility, and the underworld, and they are often regarded as protective spirits as well as potential sources of danger if disrespected.

145   The caduceus, with two snakes entwined upon a staff, is the symbol of Hermes, not of Asclepius. The top of Hermes' staff, which bears two wings, tells us so. Hermes caduceus represents the art of business and commerce, not medicine, although for many years the American Medical Association mistakenly used Hermes caduceus as its logo. That would have been appropriate if we thought of modern medicine only as a business, the business of medicine. But since the AMA wanted its logo to represent healing, in 2005 it changed its symbol to the staff and single serpent of Asclepius.

Endnotes for Chapter 14

146   This quotation is from Tim Miller, "The Alchemy of Yoga," Ashtanga Yoga Center (n.d.), https://www.ashtangayogacenter.com/the-alchemy-of-yoga.

147   For more details, see Tim Miller, "Chapter 4," Dust (May 26, 2011), https://timmiller.typepad.com/dust_by_tim_miller.

148   Spelling and translations provided by Miller in "The Alchemy of Yoga."

149   See also Richard Freeman, *The Mirror of Yoga: Awakening the Intelligence of Body and Mind* (Shambhala, 2010), 54.

150   "Talking Shop with Saul David Raye," *Yoga Journal*, August 28, 2007, https://www.yogajournal.com/lifestyle/yoga-trends/talking-shop-with-saul-david-raye.

151   Saul warned us to avoid pressing on the knee, open sores, and bones, especially ones close to the surface of the body, and to avoid going too high towards the groin. For clients with arthritis, we were advised to go very gently. He also suggested avoiding pregnant clients until we were far more experienced. Likewise, for the first few years, we should avoid working with anyone with serious medical conditions.

152   Saul explained, "In the West, we have a saying, 'No pain, no gain.' That is a terrible saying. In the East, they say, 'No pain, no pain!' Much better!"

153   From a Thai (and Ayurvedic) view, these are the *sen ittha* (the ida nadi) and *sen pingkhala* (the pingala nadi).

154   Kam Thye Chow says the heart channel of the left arm is actually part of the sen ittha and the right arm heart channel is the sen pingkhala. What Saul called the pericardium channel, Kam defines as the *sen kalathari*, although it also runs along the back and the middle of the arm.

155   Fortunately, this phase of Itamar's career did not last too long. He returned to his roots and began touring the world, releasing albums that highlighted his virtuosity. His musical styles on guitar and piano included Middle Eastern influences, flamenco, as well as jazz and classical forms. To learn more, visit www.itamarerez.com.

156   Drawings of acupressure points on "Sen" lines at Wat Pho temple in Phra Nakhon district, Bangkok, Thailand. Photograph copyright Ryan Harvey, CC BY-SA 2.0, https://commons.wikimedia.org/wiki/File:Thai_massage.jpg.

157   For younger readers who do not know what the Yellow Pages are, ask your parents.

Endnotes for Chapter 15

158   Suttee, also spelled *sati*, was the practice of a widow immolating herself on her husband's funeral pyre. This ancient idea mirrored a celestial dance between Venus as the female power and the sun as the male power. Venus as the evening star would follow the sun. Each night, Venus would set closer

and closer to the sun as it dipped below the horizon. She followed his flame into the darkness. But in a couple of weeks, Venus would reappear as the morning star just before sunrise and seem to lead the sun back to life. As in heaven, so on earth. The idea of sati was that the husband and wife should stay together, even after death, so the wife could lead the husband out of darkness and into the next life. The practice has been outlawed and is no longer practiced in modern India, although isolated cases have been reported.

159   The Magh Mela of Prayag was a precursor to the famous Kumbh Mela. It probably dates from the early centuries CE, as it is mentioned in several early Puranas. The term "Kumbh" is used to describe these pilgrimages, which probably began in the mid-nineteenth century.

160   These three horizontal lines of ash on the forehead are known as the *tripundra*. They represent Shiva but can also represent the three gunas (tamas, rajas, and satva), Shiva's three powers (will (icchāśakti), knowledge (jñānaśakti), and action (kriyāśakti)), or any of many other categories.

161   The name of this composition was the Sri-tattva-cintamani, the "Auspicious Gem of Truth," but unfortunately, it was never completed.

162   "Shivoham," sings the yogi. "I am Shiva!"

163   See Sravana Borkataky-Varma, *Menstruation: Pollutant to Potent* (Springer Science+Business Media, 2018). See also Jeffery D. Long, Rita D. Sherma, Pankaj Jain, and Madhu Khanna (eds.), *Hinduism and Tribal Religions* (Springer Nature, 2022).

164   During the Ambubachi Mela, held annually in June at the Kamakhya Temple in Assam, India, it is believed that the presiding goddess undergoes her menstrual cycle. This belief is symbolized by the temple's natural spring, which is said to turn red during this period. Some attribute this coloration to the region's iron-rich soil mixing with the water. Others suggest that deposits of cinnabar (mercury sulfide) in the surrounding mountains contribute to the red hue. Additionally, some believe that temple priests may pour vermilion into the waters to signify menstruation. B. Roy, "Ambubachi: The Festival of the Bleeding Goddess," *The Times of India* (June 22, 2021), https://timesofindia. indiatimes.com/readersblog/trivialtopics/ambubachi-the-festival-of-the-bleeding-goddess-55401.

165   Borkataky-Varma, *Menstruation: Pollution to Potent*.

166   Yoni-tattva is a mixture of semen and menstrual fluids.

167   Sahajoli mudra is the feminine version of vajroli mudra. It is a contraction of the urinary muscles as if one were to stop urinating in midstream. The Hatha Yoga Pradipika describes this quite differently than the tantric texts. The hatha yoga version is the smearing of burnt cow dung on the body. The tantric version is more akin to doing Kegel exercises.

168   This description of a woman's role as a tantric partner in the Kamakhya Temple is based upon the work of Sravana Borkataky-Varma. See specifically her study "The Ancient Elusive Serpent in Modern Times: The Practice of Kundalini in Kamakhya or the Elusive Serpent," *International Journal of Dharma and Hindu Studies* 1, no. 2 (2016).

169   These are not the eight limbs of Patanjali's Yoga Sutra. These are the seven "limbs" of yoga as described in the Gheranda Samhita. Asanas were the physical practices; mudras were the placements of the body; bandhas were the energetic valves and locks, pratyahara was the closing of the sense doors; pranayama was breathwork; dhyana was meditation; and samadhi was ecstatic trance.

170   See Hatha Yoga Pradipika 3.97.

171   Cited in the Kaulajñānanirṇaya. See Kenn Døngart, *Kundalini: The Hindu Tenets of the Serpentine Energy in Theory and Practice*, master's thesis (June 2016), 9, https://doi.org/10.1017/S0041977X11000036.

172   See Christoper Wallis, *Tantra Illuminated: The Philosophy, History, and Practice of a Timeless Tradition* (Mattamayura Press, 2013), 221. He cites the text, Sārdhatriśatikāllotara, circa 650 CE.

173   See David Gordon White, "Yoga in Early Hindu Tantra," in David Carpenter and Ian Whicher (eds.), *Yoga: The Indian Tradition* (Routledge, 2003), 150.

174   The section is called "*Sat-chakra-nirupana*: An Exposition of the Supports of the Inner Body." See Arthur Avalon (Sir John Woodroffe), *The Serpent Power: The Secrets of Tantric and Shaktic Yoga* (Luzac & Co., 1919; Dover Publications [reprint], 1974).

175   The pericarp is the outer wall of a fruit that develops from the ovary after fertilization. It surrounds and protects the seeds, often with multiple layers and textures, depending on the type of fruit. In the context of chakras, the pericarp serves as an energetic boundary encasing the core components of the lotus: its petals, bija mantra (seed sound), and presiding deities. It is often depicted as a geometric shape—such as a square (muladhara), triangle (manipura), or circle (ajna)—each symbolizing the chakra's elemental quality or function. Just as a fruit's pericarp encloses and protects the seed, the chakra's pericarp organizes and contains its energy. Some tantric texts describe it as a veil that must be pierced or purified for the chakra's full awakening. For example, the square pericarp of the muladhara represents stability and the earth element, while the hexagram of anahata symbolizes the dynamic balance of opposing forces.

176   Despite the English spelling of these bija sounds, when they are pronounced, they sound like "lum" rather than "lamb". They are pronounced lum, vum, rum, yum, hum, and aum.

177   According to Paramahansa Purnananda, within the sushumna nadi are two other channels. The first is the *vajra nadi*. Within it is the *citrini nadi*. The lotuses or chakras are inside the sushumna, and thus inside Meru as well.

According to Paul Grilley, "[the] sushumna, the central river of Prana, has four layers. These layers are nested inside each other like four Russian dolls... The first, outermost layer of Sushumna is called 'Sushumna Nadi.' Sushumna nadi stretches from the coccyx, the first chakra, to the top of the head. The second layer of Sushumna is called 'Vajra Nadi.' Vajra Nadi stretches from the second sacral vertebra, the second chakra, to the top of the head. The third layer of Sushumna is called 'Chitrini Nadi.' Chitrini Nadi stretches from the second lumbar vertebra, the third chakra, to the top of the head. The fourth layer, the innermost core of Sushumna, is called 'Brahma Nadi'." See Paul Grilley, "Chakras, Bandhas, Mudras" (unpublished manuscript, 2021), 8, https://paulgrilley.com/assets/documents/Chakras,%20Bandhas,%20Mudras%2012.1.pdf.

178   The siddhis are supernatural powers or perfections, described in yogic and tantric traditions, particularly in Patanjali's Yoga Sutra and Hatha Yoga texts. There are eight major siddhis:

1   Anima – Ability to become infinitesimally small.

2   Mahima – Ability to expand to a gigantic size.

3   Laghima – Ability to become weightless or extremely light.

4   Garima – Ability to become immensely heavy.

5   Prapti – Ability to reach anywhere instantly (teleportation).

6   Prakamya – Ability to fulfill any desire or know others' thoughts.

7   Ishatva – Lordship or control over nature.

8   Vashitva – Power to control others (hypnosis, influence).

There are 10 secondary siddhis (From the Bhagavata Purana)

1   Anurmi-mattva – Immunity from hunger, thirst, and pain.

2   Dūra-śravaṇa – Clairaudience (hearing distant sounds).

3   Dūra-darśana – Clairvoyance (seeing distant things).

4   Manojavita – Ability to travel at the speed of thought.

5   Kaama-rupa – Changing one's form at will.

6   Parakaya pravesha – Entering another's body (possession).

7   Siddha-sankalpa – Manifesting desires instantly.

8   Ajñāpratihatā – Absolute command over elements.

9   Surya-vajra – Invulnerability to harm.

10 Jalastambha – Ability to stop water flow or walk on water.

Should these be pursued? In Patanjali's Yoga Sutra, siddhis are considered distractions on the path to enlightenment. He warns against their pursuit. However, in tantra, some siddhis are tools for spiritual development.

179 In the Tirumandiram—a Tamil text attributed to Tirumular, a Tamil yogi and mystic who lived around the fifth or sixth century CE—is written: "If the timeless sage's body is burnt in fire, the entire country will suffer from that fire forever... Make a clean hole nine spans deep, spread the earth to five spans around the hole... place the body in lotus position... plant a peepul tree..." From James Mallison and Mark Singleton, *The Roots of Yoga* (Penguin, 2017), 432–4.

180 This is the preferred name used by James Mallison and Mark Singleton in *The Roots of Yoga*.

181 See Mallison and Singleton, *The Roots of Yoga*.

182 Tales have been told of yogis who could grant fertility to women unable to conceive. But a woman who conceived a son by this means would later have to give the child to the yogi, who would then offer the child up to the goddess Durga as a blood sacrifice. For a deeper review, see David Gordon White, *Sinister Yogis* (Chicago University Press, 2009).

183 While fictitious, Garima's treatment as a woman in the left-handed tantric cult in the Kamakhya temple is based on interviews with women who live there. For more on how women "miss the moksha boat," read the works of Sravana Borkataky-Varma, starting with "The Ancient Elusive Serpent in Modern Times."

Paramahansa Purnananda was a real person and the author of the *Sat-chakra-nirupana*. What little biographical information offered in the vignette is from Avalon, *The Serpent Power*. In that book, Avalon (the pen name of Sir John Woodroffe) translated not only the text but also commentaries by several people, including Shankara and Visvanatha. No details are provided about these people, so their incarnation in the vignette is purely fictional as well.

184 For example, consider the simple term, "yoga." It is such a ubiquitous word today, and yet there are many different ways to understand and interpret yoga, above and beyond the fact that as a Sanskrit word, it can have dozens of different translations. It can mean: a joining, an attaching, a way, a means, a method, a trick, a business, a profit, an undertaking, a gathering together, mixing, an assemblage, diligence, order, and even magic. In the yoga forest, yoga can be a thing or a doing or both: is yoga something you practice or something you achieve? Yes! It can lead to spiritual liberation, with several different interpretations of what that means, or to the gaining of special powers and magical abilities. It can mean the accumulation of karma, or a way to get rid of karma. These examples come from the Mallison and Singleton, *The Roots of Yoga*.

185 Mallison and Singleton, *The Roots of Yoga*. The Gheranda Samhita, a seventeenth-century hatha yoga text, describes six types of samadhi in chapter 7, verse 3. These are: *dhyana* (meditative absorption), *bhava* (devotional absorption), *laya* (dissolution), *rasananda* (bliss of devotional or aesthetic flavor), *sattvapatti* (state of purity), and *asamprajnata* (non-dual, seedless absorption).

186 Mallison and Singleton, *The Roots of Yoga*, 400.

187 Mallison and Singleton, *The Roots of Yoga*, 175.

188 David Gordon White refers to this model of the chakras as "six plus one" because the top chakra had no element associated with it; see *Kiss of the Yogini* (University of Chicago Press, 2003), 221–9.

189 See Leland, *Rainbow Body*, 30, 47.

190 Mallison and Singleton, *The Roots of Yoga*, 181.

191 Mallison and Singleton, *The Roots of Yoga*, 79.

Endnotes for Chapter 16

192 When Desikachar publicly asked his students to no longer use the term "viniyoga," he was asked whether they could call it "Desikachar yoga." He was horrified by the suggestion and said, "What I have received is from my teacher and what he received is from his teacher. There is a lineage of more than 2000 years. How can they label this Desikachar? They are murdering me because they are murdering my teacher... My father would be in tears. Whatever he invented, he never said he invented it. I know that he innovated things, but he would never say 'it is mine.' That is the Indian philosophy of humility and respect for the teacher. They always would say, 'my teacher taught this to me'."

193 Desikachar's version of the myth and its metaphors are examined in my book *Shiva Dancing at King Arthur's Court*.

194 When I met Mark Whitwell at Shiva Rea's teacher training, he mentioned he had written the English version of *The Heart of Yoga*, based on Desikachar's teachings and other writings. There does not seem to be any mention of Mark in the pages of that book, so I can only credit Desikachar for what I read. See K.V. Desikachar, *The Heart of Yoga: Developing a Personal Practice*, revised edition (Inner Traditions International, 1999).

195 Yoga Sutra 1.31.

196 See Desikachar, *The Heart of Yoga*, chapter 6.

197 These bija sounds were also used while doing the mini-sun salutations and while lying down.

Endnotes for Chapter 17

198 The book was called *Traité élémentaire de chimie* (Elements of Chemistry), published in 1789.

199 Descartes wrote: "it is not necessary to conceive of any vegetative or sensitive soul, or any other principle of movement or life, other than its blood and its spirits which are agitated by the heat of the fire that burns continuously in its heart, and which is of the same nature as those fires that occur in inanimate bodies." From René Descartes, *The World and Other Writings*, trans. S. Gaukroger (Cambridge University Press, 1998), 169.

200 See Daniel James Nicholson, *Organism and Mechanism: A Critique of Mechanistic Thinking in Biology*, PhD dissertation, University of Exeter, 2010, http://hdl.handle.net/10036/117787.

201 The phrase comes from interpretations of Aristotle's *Metaphysics*, particularly Book 8, 1045a10, where he says: "The whole is something besides the parts, and not just the sum of them all." Translated by W.D. Ross, in *The Complete Works of Aristotle*, ed. Jonathan Barnes (Princeton University Press, 1984).

202 René Descartes thought the pineal gland was the master controller of the material body, because he believed it was uniquely suited to be the seat of the soul and the point where the mind and body interact. His reasoning was that the pineal gland is singular (not divided into two hemispheres), which fit his idea that the soul must interact with the body at a single, unified point. Also it is centrally located in the brain, making it seem like an ideal candidate for coordinating bodily functions.

He theorized that the pineal gland directs the flow of "animal spirits" (a term for the fine, subtle fluids thought to carry sensory and motor information in the body). Descartes believed these spirits moved from the pineal gland into the nerves, influencing movement and perception. This idea became very influential.

203   "The animal machine is governed by three main regulators: respiration, which consumes oxygen and carbon and provides heating power; perspiration, which increases or decreases according to whether a great deal of heat has to be transported or not; and finally digestion, which restores to the blood what it loses in breathing and perspiration." Antoine Lavoisier, quoted in F. Jacob, *The Logic of Life: A History of Heredity* (Princeton University Press, 1973), 43.

204   The most prominent supporter was George Stahl, the same chemist, physician, and scientist who promoted the idea of phlogiston in the mid seventeenth century.

205   The mechanists would not agree with this logic. If a machine, say an ox cart, breaks a wheel, the machine will no longer work. This does not mean "life" has left it. If the wheel is fixed, the machine will work again. Similarly, if a human body breaks, it may no longer work. This too does not mean something vital has escaped or left the body. If the body is fixed, it should, in principle, be alive again. It is our ignorance of exactly how the body works that makes us unable to fix it and restart the process of life. This view is well described in Mary Shelley's famous novel *Frankenstein*.

206   Jacob, *The Logic of Life*, 27.

207   Nicholson, *Organism and Mechanism*, 31.

208   Théophile Bordeu (1722–1776), as mentioned in T.S. Hall, "On Biological Analogs of Newtonian Paradigms," *Philosophy of Science* 35, no. 1 (1968): 6–27; quote appears on 18.

See also this statement by Justus von Liebig, German chemist (1803–1873): "It is as legitimate to ascribe a vital cause as it is to ascribe a gravitational force. Science studies the laws of the vital force, not the vital source itself, just as the laws of gravity are not an explanation of gravity but of its operation. We know about gravity through its operation." Cited in I. Coulter, P. Snider, and A. Neil, "Vitalism – A Worldview Revisited: A Critique of Vitalism and Its Implications for Integrative Medicine," *Integrative Medicine* 18, no. 3 (2019): 60–73.

Endnotes for Chapter 18

209   For more on Sarah Powers's biography, see her book *Insight Yoga: An Innovative Synthesis of Traditional Yoga, Meditation, and Eastern Approaches to Healing and Well-Being* (Shambhala Publications, 2008).

210   Again, for deeper insight into Sarah's teaching see *Insight Yoga* and her second book, *Lit from Within: Yoga, Teachings, and Practices to Illuminate Our Inner Lives* (Shambhala Publications, 2021).

211   I was to learn later, it was more complicated than that. Where the foot will point when the femur is in a neutral orientation in the hip socket depends upon many factors, including tibial torsion, femoral torsion, and the degree of anteversion of the hip socket. These are described in detail in the book *Your Body, Your Yoga*.

Endnotes for Chapter 19

212   The first stage is called *Brahmacharya*. The second stage is called *Grihastha*. The third stage is *Vanaprastha*. The final stage is *Sannyasa*.

213 Why Madras? It is not certain why this name was chosen, but it was probably due to the Anglicization and shortening of the name of a smaller village nearby called Madraspattinam.

214 According to one biography, Charles Leadbeater was advising his young students to practice masturbation in order to reduce their sexual urges and maintain celibacy, which was essential for spiritual progress. See Gregory John Tillett, *Charles Webster Leadbeater 1854–1934: A Biographical Study* (Leadbeater.org, 2008), https://web.archive.org/web/20170703063510/http://leadbeater. org/tillettcwlchap10.htm.

215 Most of the teachings shared in this section are taken from C.W. Leadbeater, *The Hidden Side of Things* (Theosophical Publishing House, 1913).

216 There are six darshanas of Indian philosophy: Nyaya, Vaisheshika, Samkhya, Yoga, Mimamsa, and Vedanta. Each is a classical school of thought that provides different perspectives on understanding reality, knowledge, the self, and the path to liberation, while sharing common roots in the Vedic tradition.

217 See René Guénon, *Theosophy: History of a Pseudo-Religion* (Sophia Perennis, 2004). This book is a critical analysis of the Theosophical Society and its teachings, originally published in French in 1921 and later translated into English by Alvin Moore, Jr., Cecil Bethell, Hubert Schiff, and Rohini Schiff.

218 Leland, *Rainbow Body*, 198.

Endnotes for Chapter 20

219 See Ted Kaptchuk, *The Web That Has No Weaver*, 2nd edition (Contemporary Books, 2000) 43.

220 *Jing* is commonly translated as "essence" in Daoist and Traditional Chinese Medicine literature. However, I use "vitality" instead to avoid confusion with the concept of soul or core identity. While jing is indeed foundational, it refers to the stored vitality that fuels development, reproduction, and longevity—not the essence of who we are in a metaphysical or psychological sense.

221 Here, "essence" is used in the traditional Daoist/TCM sense to indicate a more concentrated or subtle expression of energy—not to be confused with the idea of "soul" or metaphysical essence as defined elsewhere in this book.

222 Paul Grilley, *Yin Yoga: Principles and Practice*, 2nd ed. (White Cloud Press, 2012), 28.

223 Chapter 3 of Yoga Sutra lists the siddhis, which include clairvoyance, telepathy, levitation, knowledge of past lives, invisibility, and control over bodily functions.

224 See Bikram Choudry, *Bikram's Beginning Yoga Class* (Penguin Putnam, 1978).

225 Hiroshi Motoyama, *Theories of the Chakras: Bridge to Higher Consciousness* (Theosophical Publishing House, 1981), 248.

226 For more on Motoyama Kinue and the founding of the Tamamitsu Church, see "Tamamitsu Jinja," in Kokugakuin University's *Encyclopedia of Shinto*, https://dmuseum.kokugakuin.ac.jp/ eos/detail/id=9760.

227 Hiroshi Motoyama, *Awakening of the Chakras and Emancipation*, English edition (Human Science Press, 2003), 83–85.

228 Motoyama, *Theories of the Chakras*, 8.

229 Powers, *Insight Yoga*, 9.

230 Grilley, *A Yogi's Guide to Chakra Meditation*, 12–16.

231 Motoyama, *Theories of the Chakras*, 23.

232   Paul Grilley, drawing from Dr. Hiroshi Motoyama's integration of yoga and subtle physiology, describes prana as "intelligent energy" with two interactive aspects: *shiva-prana*, the guiding intelligence, and *shakti-prana*, the animating force. These two flow down the central channel (*sushumna*) of the spine, differentiating the chakras into specific psychic and physiological functions. Grilley emphasizes that the fusion and reversal of these pranas up *sushumna*—a process aided by pranayama, bandhas, and mudras—generates increasingly subtle forms of energy known as "nectar," which open deeper layers of consciousness and ultimately lead the practitioner beyond the physical, astral, and causal bodies to the realization of *Purusha*, or pure awareness. See Grilley, *Chakras, Bandhas, Mudras*, 2, https://paulgrilley.com/assets/documents/Chakras,%20Bandhas,%20Mudras%2012.1.pdf.

233   Motoyama, *Awakening*, 94.

234   Sarah Powers describes shoshuten in *Insight Yoga with Sarah Powers* (DVD) (Pranamaya, 2005).

235   See Motoyama, *Awakening*, 119. For more, visit: https://yinyoga.com/yinsights/the-microcosmic-orbit.

236   Richard Wilhelm, *The Secret of the Golden Flower: A Chinese Book of Life*, trans. C.F. Baynes (Harcourt, 1962; originally published 1929).

237   The AMI originally was named Apparatus for Measuring the Function of the Meridians and Corresponding Internal Organs. Hiroshi Motoyama, *Science and the Evolution of Consciousness* (Autumn Press, 1978), 116–18.

238   Motoyama, *Science*, 116–18.

239   Motoyama, *Science*, 116.

240   See L. Turner, W. Linden, A. Talbot Ellis, and R. Millman, "Measurement Reliability for Acupoint Activity Determined with the Prognos Ohmmeter," *Association for Applied Psychophysiology and Biofeedback* 237 (2010): 251–6.

241   Motoyama, *Theories of the Chakras*, 271–279. See also Popp, Fritz-Albert, Qiao Gu, and Bernd Li. "Human Ultra-Weak Photon Emission as a Non-Invasive Spectroscopic Tool for Diagnosis of Internal States – A Review." January 2021*Journal of Photochemistry and Photobiology B Biology* 216(1):112141. DOI: 10.1016/j.jphotobiol.2021.112141

242   Motoyama, *Theories of the Chakras*, 271–9.

243   Motoyama, *Theories of the Chakras*, 259–61.

244   Motoyama speculated that Leadbeater may have been observing only the etheric layer; *Theories of the Chakras*, 238–9.

245   Robert O. Becker and Gary Selden, *The Body Electric: Electromagnetism and the Foundation of Life* (William Morrow and Company, 1985).

246   Gerald H. Pollack, *Cells, Gels, and the Engines of Life: A New, Unifying Approach to Cell Function* (Ebner and Sons Publishers, 2001).

247   James L. Oschman, *Energy Medicine: The Scientific Basis* (Churchill Livingstone, 2000).

248   H.M Langevin and J.A. Yandow, "Relationship of Acupuncture Points and Meridians to Connective Tissue Planes," *Anatomical Record* 269, no. 6 (2002): 257–65, doi.org/10.1002/ar.10185.

249   Some traditions also describe sinew meridians, which run within muscles and tendons, unlike acupuncture meridians which run around them. These sinew channels, considered part of the body's defensive system (*wei chi*), form a continuous network without discrete muscle boundaries.

250 Jaap van der Wal, "The Architecture of Connective Tissue as a Functional Substrate for Proprioception in the Locomotor System," paper presented at the *Second International Fascia Research Congress*, Amsterdam, Netherlands, October 27–30, 2009.

251 Jaap van der Wal, "Fascia, Fabrica or Fabric – On the Origin of Fascia," May 2020, https://www.embryo.nl/wp-content/uploads/2023/09/Van-der-Wal-Fascia-Fabrica-or-Fabric-EN-2020-1.pdf.

252 Di X, et al. "Cellular Mechanotransduction in Health and Disease: From Molecular Mechanisms to Therapeutic Targets," *Signal Transduction and Targeted Therapy* 8 (2023): 282, https://doi.org/10.1038/s41392-023-01501-9.

253 Langevin and Yandow, "Relationship of Acupuncture Points."

254 Helene Langevin, "The Science of Stretch," *The Scientist*, May 2013, https://www.the-scientist.com/the-science-of-stretch-39407.

255 Sarah M Corey, Margaret A. Vizzard, Nicole A. Bouffard, Gary J. Badger, and Helene M. Langevin, "Stretching of the back Improves Gait, Mechanical Sensitivity and Connective Tissue Inflammation in a Rodent Model," *PLoS One* 7, no. 1 (2012): e29831.

256 L. Berrueta, J. Bergholz, D. Munoz, I. Muskaj, G.J. Badger, A. Shukla, H.J. Kim, J.J. Zhao, and H.M. Langevin, "Stretching Reduces Tumor Growth in a Mouse Breast Cancer Model," *Scientific Reports* 8, no. 1 (2018): 7864.

257 This is known as the *resting membrane potential*. Values vary by cell type: neurons typically range from –60 to –70 mV, while muscle cells rest around –85 mV.

258 Other contributors include *morphogens*, specialized signaling molecules (e.g., Wnt, Nodal, BMP) that help establish gradients of information in the embryo—indicating where the head, feet, back, front, and sides will form.

259 M. Levin, "Molecular Bioelectricity in Developmental Biology: New Tools and Recent Discoveries," *BioEssays* 34, no. 3 (2012): 205–17, https://doi.org/10.1002/bies.201100136.

260 M.H. Shamos and L.S. Lavine, "Piezoelectricity as a Fundamental Property of Biological Tissues," *Nature* 213 no. 5073 (1967): 267–9. https://doi.org/10.1038/213267a0. This foundational paper confirmed the piezoelectric nature of collagen-based tissues in the human body, including bone, tendon, and skin.

261 E. Fukada and I. Yasuda, "On the Piezoelectric Effect of Bone," *Journal of the Physical Society of Japan* 12, no. 10 (1957), 1158–62. A classic study that directly demonstrated the piezoelectric effect in bone, laying the groundwork for understanding how mechanical stress translates to osteogenic signaling (Wolff's Law).

262 R.K. Aaron and D.M. Ciombor, "Therapeutic Effects of Electromagnetic Fields in the Stimulation of Connective Tissue Repair," *Journal of Cellular Biochemistry* 51 no. 4 (1993), 387–93. This research supports the idea that electrical currents generated in collagen-rich tissues aid in healing and repair

263 S. Gudi, C.B. Clark, and J.A. Frangos, "Fluid Flow Rapidly Activates G Proteins in Human Endothelial Cells: Involvement of Mechanosensitive Elements," *Circulation Research* 79 no. 4(1996), 834–9. Describes how blood vessel endothelial cells use mechanosensitive elements to regulate vascular tone and stiffness in response to fluid pressure, likely involving piezoelectric-like mechanisms.

264 S.S. Ranade, Z. Qiu, S. Woo, S.S. Hur, S.E. Murthy, S.M. Cahalan, J. Xu, J. Mathur, M. Bandell, B. Coste, Y.J. Li, S. Chien, and A. Patapoutian, "Piezo1, a Mechanically Activated Ion Channel, Is Required for Vascular Development in Mice," *Proceedings of the National Academy of Sciences* 111 no. 28(2014), 10347–52. Identifies Piezo1 as a key mechanosensitive channel essential for

cardiovascular development, highlighting how biological systems respond to physical forces at the molecular level.

265 S. Guerin, S.A.M. Tofail, and D. Thompson, "Organic Piezoelectric Materials: Milestones and Potential," *NPG Asia Materials* 11 no. 1 (2019), 1–5. https://doi.org/10.1038/s41427-019-0110-5. A review of the growing evidence for piezoelectricity in organic (living) tissues and materials, asserting that most biological tissues may exhibit inherent piezoelectric properties.

266 S.R. Pollack and A.L. Boskey, "The Electrical Properties of Bone and Their Functional Significance," *Journal of Biomechanics* 9 no. 6 (1976), 377–91. This study outlines the distinction between piezoelectric signals (electron-based and transient) and strain-generated electrical potentials (SGEPs), which involve the movement of ions under sustained stress.

267 Three processes occur when tissue is damaged: (1) inflammation begins within minutes and lasts a few days; (2) new tissue forms over several days; and (3) tissue reformation unfolds over a few weeks. Platelets release growth factors, activating fibroblasts and white blood cells. These cellular processes appear to be guided by injury currents. See B. Reid and M. Zhao, "The Electrical Response to Injury: Molecular Mechanisms and Wound Healing," *Advances in Wound Care* 3, no. 2. (2014): 184–201, https://doi.org/10.1089/wound.2013.0442.

268 Various electrical therapies—direct current, pulsed fields, alternating fields—have shown potential in promoting healing in chronic wounds. Though clinical protocols are still evolving, the area holds promise for regenerative medicine; Reid and Zhao, "The Electrical Response."

269 Bioelectric processes are central not only to animal cells but also to plant regeneration. Momoko Ikeuchi, Yoichi Ogawa, Akira Iwase, and Keiko Sugimoto, "Plant Regeneration: Cellular Origins and Molecular Mechanisms," *Development* 143 (2016): 1442–51, https://doi.org/10.1242/dev.134668.

270 R.C. Strohman, "Ancient Genomes, Wise Bodies, Unhealthy People: Limits of a Genetic Paradigm in Biology and Medicine," *Perspectives in Biology and Medicine* 37 no. 1 (1993): 112–45, https://doi.org/10.1353/pbm.1994.0003.

271 S.E.B. Tyler, "Nature's Electric Potential: A Systematic Review of the Role of Bioelectricity in Wound Healing and Regenerative Processes in Animals, Humans, and Plants," *Frontiers of Physiology* 8 (2017), 627, https://doi.org/10.3389/fphys.2017.00627.

272 Cells communicate constantly. Some signals affect the same cell (autocrine) and others nearby cells (paracrine), while still others travel far via the bloodstream (endocrine). There are physical surface-to-surface exchanges (juxtacrine), and exosomal messages are carried by tiny vesicles; see Reid and Zhao, "The Electrical Response."

273 J. Oschman, *Energy Medicine in Therapeutics and Human Performance* (Butterworth-Heinemann, 2003).

274 O. Kučera and M. Cifra, "Cell-to-Cell Signaling Through Light: Just a Ghost of Chance?" *Cell Communication and Signaling* 11 (2013): 87, https://doi.org/10.1186/1478-811X-11-87.

See also N. Liu, W. Zhuo, and J. Dai, "Intracellular Simulated Biophoton Stimulation and Transsynaptic Signal Transmission," *Applied Physics Letters* 121 no. 20 (2022): 203701, https://doi.org/10.1063/5.0128956.

275 Oschman speculates even more boldly that one day, we may uncover quantum forms of communication, but he is not the first to propose this. Sir Roger Penrose, a Nobel prize winner in physics, and his colleague Stuart Hameroff contentiously proposed that consciousness is a consequence of quantum processes within the neurons' microtubules. See S. Hameroff and R. Penrose, "Consciousness in the Universe: A Review of the 'Orch OR' Theory," *Physics of Life Reviews* 11 no. 1 (2014): 39–78, https://doi.org/10.1016/j.plrev.2013.08.002.

276 SQUIDs allow the detection of magnetic fields as weak as a femtotesla (10^{-15} T).

277 D. Cohen, "Magnetoencephalography: Detection of the Brain's Electrical Activity with a super-conducting Magnetometer," *Science* 175 no. 4022 (1972): 664–6.

278 D. Cohen, E. Edelsack, and J. Zimmerman, "Magnetocardiograms Taken Inside a Shielded Room with a Superconducting Point-Contact Magnetometer," *Applied Physics Letters* 16 (1970): 278–80, https://doi.org/10.1063/1.1653195.

279 Robert O. Becker and Gary Selden, *The Body Electric: Electromagnetism and the Foundation of Life* (William Morrow & Co., 1985).

280 M.S. Markov, "Pulsed Electromagnetic Field Therapy: History, State of the Art and Future," *Environmentalist* 27 (2007): 465–75. C.A. Bassett, R.J. Pawluk, and A.A. Pilla, "Acceleration of Fracture Repair by Electromagnetic Fields," *Annals of the New York Academy of Sciences* 238 (1974): 242–62, https://doi.org/10.1111/j.1749-6632.1974.tb26794.x.

281 L.Y. Sun, D.K. Hsieh, P.D. Lin, H.T. Chiu, and T.W. Chiou, "Pulsed Electromagnetic Fields Accelerate Osteogenic Gene Expression in Human Stem Cells," *Bioelectromagnetics* 31 no. 3 (2010): 209–19.

282 L. Caliogna, M. Medetti, V. Bina, A.M. Brancato, A. Castelli, E. Jannelli, A. Ivone, G. Gastaldi, S. Annunziata, M. Mosconi, and G. Pasta, "Pulsed Electromagnetic Fields in Bone Healing," *International Journal of Molecular Sciences* 22 no. 14 (2021): 7403. Richard Hoover, "PEMF Waves & Frequencies: Understanding Their Impact on Health and Wellness," PEMF Advisor, https://www.pemfadvisor.com/pemf-waves/.

283 Richard Hoover, "PEMF Frequency Chart: Understanding the Benefits of Each Frequency," PEMF Advisor, https://www.pemfadvisor.com/pemf-waves/frequency-chart.

284 Seto's team used a magnetometer with two coils and 80,000 wire turns—sufficient to measure small but not ultra-faint magnetic fields.

285 Seto A et al. "Detection of Extraordinary Large Biomagnetic Field Strength from Human Hand During External Qi Emission," *Acupuncture and Electrotherapeutics Research* 17 no. 2 (1992): 75–94.

286 A.L Baldwin, W.L. Rand, and G.E. Schwartz, "Practicing Reiki Does Not Appear to Routinely Produce High-Intensity Electromagnetic Fields from the Heart or Hands of Reiki Practitioners," *Journal of Alternative and Complementary Medicine* 19 no. (2013): 518–26. https://doi.org/10.1089/acm.2012.0136.

287 W.O. Schumann, (1952). "*Über* die strahlungslosen Eigenschwingungen einer leitenden Kugel, die von einer Luftschicht und einer Ionosphärenhülle umgeben ist," *Zeitschrift für Naturforschung A* 7 no. 1 (1952): 149–54. H.L. König, Electromagnetic Standing Waves in the Earth-Ionosphere Cavity," (1954), cited in C. Polk, "Schumann Resonances," in *Handbook of Atmospheric Electrodynamics*, volume 1 (CRC Press, 1982).

288 L.C. Matos, J.P. Machado, F.J. Monteiro, and H.J. Greten, "Perspectives, Measurability and Effects of Non-Contact Biofield-Based Practices: A Narrative Review of Quantitative Research," *International Journal of Environmental Research and Public Health* 18 no. 12 (2021): 6397. https://doi.org/10.3390/ijerph18126397.

289 See the Cochrane Collaboration report: Xavier L. Griffin, Matthew L. Costa, Nick Parsons, and Nick Smith, *Electromagnetic Field Stimulation for Treating Delayed Union or Non-union of long Bone Fractures in Adults*, Cochrane Database of Systematic Reviews (John Wiley & Sons, 2011), https://doi.org/10.1002/14651858.CD008471.pub2.

290 Biofield is a term used for electrical and magnetic fields surrounding and within the body. Sometimes energy medicine is also known as *biofield therapy*. See Matos et al. 2021.

291 For a skeptic's view of the work cited in James Oschman's books, see H. Hall, "Energy Medicine: The Scientific Basis" [Review of the book *Energy Medicine: The Scientific Basis*, by J. L. Oschman], *Skeptic*, 11 no. 3 (2005): 89–93.

292 See Griffin et al., 2011.

293 The original Latin phrase attributed to Paracelsus (1493–1541), a Swiss physician, alchemist, and pioneer of early toxicology, is: "*Omnia sunt venena, nihil est sine veneno. Sola dosis facit venenum.*" It can be translated as, "All things are poison, and nothing is without poison; only the dose makes a thing not a poison."

Endnotes for Chapter 21

294 Luciano Bernardi, Peter Sleight, Gabriele Bandinelli, Simone Cencetti, Lamberto Fattorini, Johanna Wdowczyc-Szulc, and Alfonso Lagi, "Effect of Rosary Prayer and Yoga Mantras on Autonomic Cardiovascular Rhythms," *British Medical Journal* 323 no. 7327 (2001): 1446–9, https://doi.org/10.1136/bmj.323.7327.1446.

295 Bernardi et al., 2001.

296 Peripheral chemoreceptors (carotid, aortic bodies) detect O_2/CO_2; central chemoreceptors near the brainstem respond to pH changes tied to CO_2. See "Neural Mechanisms (Respiratory Center)," in *Boundless Anatomy and Physiology*, Nursing Hero, n.d., https://courses.lumenlearning.com/boundless-ap/chapter/respiration-control.

297 Hypoxemia (low O_2 in blood) can cause hypoxia (low O_2 in tissues). Hyperventilation at high altitudes reduces CO_2 (hypocapnia), causing alkalosis, dizziness, or syncope (fainting).

298 Normally, our blood pH levels are on the order of about 7.35 to 7.45. Acidosis can result from very slow breathing, causing excess CO_2, lowering blood pH (<7.35), and disrupting enzymes, protein structures, electrolyte balance, and heart function.

299 Alkalosis (pH >7.45) from hyperventilation impairs oxygen release (due to the Bohr effect), lowers calcium levels, and may trigger spasms, nausea, or arrhythmias.

300 The average person breathes about 15 times per minute, but there is substantial variation between people. See L. Bernardi, A. Gabutti, C. Porta, and L. Spicuzza L, "Slow Breathing Reduces Chemoreflex Response to Hypoxia and Hypercapnia, and Increases Baroreflex Sensitivity," *Journal of Hypertension* 19 no. 12 (2001): 2221–9, https://doi.org/10.1097/00004872-200112000-00016.

301 See Bernardi's presentation at the Mount Everest Foundation: "Yoga, Oxygen and Respiration," https://www.mef.org.uk/expeditions/altitude-physiology-expedition-apex-6.

302 For supporting research, I suggest several studies: Luciano Bernardi, Cesare Porta, Lucia Spicuzza, Jerzy Bellwon, Giammario Spadacini, Axel W. Frey, Leata Y. C. Yeung, John E. Sanderson, Roberto Pedretti, and Roberto Tramarin, "Slow Breathing Increases Arterial Baroreflex Sensitivity in Patients with Chronic Heart Failure," *Circulation* 105, no. 2 (January 15, 2002): 143–45, https://doi.org/10.1161/HC0202.103311; Luciano Bernardi, P. Sleight, G. Bandinelli, S. Cencetti, L. Fattorini, J. Wdowczyc-Szulc, and A. Lagi, "Effect of Rosary Prayer and Yoga Mantras on Autonomic Cardiovascular Rhythms: A Comparative Study." *British Medical Journal* 323, no. 7327 (December 2001): 1446–49, https://doi.org/10.1136/bmj.323.7327.1446; C. N. Joseph, C. Porta, G. Casucci, N. Casiraghi, M. Maffeis, and M. Rossi, "Slow Breathing Improves Arterial Baroreflex Sensitivity and Decreases Blood Pressure in Essential Hypertension," *Hypertension* 46, no. 4 (October 2005): 714–18, https://doi.org/10.1161/01.HYP.0000179581.68566.7D

303 The vagus nerve regulates the heart, breath, and most upper abdominal organs. It does not affect the lower intestines, bladder, or reproductive organs.

304 Normal arterial O_2 saturation: ~97.5%; venous: ~75%. See J.B. West and A.M. Luks, *West's Respiratory Physiology*, 10th ed. (Lippincott Williams and Wilkins, 2015).

305 If we breathe in pure oxygen, we can quickly increase O_2 saturation in the blood to 100%, but then the hemoglobin is full and cannot take on any more. This is not quite the end of the story, however, because if we breathe in air under pressure, some oxygen will dissolve into the blood plasma. This can be a problem for some people, such as divers who come up too fast from deep waters. Without the continued pressure holding gas in the plasma, it starts to bubble out causing the dreaded condition known as "the bends."

306 A 10-second breath (~6/min) improves gas exchange by ~21% over a typical five-second breath, due to reduced dead space. Dead space is the area in the mouth and the throat where air resides but does not reach the lungs; no gas exchange occurs in this space.

307 For Bernardi's full lecture slides, see https://cdn.ymaws.com/www.iayt.org/resource/resmgr/docs_syr2017/Slides-post-conference/BERNARDI.pdf.

308 Heather Mason, Matteo Vandoni, Giacomo deBarbieri, Erwan Codrons, Veena Ugargol, and Luciano Bernardi, "Cardiovascular and Respiratory Effect of Yogic Slow Breathing: What Is the Best Approach?" *Evidence-Based Complementary and Alternative Medicine* 2013; 2013:743504, https://doi.org/10.1155/2013/743504.

309 Laborde et alia found minor benefits of 1:1.2 over 1:1 or 0.8:1 for vagal tone; see Sylvain Laborde, Maša Iskra, Nina Zammit, Uirassu Borges, Min You, Caroline Sevoz-Couche, and Fabrice Dosseville, "Slow-Paced Breathing: Influence of Ratios and Pauses," *Sustainability* 13 (2021): 7775. Found https://doi.org/10.3390/su13147775.

310 For further reading, see my book *Your Spine, Your Yoga*, 213–21.

311 Musicians and singers often hyperventilate during performances, leading to anxiety or respiratory symptoms. See Regina Studer, Brigitta Danuser, Horst Hildebrandt, Marc Arial, and Patrick Gomez, "Hyperventilation Complaints in Music Performance Anxiety Among Classical Music Students," *Journal of Psychosomatic Research* 70, no. 6 (2011): 557–64, https://doi.org/10.1016/j.jpsychores.2010.11.004; M. Teirilä, *Physiology of Wind-Instrument Playing* (University of Jyväskylä, 1998).

312 Hatha Yoga Pradipika 2.15.

Endnotes for Chapter 22

313 The Prognos is an electrodermal diagnostic tool similar to Dr. Motoyama's AMI device. For product information, see https://www.medprevent-systems.net/en/products/prognos (accessed Jan 27, 2025). For reviews of its reliability, see: Agatha P. Colbert, Richard Hammerschlag, Mikel Aickin, and James Mcnames, "Reliability of the Prognos Electrodermal Device," *Journal of Alternative and Complementary Medicine* 10 no. 4 (2004): 610–16, https://doi.org/10.1089/acm.2004.10.610; L. Turner, W. Linden, A. Talbot Ellis, and R. Millman, "Measurement Reliability for Acupoint Activity Determined with the Prognos Ohmmeter," *Applied Psychophysiology and Biofeedback* 35 no. 3 (2010): 251–6, https://doi.org/10.1007/s10484-009-9127-9.

Index

Page numbers followed by "n" indicate notes.
Numbers in *italics* indicate photos or illustrations.

B

Babylon, 81

bahya (bahir) kumbhaka, 36, 40

bandhas, 43–44, 65, 68

Bangalore, India, 48

Bangladesh, 175

Banyen Books (Vancouver, Canada), 89

baroreflex, 203

Barr, Susan, 89, 207

Basmu, 215n24

Bassett, Andrew, 195

Basti, 217n50

Batts, Diana, 208–209

Beatles, 37

Becker, Robert O., 187, 191, 195–196

Beckwith, Jim, 119

belly button rings, 117

bends, 236n305

Bernardi, Luciano, 201–202, 204–205

Besant, Annie, 164–165, 174

Bhagavata Purana, 226–227n178

Bhajan, 216n44

Bhakti, 87–93

bhakti yoga, 92–93

bhastrika ("breath of fire"), 41–42, 216n44

bhuta, 166, *167*

bhuttas, 59

Bible, 32

bija sounds, 146

bindu, 138–139

bioelectricity, 186, 191, 193, 198, 233n269

biofield therapy, 234n290

biophotons, 186–187

Birch, Beryl Bender, 117

Blavatsky, Helena, 164, 175

Blood, 180

bodhisattva, 222n119

body piercings, 117

Bohr effect, 235n299

Bordeu, Théophile, 229n208

Borkataky-Varma, Sravana, 225n168

Bosque Del Cabo Resort (Costa Rica), 63–65, 70

Boyle, Hugh, 142, 153

Brahe, Tycho, 123

Brahmacharya, 229n212

brahmamuhurta, 124

brahman, 59, 61, 81, 218n61

Brahmanas, 61

Brahmins, 218n60

Braulio Carrillo National Park, 70–71

breathing
  abdominal, 38
  alternate nostril, 39–40, 216n38
  bhastrika ("breath of fire"), 41–42, 216n44
  chakra, 42
  diaphragmatic, 38
  guidelines and cautions, 37–38
  nasal, 204
  paradoxical, 38
  as path to stillness, 36
  physiology of, 202
  rate of breath, 201–204
  safe, 37–38
  to stimulate chi, 155–156
  training the breath safely, 203–205
  ujjayi, 66–70, 121, 204
  yogic, 38

Brihadaranyaka, 61–62, 107

British East India Company, 163–164

brow center, 170

Bruno, Giordano, 85

Buddha, 60

buddhi, 58–59, 166, *167*

Buddhism, 61, 97, 103, 110, 115, 144, 222n119

Mahayana, 106, 222n119

Burma, 175

C

caduceus, 28, 224n145

Calcutta, India, 51

caloric, 150

Cambrian explosion, 119

Campbell, Joseph, 23, 43, 142

Candida, 89

carbon dioxide (CO_2), 42, 149, 202

Cartesian machines, 152–154

Cassiopeia, 123

Catholic Church, 109, 223n138

causal dimension, 184

Cavendish, Henry, 149

Center for Integrated Human Studies (CIHS), 10

Ceylon, 175

chakra breathing, 42

Chakra Instrument, 186–187

chakra meditation, 185

chakras, 28, 131–132, 138–139, 168–172
  vs. force centers, 168–170
  Leadbeater on, 175–176
  Motoyama on, 183–187
  strategies to avoid imbalances, 185
  Western model, 176

Chandogya, 61–62

Chandogya Upanishad, 107

Chandra, 134

Chandragupta II, 97

channels of life, 83–84. *see also* meridians; nadis

chanting, 201–202

Charaka Samhita, 99, 108, 223n137
chelas, 128
chemistry, 149, 153
chemoreceptors, 202
chemoreflex response, 203
Chennai, India, 51
chi (life force, 氣), 6, 102–103, 117, 179–181, 213n6
    conceptual evolution, 183
    forms of, 157
    measuring, 186–187
    original or prenatal, 116, 180
    reservoirs of, 182
    sources of, 180
    ways to stimulate movement of, 155–156
Chinese medicine, 102–103, 115, 183, 213n7
Choudhury, BIkram, 182
chyle, 222n121
cin mudra, 143
citrini nadi, 226n177
City Yoga (Vancouver, Canada), 63–65, 117, 209
cleansing practices *(shat kriyas)*, 217n50
cleavage planes, 187
cloth swallowing *(vastra dhauti)*, 217n50
coffee enemas, 43
Cohen, David, 195
compression, 160
Confucianism, 61
connective tissue, 186
Cosmic Ocean, 144
Coward, Noel, 48
crown center, 170
cytoskeleton, 189, 193

D

Dalits, 218n60
Dao, 102–103
Daoism, 61, 102–103, 106–108, 157, 180, 185, 230n221
darshanas, 230n216
de qi, 189
de Staël, Germaine, 147–152
dead space, 236n306
Decker, Julian, 117
deep fascia, 187
Dehradun, 47–49
delayed ensoulment, 84
Democritus, 77, 148–149
Dennison, Mike, 63–64, 111, 117
Descartes, René, 152–154, 228–229n202, 228n199
Desikachar, Kausthub, 142–143
Desikachar, Lakshmi, 142
Desikachar, Shraddha, 142
Desikachar, T.K.V., 69, 91, 110, 139, 142–146, 219n90, 228nn192–193
devadatta vayu, 221n114
Devakinanda Gopala, 118
Devi, 135
dhamanis, 223n137
dhananjaya vayu, 221n114
Dhanvantari, 99, 101–103, 222n121
dharma, 30, 98
dhatus, 100–102, 222n121
dhatvagnis, 222n121
Dhauti, 217n50
dhyana, 127
diaphragmatic breathing, 38
digestion, 222n121
Divodasa (character), 99–103
divya deha, 135
doshas, 100–102
dragon pose (low lunge), 121
drishti, 65–66

E

ear piercings, 117
earth, 150
Earth, 196–197
Ecclesiastes, 107
ecstasy, 214n15
Eden, 110
Egypt, 81–82, 214n16
electrical therapy, 233n268
electricity, 150–151, 168–169, 190–191
    bioelectricity, 193, 198, 233n269
    electrical currents, 190–191, 193
    piezoelectricity, 191–193
electrolytes, 209
electromagnetism, 194
electrotaxis, 194
Empedocles, 78, 80
enemas, coffee, 43
energy
    of communication, 194
    ways to mobilize, 155–156
energy lines, 89–91
Energy Medicine, 177, 179–199, 234n290
Enki, 32, *33*, 82
Enlil, 32
ensoulment, 83–84
Epicurus, 148–149
epimysium, 187
Erez, Ifat, 22. see also Shakti Mhi
Erez, Itamar, 22, 119
essence, 230n221
ethics, 171–174
Eve, 31
evolutes, 100–101
exhalation, 146
exosomes, 194

today, 199
traditional
    understanding of, 177
views of, 138–139
ways to stimulate
    movement of,
    155–156
Prana Urban Monastery,
    209–210
Prana Yoga and Zen Centre
    (Vancouver, Canada), 21,
    88, 119, 142, 209–210
pranava, 144
pranayama, 5, 112
    components of, 39
    Desikachar on, 145–146
    Iyengar on, 216n35
    key aspects of, 39
    Shakti's practices, 35–
        42, 216n41, 217n48
    Sivananda practices,
        216n41
    sitali, 66–67
    Sivananda tradition, 39
    stages of, 39
    ujjayi, 66–70, 121, 204
    in the woods, 39–41
prasarita padottanasana
    (wide-legged forward
    fold), 122
pratyahara, 127, 179
Prayag, 124
prayer beads, 201
preformation, 78
Premal, Deva, 119
prenatal chi, 180
pressure
    acupressure, 189–190
    electricity from,
        191–193
Priestley, Joseph, 149
priests and priestesses,
    25–29, 31–34
Prognos, 208, 236n313
proto-Indo-Europeans, 60
proto-yogis, 16
psyche, 6, 82–83

psychic healing, 183
psychotherapy, 179
Ptolemy, 74, 84
pulsed electromagnetic field
    therapy (PEMF), 195–197
Pura Vida Resort (Costa
    Rica), 63, 70–71
puraka, 36
Purnananda, Paramahansa,
    124–125, 129–131, 136
purusha, 55, 59–62, 134,
    218n61
    consciousness, 166–
        167, *167*
    soul, 137
Pythagoras, 80–81
Pythagoreans, 79–80, 83

Q

qi. see chi
qi gong, 190
Qigong, 196

R

Radha, 118
Rahula, Yoga Vachara, 114
raja yoga, 137, 175
rajas, 101
rakta, 101
Ram, 118
Rama Tirtha, 175
Ramayana, 52, 144
rasa, 101, 104–105
rasayana, 104–105
Ratnasara, *120*
Raye, Saul David, 114–117,
    121, 182, 196
Rea, Jai, 68–69
Rea, Shiva, 68–69, 117
rebirth, 30–31
rechaka, 36
recovery, 207–210
regeneration, 191
Reiki, 196

reincarnation, 30, 61,
    222n119
Renaissance, 152
resting membrane potential,
    232n257
restorative yoga, 121
retas, 101
Rig Veda, 60
Rigveda, 218n60
Rooftop Meetings, 164
root force center, 169
rosaries, 201
Rousseau, Jean-Jacques, 151
Royal Society of London, 85
rta, 104
Rudra, 131–132
Rumford, Count (Sir
    Benjamin Thompson),
    147–152

S

sacral (svadhisthana) chakra,
    170
sacrifice, 105
Sada-Shiva, 132
sadhana, 124
safe breathing, 37–38
sahajoli mudra, 126,
    225n167
salamanders, 191
salambasarvangasana
    (shoulder stand), 65
Saltonstall, Ellen, 202
samadhi, 37, 127, 137, 139,
    227n185
samakonasana, 160
samana, 101
Samkhya, 57–62, 83, 166–
    168, *167,* 218n61
samsara, 66, 222n119
samtosha (contentment),
    208
Sannyasa, 229n212
Santa Barbara Yoga Center,
    121

Sri Yantra, 69, *69*
Sri-tattva-cintamani,
   225n161
St. Paul's Hospital
   (Vancouver), 113
St. Peter's Basilica, 96
Stahl, George, 150, 153,
   229n204
standing forward fold
   (uttanasana), 121
Stang, Fiona, 63–64, 117
star pose, 91
Stomach meridian, 116,
   181, 188
stomach washing *(vamana
   dhauti),* 217n50
Stowe, Irving and Dorothy,
   141
strain-generated electrical
   potentials (SGEPs), 192–
   193, 233n266
streaming potentials,
   192–193
strength training, 91
Stringer, David, 118
Strohman, Richard, 193
Stryker, Rod, 37, 117
Sumer, *31,* 33–34, 82,
   214n21, 215n24
      creation story, 215n28
      fictional vignette, 25–29
Sunshine Belt, 45
superconducting quantum
   interference devices
   (SQUIDs), 195, 233n276
superficial fascia, 187
Sushruta Samhita, 99, 108,
   223n137
sushumna, 28, 138, 231n232
sushumna nadi, 83, 116,
   226n177
Susmita, 105
suttee (sati), 124, 224n158
svadhisthana (sacral) chakra,
   131, 170, 172, 186
Svadhyaya, 112
Svetaketu, 53–57, 61–62, 81

Swenson, David, 44, 62–66,
   68–70, 88, 117, 219n74
symbols, *27,* 29–33, *31, 33,*
   109
The Symbols of Yoga
   workshop (2003), 142
Symposium on Yoga
   Therapy and Research
   (SYTAR), 201–202

T

t'ai chi, 190
Taklushmon, 114
Tamamitsu Church, 183,
   230n226
Tamamitsu Shrine (Tokyo),
   183
tamas, 101
Tandava, 109–110, 125–126
tanmatras, 58–59, 166–167,
   167
tantra yoga, 106, 133, 137
tantric anatomy, 83
tantric yoga, 137
Tarka (character), 13–15
Taxila, 95–107
tension, 160
Thai yoga massage, 115–
   116, *119,* 121
Thai yoga therapy, 92,
   114–121
Thales of Miletus, 75–76,
   81, 83
Theodosius, 99
Theophrastus, 74–80, 84
Theosophical Society, 161,
   164–175, *174,* 183
Theosophy, 163–177, *167,*
   175–176
therapeutic touch, 194–195
Thich Nhat Hanh (Thay),
   208–209
Thompson, Benjamin
   (Count Rumford),
   147–152

three-part yogic breath, 38
throat center, 170
thumbing, 116, 121
tibial torsion, 160–161
Timaeus (Plato), 77
Tirumandiram, 227n179
Tirumular, 227n179
torsion, tibial, 160–161
Traditional Chinese
   cosmology, 221n116
Traditional Chinese
   Medicine, 157, 213n7,
   221n117, 230nn220–221
trance, 214n15
transmigration, 30
transubstantiation, 109,
   223n138
Trataka, 217n50
Triple Burner meridian, 181
tripundra, 225n160
Tufts University, 191
two-seed theory, 78–79

U

udana, 101
Uddalaka Aruni, 61–62,
   218n67
uddiyana bandha, 45, 65,
   217n55
ujjayi pranayama, 66–70,
   121, 204
Upanishads, 61–62, 173,
   218n61
Ur, 30, 215n23
Urinary Bladder meridian,
   116, 158, 181, 188
Ur-Ningirsu (character),
   27–29
US Food and Drug
   Administration (FDA),
   195, 197
Usimu, *33*
utkranti, 138
Uttal, Jai, 119

Other Books by Bernie Clark

Whether you're drawn to the physical practice of yoga, the depths of philosophy, or the mysteries of myth and meaning, Bernie Clark's other books offer something for every curious mind and embodied spirit.

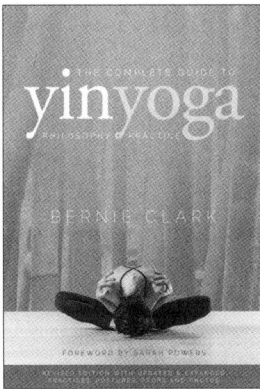

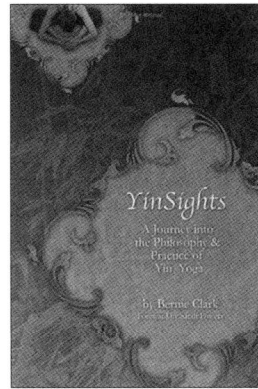

The Complete Guide to Yin Yoga
The Philosophy and Practice of Yin Yoga

Now in its second edition, this widely respected guide offers a comprehensive look at the philosophy and practice of Yin Yoga. It includes over two dozen postures, with detailed guidance on how to enter and exit each pose, their benefits, contraindications, and suggested variations. Unlike more active styles, Yin Yoga emphasizes long-held, passive poses that stress the body's deeper layers—ligaments, joints, and fascial networks—as well as the energetic pathways known as meridians. The practice encourages a meditative inward journey, bridging yoga and mindfulness. Expanded content includes in-depth discussions of the physiological, energetic, and emotional effects of the practice, along with new photographs showcasing a diversity of practitioners.

Yinsights: A Journey into the Philosophy and Practice of Yin Yoga

Bernie's first book on Yin Yoga (2007) is a blend of Eastern philosophy, scientific research, and personal reflection. *Yinsights* takes readers beyond the poses, into the deeper dimensions of Yin Yoga. The book explores concepts from Taoism, traditional Chinese medicine, and mindfulness meditation, weaving together the physical, energetic, and contemplative layers of practice. A perfect read for those seeking both intellectual clarity and embodied wisdom.

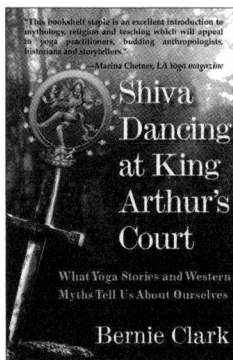

Shiva Dancing at King Arthur's Court

What Yoga Stories Tell Us About Ourselves

Originally published under the title *From the Gita to the Grail*, this unique work travels through time and tradition to examine the symbolic threads linking Eastern and Western wisdom. Through mythic storytelling, philosophical analysis, and comparative inquiry, Bernie explores the shared human longing for meaning, transformation, and transcendence. Whether it's Shiva's cosmic dance or the quest for the Holy Grail, the myths we carry reveal the inner journeys we live.

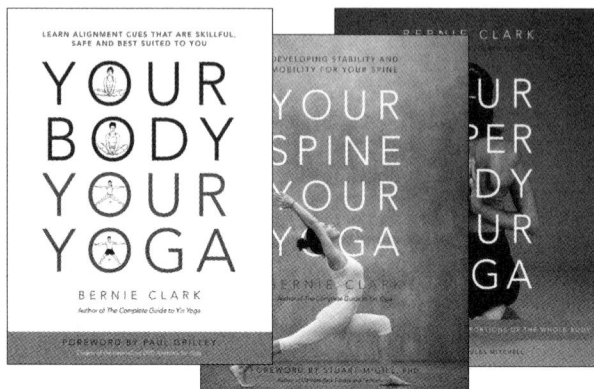

Your Body, Your Yoga Trilogy

This pioneering three-book series explores how individual anatomical variation affects yoga practice, and why one-size-fits-all alignment doesn't work. Based on a functional approach to movement, the trilogy is structured into five volumes spanning the three books. The books offer practical insights into how bones, joints, and ranges of motion differ from person to person and affect the experience of yoga postures.

- Volume 1, in *Your Body, Your Yoga*, the first book of the trilogy, addresses the central question: "What stops me?" It provides an in-depth explanation of the physiological barriers to movement—primarily tension and compression—and how they arise.
- Volume 2 in *Your Body, Your Yoga* explores the anatomical variations of the lower body.
- Volume 3 in *Your Spine, Your Yoga* explores the axial body.
- Volume 4 in *Your Upper Body, Your Yoga* explores the shoulders, arms, and hands.
- Volume 5, included in the third book, examines asymmetries, proportions, and how individual structure influences balance, orientation, and the ability to perform postures.

Together, these books empower practitioners and teachers to move beyond dogma and embrace yoga as a personal, adaptive exploration.

All titles are available through booksellers worldwide and at **www.yinyoga.com**.

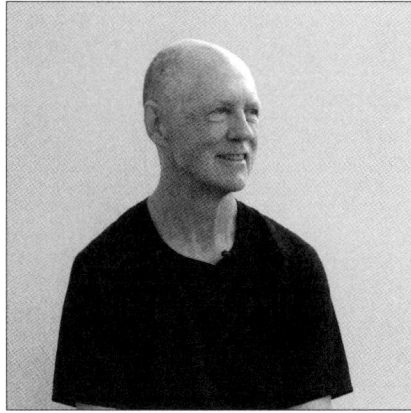

About the Author

Bernie Clark has been a dedicated student of science, mythology, and the contemplative traditions for over four decades. Best known for his pioneering work in yin yoga and his widely respected books on anatomy and practice, Bernie brings a unique blend of intellectual rigor, deep inquiry, and storytelling to all his writings.

Before turning to teaching full-time, Bernie had a successful career in science and technology, where his fascination with systems and structure laid the foundation for his later explorations of the body, breath, and mind. His teaching is informed not only by years of practice and study in yoga, meditation, and philosophy, but also by a lifelong curiosity about the human experience.

In *Prana*, Bernie turns his attention to one of yoga's most elusive and profound concepts—breath as life force—tracing its meaning across cultures, eras, and disciplines. Blending personal story with philosophical reflection, ancient wisdom, and modern science, he invites readers into a multidimensional investigation of what it means to be alive.

Bernie lives and teaches in Vancouver, Canada and shares his teachings through trainings, writings, and the website **www.yinyoga.com**.